# Health and Consciousness through Ayurveda and Yoga

## by Dr. Nibodhi Haas

The information and ideas expressed in this book are solely the responsibility of the author and do not reflect the opinion of Amma, the M.A. Math, M.A. Center or any of their affiliates.

Mata Amritanandamayi Center, San Ramon
California, United States

Health and Consciousness through Ayurveda and Yoga
By Dr. Nibodhi Haas

Published by:
    Mata Amritanandamayi Center
    P.O. Box 613
    San Ramon, CA 94583
    United States

In India:
    www.amritapuri.org
    inform@amritapuri.org

In Europe:
    www.amma-europe.org

In US:
    www.amma.org

The information in this book is for educational purposes only. It is not
intended to diagnose, prevent or treat any disease or disorder.

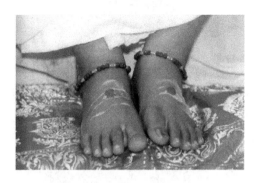

# Offerings

Any omissions in this text are entirely the responsibility
of the author. All truth and benefit that might be received
from this book are solely due to the Guru's grace.

I offer this book, my words, my actions and my life at the sacred
Lotus Feet of my beloved Satguru Sri Mata Amritanandamayi
Devi, for it is Her grace alone that allows all of this to be possible.

MATARANI KI JAI!

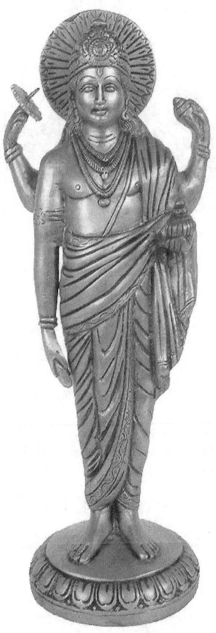

Lord Dhanvantari. He is regarded as the source of
Ayurveda. Dhanvantari is depicted as Vishnu with four
hands, holding medical herbs in one hand and a pot
containing rejuvenating nectar called amrita in another.

Om namo bhagavate vasudevaya danvantraye
amrita kalasa hasthaya, sarvamaya vinasanaya
trilokya nathaya sri maha vishnave namah

Salutations to Vasudeva, Lord of the universe, who has incarnated
in the form of Dhanvantari, who holds the pot of ambrosia in
his hands, who removes all disease, who is the Lord of the three
worlds and who is none other than Lord Vishnu himself.

# Contents

# Contents

# Preface

*adhyatma-vidya netanum*
*saddharmacharanattinum*
*bhukti mukti prade devi*
*sashtangam pranamichidam*

I prostrate before the goddess who grants both *bhukti*
and *mukti* (worldly enjoyments and spiritual salvation),
with the supplication that I gain in spiritual knowledge and
will be able to uphold *dharma* (righteousness).

A seed has been planted inside your heart and love is
the water that feeds. With love eternally it will grow; the
Divine Mother, She makes it so. Be in the now, you will
find, and be in the heart, you will see. Allow this love
that grows so deep inside, for within there lies a seed.
                                        ~ *Traditional South American hymn*

We are currently living in the *Kali Yuga* (the dark age of materialism). Dharma is at an all-time low. We are surrounded on all sides
by war, violence, disease, hostility, famine, overpopulation and
environmental destruction. Amma says repeatedly, "The world is
caught in the grip of an octopus of fear." People are becoming more
and more isolated from themselves and each other. The balance of
nature is greatly disturbed. The seasons rarely come on time. There
are droughts, floods, storms, earthquakes and tsunamis causing
great destruction.

There was a time when humans and nature co-existed in perfect
harmony. Now, our ignorance and our separation from our true Self
and from nature have greatly disturbed that balance.

The intention of this book is to provide a basic introduction to the
ancient systems of Ayurveda and yoga, as well as further exploration

13

of how they can be used for restoring the lost dharma within ourselves and in nature. Through Ayurveda and yoga we can manifest our highest aspirations and live a peaceful, harmonious and balanced life. We can learn to live in rhythm with the cycles of nature, both within and around us. We can uphold dharma and restore the beauty of God's divine creation here on Mother Earth, and we can awaken to the splendor and glory of the love deep within us.

Only love can heal and restore the lost harmony in this world. Love is the answer to every single question. Love is the solution to all problems. Amma often says, "Love is the only medicine that can truly heal the wounds of the world." Ayurveda and yoga are pathways to awakening this divine love that is hidden deep within each one of us.

May this offering be a manifestation of that Supreme Unconditional Love. May it be a small lamp to light the way through the *Kali Yuga*. May it serve as a small tool in the garden of life, and may the seeds of consciousness be firmly planted in the soil of love.

*Om asato ma sat gamaya*
*tamaso ma jyotir gamaya*
*mrtyor ma amritam gamaya*

Lead us from untruth to truth,
from darkness to light,
and from death to immortality.

*Om lokah samastah sukhino bhavantu*
May all beings in all the worlds be happy.

*Om shanti shanti shanti*
May there be peace, peace, peace. May peace prevail.

*May the tree of our life be firmly rooted in the soil of love.*
*Let the good deeds be the leaves on that tree;*
*May words of kindness form its flowers;*
*May peace be its fruit.*
*Let us grow and unfold as one family, united in love*
*So that we may rejoice and celebrate our oneness*
*In a world where peace and contentment prevail.*

*~ Amma*

# Introduction

*Everything will be known spontaneously if you do sadhana [spiritual practice]. Understand who you are. Know the Self. Then you can lead a life without attachment to anything. Such a state of mind will come if you do sadhana sincerely.*

*~ Amma*

*In the beginning was but the absolute Self alone.*

*~ Aitareya Upanishad 1.1*

Ayurveda, the "science of life," is the ancient wisdom science of living in harmony with each other and our environment. It is a part of the spiritual tradition of *Sanatana Dharma*, or the Eternal Truth.

Because Sanatana Dharma transcends all boundaries of caste, creed, nationality and religion, it is applicable to all people of all places and times. The knowledge of Ayurveda was given to us by the ancient *rishis* (seers). It expounds spiritual insights for living happy, healthful and peaceful lives, while seeking the ultimate goal of Self-realization. Ayurveda also incorporates the mystical science of yoga and *Vedanta* (the philosophy of non-dual or unified consciousness). The knowledge of Ayurveda is found in all of the four *Vedas*. The main ayurvedic text, the *Charaka Samhita*, describes the nature of the universe with all its manifestations, and how to bring ourselves into harmony with it. The sayings "We are the microcosm of the macrocosm" and "As above, so below" eloquently explain the universal truth that the whole universe is interconnected and interdependent.

Ayurveda is the traditional natural healing system of India. The concept of Ayurveda is not just focused on medical treatment or diagnosis of a diseased condition; it is a set of practical, simple

16

guidelines for living a long and healthful life. Through these principles, we can bring our bodies and minds into perfect balance. Ayurveda has a theoretical basis, but is also completely practical in nature. The word "Ayurveda" is composed of two words – *ayus* and *veda*. *Ayu* means "life" and veda means "science." Together, the words mean "the knowledge of life." In Ayurveda, the process of ayu is considered as a combined experience of body, senses, psyche/mind and soul. Ayu represents all aspects of life, including death, dying and immortality.

The science of Ayurveda has developed over thousands of years. Today, it is at the forefront of body-mind-spirit medicines. Ayurveda has expanded far beyond its traditional base in India and is gaining recognition throughout the world. With its profoundly comprehensive understanding of life and consciousness, it is becoming the medicine of the present and future.

The main aims of Ayurveda are the prevention, treatment and cure of disease, as well as the promotion of health on four levels: physical, mental, emotional and spiritual. There is also a direct correlation between Ayurveda and yoga. The science of yoga also originates from the Vedas and was revealed by the ancient rishis. As with Ayurveda, the goal of yoga is union with the Divine. The word "yoga" means "to unite" or "to join together." The principles of yoga and Ayurveda are the same and have similar systems of healing the body, mind and spirit. Yoga was first expounded by the sage Patanjali, who gave us the *Yoga Sutras*. Patanjali is said to have also been proficient in Ayurveda. Ayurveda and yoga are first and foremost spiritual sciences. They are maps to guide us along the spiritual journey.

Ayurveda and yoga teach us how to create balance in order to attain perfect health. As we come to better understand the union of our body, mind and soul, we are able to extend our life span and enhance our well-being. The deeper purpose of this science, however, is to provide the opportunity for Self-realization, to know the true Self, *sat-chit-ananda* (Existence-Consciousness-Bliss). We must recognize that our bodies and minds are constantly changing in this world of duality. Our task is to discover the veiled part of us that is always there – the knower, the seer, the infinite, unchanging Source. With diligence, perseverance and patience, we can wake up from *maya* (the dream/illusion) and become free of suffering. And as we awaken to our true Self, we create freedom in our body-mind-spirit. Ayurveda recognizes that we came to this earth to remember who we really are and to follow that dharma, to learn to take care of this physical existence while seeking *moksha* (liberation). When harmony of body, mind and spirit is established, we become free.

Ayurveda offers clear direction for managing treatment specific to each individual:

- Ayurvedic theory, with its profound understanding of causal factors in disease manifestation, includes analysis and diagnosis of the individual constitution.
- Ayurveda can be used to structure holistic models of the physical, mental, emotional and spiritual state of each person, and to create a vision or goal for a balanced state of being.
- Ayurveda offers specific recommendations to each individual on lifestyle, diet, exercise, yoga, herbal therapy and spiritual practices to restore and maintain balance in body and mind.

"Lead me from death to immortality" is a prayer originating from the Brihadaranyaka Upanishad. The Kaivalya and Katha Upanishads clearly describe the methods by which this immortality can be attained.

The Kaivalya Upanishad verse 1.2 states, "Through renunciation alone is immortality attained". While in the Katha Upanishad 2:3:14 -15 says, "The mortal in whose heart desire is dead becomes immortal. The mortal in whose heart the knots of ignorance are untied becomes immortal. These are the highest truths taught in the scriptures."

When the worldly, limited desires in our consciousness die, our already existent immortality awakens. We "become" immortal, but in ultimate reality we have always been and always will be immortal.

This immortality is not that of the physical body; it is the infinite, unchanging Self. The spiritual paths of Ayurveda and Yoga are a direct and tangible means to assist us in the journey from death to immortality.

*No one is ours and there is nothing to call our own. In our last days, only the true Self will remain with us. We can take nothing with us during the last journey. Why then this madness for earthly possessions? That which truly exists is within us. To see That, we must go within. There is not even a trace of sorrow there. There the true Self shines in its own glory. The awakening of the inner Self and true knowledge comes only when egoism is completely gone. We go from untruth to Truth when we love and serve all living beings.*

*~ Bandham Illa, Bhajanamritam, Vol.1*

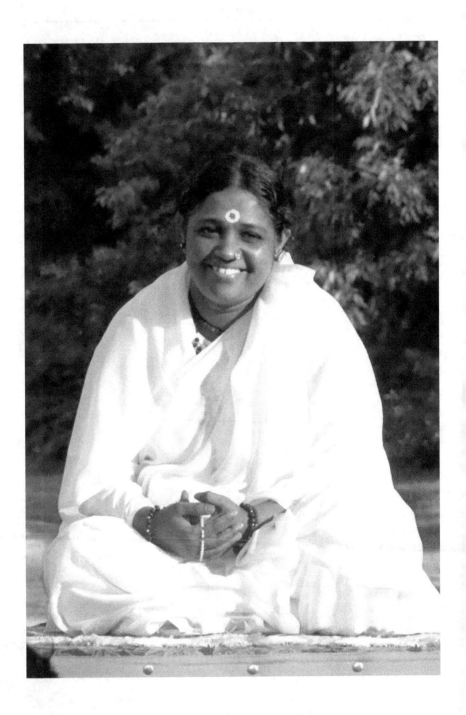

# Sri Mata Amritanandamayi Devi

*The world should know that a life dedicated to selfless love*
*and service is possible. Love is our true essence. Love has*
*no limitations of caste, religion, race or nationality. We*
*are all beads strung together on the same thread of love.*

*~ Amma*

Through Her extraordinary acts of love and self-sacrifice, Mata
Amritanandamayi, or Amma (Mother) as She is known, has endeared
Herself to millions of people around the world. Tenderly caressing
everyone who comes to Her, holding them close to Her heart in a
loving embrace, Amma shares boundless love with all, regardless of
their beliefs, who they are or why they have come to Her. In this
simple yet powerful way, Amma is transforming the lives of countless people, helping their hearts to blossom, one embrace at a time.
In the past 37 years, Amma has physically hugged more than thirty
million people from all parts of the world.

Her tireless spirit of dedication to uplifting others has inspired a
vast network of charitable activities through which people are dis-
covering the sense of peace that comes from selflessly serving others.

Amma's teachings are universal. Whenever She is asked about
her religion, She replies that Her religion is love. She does not ask
anyone to believe in God or to change their faith, but only to inquire
into their own real nature and to believe in themselves.

Among the wide array of charitable projects that have been
inspired by Amma are free homes for the poor, disaster relief work,
an orphanage, free food, medicine and pensions for destitute women,
sponsored weddings for the poor, free legal aid, prisoner's welfare
programs, extensive healthcare programs that include multi-specialty
hospitals and medical camps which offer free healthcare to the poor,
and many schools, colleges and educational programs.

For more information on Amma's charitable activities, please visit:

www.embracingtheworld.org
www.amritapuri.org
www.amma.org

# Chapter 1

# Sankhya Philosophy

*The Creator and the created are one and the same. There
is no separate Creator from the creation. The Creator
Him- or Herself has become the whole of creation.
There is no separation. So from this point of view, it is
like the waves in the ocean. The waves are not different
from the ocean. Even though the waves have different
shapes, lengths and heights, they are not actually different
from the ocean. The ocean itself becomes the waves.*

*~ Amma*

*Only that Illumined One who keeps seducing
the formless into form had the charm to win my heart.
Only the Perfect One who is always laughing
at the word Two can make you know of love.*

*~ Hafiz*

Due to intense sadhana (spiritual practices) and prayer, the Universal
Truth or Ultimate Reality dawned within the minds of the rishis.
The *Sankhya* philosophy, the foundation for Ayurveda and yoga, was
given by the enlightened rishi Kapila. Sankhya has two meanings.
The word *sankhya* translates as "to know truth" or "to understand
truth." *San* is truth and *khya* means to realize. Sankhya also means
"number" or "to measure." The system gives an enumeration of
twenty-four principles of the universe.

# Sankhya Philosophy:
# 24 Principles of Creation (Tattvas)

1. *Purusha* (Universal Consciousness) and *Prakriti* (Divine Manifestation or nature)
2. *Mahat* (Cosmic or Universal Intelligence) and *Buddhi* (differentiated individual intellect)
3. *Ahamkara* (Ego)
From ahamkara the three *gunas* (universal qualities) manifest: *sattva, rajas, tamas*
4. *Manas* (mind)

## Pancha Jnanendriyas (Five Sensory Organs)

5. Hearing
6. Touch
7. Vision
8. Taste
9. Smell

## Pancha Karmendriyas (Five Organs of Action)

10. Speech
11. Grasping
12. Walking
13. Procreation
14. Elimination

## Tanmatras (Objects of Perception)

15. Sound (*Shabda*)
16. Touch (*Sparsha*)
17. Form (*Rupa*)
18. Taste (*Rasa*)
19. Smell (*Gandha*)

## Mahabhutas (The Elements)

20. Ether/Space (*Akasha*)

21. Air (*Vayu*)
22. Fire (*Agni*)
23. Water (*Apas*)
24. Earth (*Prithvi*)

## Purusha and Prakriti

The Sankhya philosophy enumerates the *tattvas* (twenty-four divine principles) that support the universal manifestation. The most important principles are those of purusha and prakriti. Everything emerges from prakriti and then is infused with purusha. Purusha (represented by *Shiva*, the Divine Masculine) and prakriti (represented by *Shakti*, the Divine Feminine) together form the fundamental basis of all manifestation. Prakriti and purusha are *anadi* (beginningless) and *ananta* (infinite). Purusha is pure consciousness, all-pervading and eternal. Prakriti is the doer and enjoyer. The true Self, *Atma*, when joined with the five great elements (*pancha mahabhutas*), becomes matter and thus assumes life. The pancha mahabhutas are the basic elements required for the formation of all the bodily tissues and sensory and motor organs, including the mind.

Purusha is pure consciousness, the Divine Self without a second. It is self-existent, without the identity of individuality. It is conscious beingness, the principle of spiritual energy. Prakriti, the first cosmic principle, is the original pure creative energy (*parashakti*) of purusha. Purusha is the unmanifest consciousness. Prakriti is the manifestation of consciousness. While purusha exists solely in and of itself, prakriti exists because of purusha. Purusha can also be called the unknowable. It is the state beyond all fluctuations of manifestation. It is the pure unmanifest, formless awareness that is beyond attributes, cause and effect, time and space. Purusha is the supreme Self, or Atman, that is beyond body consciousness. When the individual soul (*jiva*) returns to its original state (the supreme Self or Atman), the concepts of "I" and "mine" disappear. Purusha, or the Self, is beyond prakriti. It is subtle and omnipresent. It is beyond mind, intellect and the senses. It is the eternal seer, the witness.

Prakriti is the manifested, knowable source of all creation that can be experienced with attributes, name and form – that which is in time and space. Prakriti means "the first creation" or "to come into creation." It also means "that which is primary, which precedes what is made." It comes from *pra* (before) and *kri* (to make or to do). Prakriti is the root cause of the universe and is called *pradhana*, or prime. All effects are founded on this principle. As such, it represents how we initially come into life before any fluctuations or modifications have taken place. Prakriti is the basis of existence. She is the Mother of the Universe. She does not create for Herself, but for Her children. All objects are for the enjoyment of the soul. Prakriti creates only when She comes into union with purusha. This dance is created for the emancipation of each individual soul.

Prakriti represents the primordial will and its creative potential. It has form and attributes and can be named. It is the conscious will or choice to create. Prakriti is eternal, all-pervading and immovable. Prakriti is independent and uncaused, while the products are caused and dependent. Divine will manifests through the activity of its own constituent gunas of mind: sattva, rajas and tamas. The gunas will be discussed in more detail later.

In the *Sri Lalita Sahasranama* (*The Thousand Names of the Divine Mother*) there is a verse that describes the union of purusha and prakriti, *Siva-Saktyaika-Rupini* (verse 999). This verse translates as "She who is the union of Shiva and Shakti, purusha and prakriti." Shiva, or purusha, is considered to be masculine in nature, and Shakti, or prakriti, is feminine. The ultimate truth is that neither is possible without the other, and in reality neither is masculine or feminine. Even to mention the word "other" is negating the totality of their union.

In Hinduism there is a deity called Ardhanarishvara, who is the union of Shiva and Shakti as one being. Ardhanarishvara is the personification of this truth. Without Shiva, Shakti would have no consciousness to manifest, no awareness of Self. Without Shakti, Shiva would have no energy to manifest, thus becoming *shava,* a corpse. From the union of pure consciousness and pure creativity comes the manifestation of the universe. The *Tao Te Ching* states, "Out of nothing comes the One. Out of One comes the Two. Out of Two comes the Three. Out of Three comes all things." The one represents the undividable truth. The two is the union of Shiva and Shakti. The three are the three gunas. Amma has described the greater significance of the deep connections within creation this way: "In order to feel real love and compassion, one must realize the oneness of the life force that sustains and is the substratum of the entire universe. Everything is pervaded by consciousness. It is that consciousness that sustains the world and all the creatures in it. To worship everything, seeing God in all, that is what religion advises."

## Mahat and Buddhi

Purusha and prakriti gave birth to *mahat,* Divine Consciousness/Cosmic Intelligence. Mahat means "great" and applies to the whole of creation. Creation is a wondrous, mystical dance of the union of form and formlessness. Mahat is perfect. It is universal, the ideal creation, transcendental beyond time and space. Divine Consciousness comes down to the level of individual manifestation and becomes discrimination. Discrimination is the conscious awareness of truth and untruth, right and wrong, eternal and transient. Through the power of discrimination, the Divine Mind merges back into Itself.

When mahat becomes individualized it is known as *buddhi,* the intellect with the power of thought and reason. Mahat joined with buddhi becomes a jiva, the individual consciousness. The jiva is the soul in union with the senses. It is housed in the body and is empowered by ego. It is associated with ignorance and karma. It is subject to pleasure and pain, to actions and their fruits, and constantly repeats the cycle of birth and death (reincarnation).

The intellect, or the buddhi, is the most important of all the manifestations of prakriti. The senses offer their objects to the intellect. The intellect is the instrument that is the medium between the sense organs and the Self. All of the concepts and projections that arise from sensation, reflection or consciousness are recorded and stored in the intellect before they can be known to the Self. The intellect discriminates between purusha and prakriti, between the real and the unreal, between truth and untruth.

Amma says, "Train the mind using the weapons of discrimination and detachment in order to convince yourself that the body is non-eternal. What is the body after all, except a bag of excrement, flesh and blood? This is the thing that you dress with beautiful clothes and golden ornaments. Try to pierce through and see the real thing, which makes it beautiful and shining. That is the Supreme Consciousness."

## Ahamkara

From mahat and buddhi, *ahamkara* (ego) is formed. Ahamkara translates as the individual consciousness, the feeling that "I" exist. It is through the manifestation of ego that consciousness, veiled by *maya* (illusion), starts to take on false identities. It is this that creates the perception of limited individuality. The limited, individuated mind is born of ahamkara. It carries out the orders of the ego's will through the organs of action (*karmendriyas*). As an individual consciousness, the ego separates and divides things. It is the part of creation that is maya, acting as a veil over the supreme nature of reality. As the ego continues to divide, all things in the transient world come into manifestation. The intellect, the mind and the ego are like gatekeepers, and the five senses or organs of perception (*jnanendriyas*) are the gates. Ahamkara is the process of all division. It determines "this is this" and "that is that." It is from ahamkara that all diseases manifest. The wrong use of the karma and jnanendriyas creates an imbalance in our body, mind and soul. This wrong use leads to disease, death and destruction. It is the cause of war and poverty. We must learn the proper use of the indriyas and live in harmony with Mother Nature and humanity.

Amma gives numerous examples to describe the nature of ahamkara. She says, "The ego creates division. It can be compared to the walls that delineate the divisions of a house. If you demolish the walls, the house disappears and again you have only space. Remove the ego and you will again become space. The shell around the seed has to break before the tree can emerge. You have to get rid of the ego before you gain knowledge. When there is a curtain over the window, we cannot see the blue sky. If we remove the sense of 'I' from our mind, we will be able to see the light within us."

## Manas

Ahamkara gives way to manas, which is the mind bound by time, space, name and form. It operates completely through the world of the senses. As such, the mind is both an organ of sensation and of action. The senses receive numerous impressions from the external world. The mind then agrees with the senses, and the impressions are perceived and formulated into concepts. The mind thinks, the intellect determines, and ego becomes conscious and projects itself back onto the world. The gunas (universal qualities) and tanmatras (objects of perception) are also manifestations of manas. Manas manifests from the sattvic and rajasic properties of the ahamkara. It has the ability to discriminate and create a peaceful, sattvic existence. It is also necessary for action to occur. There is a great saying: "The mind makes a horrible master but an excellent servant."

# The Three Gunas

*Om iccha sakti jnana sakti kriya sakti svarupinyai namah*

I worship Her who is the form of the powers of will, knowledge and action.
~ *Sri Lalita Sahasranama, verse 658*

The three gunas, known as sattva, rajas and tamas, are the universal
qualities of the fluctuations in the mind. They each manifest on a
universal cosmic level and on an individual level, including in our
own bodies and in all of nature. The three gunas are never separate;
they support and intermingle as intimately as the flame, oil and
wick of a lamp. They form the very substance of prakriti. All objects
are composed of the three gunas, which act on one another. In the
*Chandogya Upanishad* it is said that the sound *aum* is the totality of
the three gunas. *A* is the state of sattva, and is the waking state or
the subjective consciousness. It is represented by Brahma, the Creator. *U* is rajas and the dream state. It is represented by Vishnu, the
Preserver. *M* is tamas, the yogic sleep state of undifferentiated awareness, represented by Shiva, the Destroyer or the great Transformer.

*Om trigunayai namah*

I bow to Her who is endowed with
the three gunas of sattva, rajas and tamas.
~ *Sri Lalita Sahasranama, verse 984*

The gunas are the primary original qualities or states of mind. These
vibrational frequencies and attitudes are found in the mind as well
as in all of creation. The three qualities of the mind are directly
connected with the doshas. It is the gunas that attach the consciousness to the physical body. The mental nature of a person can
be categorized according to these gunas. The three gunas are *sattva*
(pure or essence), *rajas* (movement) and *tamas* (inertia). The three
gunas are found in all of nature as well as in the mind. Ayurveda

offers a clear description of people on the basis of their psychological constitution (*manas prakriti*). All individuals have a combination of the three, wherein the predominant guna determines an individual's mental nature.

When in balance, the three gunas maintain a healthy state of mind and, to some extent, of body as well. The three gunas are the very fabric of creation as they permeate through all living and non-living, tangible and intangible things. An object's predominant guna determines the vibrations it emits and its behavior. Disturbances to the harmony of the gunas result in different types of mental disorders. The development of a sattvic mind is goal of yoga and Ayurveda.

The three gunas manifest in our body, mind and consciousness. As they are more subtle than the doshas, disturbances in the gunas create disturbances in the gross body. The gunas make up our mental disposition and spiritual inclinations. Everyone has some proportion of sattva, rajas and tamas. The key is to keep them balanced and in harmony with each other and with the manas prakriti. The goal of yoga is to balance and control tamas, rajas and sattva within one's consciousness.

## Sattva

*Om Maha-Sattvayai Namah*

I bow to Her who possesses great sattva.
~ *Sri Lalita Sahasranama, verse 216*

Often considered to be the pure state of mind or consciousness, sattva is a clear, light, innocent and undisturbed inner state of being. Content and divine in nature, sattva is the union of the heart and mind. It is virtuous, patient and compassionate – the mind in its natural state of pure being.

A sattvic mind reflects clarity of perception and peace of mind. One endowed with a sattvic nature is free from suffering and is a beacon of light for the world. Sattvic types are always engaged in good actions and work toward the betterment of humanity.

As we increase the amount of the sattva guna within us, our spiritual vibration and the positive aspects of our personalities are greatly enhanced. One who is endowed with sattva has control over emotions, thoughts and actions. They posses all virtues and will adhere to dharma. They are lawful, tolerant and serene. They possess a stable intellect and are not egotistical. A sattvic person is a living example to the world. By their own example, they serve society and assist others to grow spiritually by increasing their awareness and compassion.

Manas (the mind) as well as the *pancha jnanendriyas* (five sensory organs) and the *pancha karmendriyas* (five organs of actions) manifest from the union of sattva and rajas.

## Rajas

*Om manomayyai namah*

I bow to Her who is in the pure form of the mind.
~ *Sri Lalita Sahasranama, verse 941*

Rajas is the nature of movement and action. It has the power of observation. Rajas is the active force that moves sattva into action. With rajas present, the pure mind is disturbed, agitated and active. With the mind's gaze looking outward, we start desiring; thus, rajas is the essence of desire. The most active of the gunas, rajas characterizes motion and stimulation. All desires and aspirations are a result of rajas. It influences all endeavors, including the logical, rational, thinking mind. It creates indecisiveness, unreliability, hyperactivity and anxiety. Rajas generates lust and greed for money, material luxuries and comfort. When one has desire, attachment follows. These attachments are the cause of all suffering. Rajas is self-serving and considers its own interests first, at any cost. When desires are not fulfilled, more suffering results.

Rajas, when balanced with sattva, manifests love and compassion. When disturbed it brings anger, rage, hostility and disease. Rajas is the manifestation of ego or individualization. The five organs of action (mouth, hands, feet, reproductive organs and eliminatory organs) come from rajas. The mind is also the active principle of rajas.

## Tamas

*Om tamopahayai namah*

I bow to Her who removes the ignorance of tamas.
*~ Sri Lalita Sahasranama, verse 361*

Tamas is the nature of destruction, dissolution and darkness. Tamas is the inability to perceive light or consciousness. Excess tamas is inertia. Tamas is characterized by heaviness and resistance. Delusion, laziness, apathy and drowsiness are caused by it. Sedative in nature, tamas causes pain and suffering and leads to depression.

Tamas manifests as blocked emotions. Tamas is the nature of destruction, degeneration and death. It is unfulfilled desire suppressed in the recesses of the subconscious mind. The presence of tamas creates vindictiveness, violence, hatred, criminality and psychopathic behavior. Its nature is animalistic, delusional, self-serving, materialistic and demonic. Because tamas contains all the doshas, it rules over the earth and the five elements.

The three gunas are contained within every being. One of the three gunas is generally predominant in a person. A sattvic person is virtuous and leads a pure and pious life. When sattva prevails, one is calm and tranquil. One reflects and meditates. A rajasic person is passionate and active. When rajas prevails, one performs a variety of worldly activities. A tamasic person is dull and inactive. When tamas prevails, one becomes lazy and careless. Tamas generates delusion. Sattva makes one divine and noble, rajas makes one selfish, and tamas makes one animalistic and ignorant. For example, a sage or saint is usually sattvic, while a soldier, politician or businessperson is rajasic.

As human beings, we have the great blessing to be able to consciously alter the gunas in our bodies and minds. Until enlightenment, we cannot separate or remove the gunas by ourselves. Yet through conscious action and awareness, lifestyle practices and thoughts, the gunas may be acted upon in order to increase or decrease them.

Sattva is the pure manifestation of the cosmic and individual mind. Sattva is pure light, dharma, consciousness, creativity and the power of observation. Sattva gives the power of discrimination, knowledge and the ability to know the truth. The pure state of sattva manifests as peace, harmony, contentment, compassion, unconditional love, selflessness, devotion and faith. Sattva is equilibrium. When sattva prevails, there is peace and tranquility. When sattva is predominant, it overpowers rajas and tamas.

Rajas is the active, vital, ever-changing, moveable principle. Rajas provides the shakti (energy) for creation to be perceived. We find rajas in the changeability of the mind and thoughts that shift from one end of the spectrum to another without rest. Activity that is expressed as likes and dislikes, love and hatred, attraction and repulsion, is rajas. It is the energy that observes and perceives through the intellect. Without rajas, sattva is unmoveable. Shiva lies in a tranquil, meditative, unmovable, blissful state without rajas to force Him into action. Rajas is necessary for creation. Through rajas one experiences the senses, the world and individuality. It is the energy that makes one desirous and seek sense pleasure. Rajas is also the energy that gives us the ability to discriminate between the eternal and non-eternal. When rajas is dominant, it overpowers sattva and tamas. When in harmony, it destroys tamas and activates sattva.

Amma has described the proper use of rajas for us. She says, "Everyone is madly running around looking for peace. Peace should come from within. What is to be done in order to obtain this peace? We should live our lives understanding and discriminating between the eternal and non-eternal. That is the only way. We will get peace only through the knowledge that God alone is eternal."

Tamas is inertia, darkness, confusion and maya. Tamas is a destructive power. It is the dense matter of the universe. Tamas is that binding force that tends toward lethargy, sloth and foolish actions. It causes delusion and non-discrimination. Time and space, which are non-eternal, are said to be ruled by tamas. Tamas is the process of decay and is responsible for death and disease. From a balanced state, tamas is responsible for sleep, hybernation and rebirth. It is the pull of the unmanifest calling us back to our original state. Tamas is the process of trees shedding their leaves in the fall. The leaves die and decay in the earth only to provide fertilizer for new birth and rejuvenation of life in the springtime.

## Tanmatras

The gunas manifest as *tanmatras* (the five sensory perceptions), jnanendriyas (the five sense organs), karmendriyas (the five organs of action), and *pancha mahabhutas* (the five elements). *Sattvaguna* is responsible for the five sense organs, the five motor organs and mind/consciousness. *Tamasguna* is responsible for the five sensory perceptions and the five elements. *Rajasguna* connects sattvaguna and tamasguna.

The tanmatras or senses are manifest in all life forms in all of creation. The tanmatras and indriyas emerge out of unmanifest matter, prakriti. These are the subtle forms of the five elements in their vibrational state of being. The tanmatras are *shabda* (sound), *sparsha* (touch), *rupa* (form or sight), *rasa* (taste) and *gandha* (smell). These subtleties are responsible for our ability to sense and objectify the external world. Shabda relates to the ether element, sparsha to air, rupa to fire, rasa to water and gandha to earth.

The tanmatras directly relate to the mahabhutas. Everything in this entire universe consists of different combinations of these five elements: ether, air, fire, water and earth. They represent the ether, gaseous, radiant or light, liquid and solid forms that make up the physical universe, including our bodies. Each element corresponds and relates to one of the tanmatras in a dynamic, creative way. Ether corresponds to sound/hearing; air to touch; fire to sight; water to taste; and earth to smell.

The tanmatras and the five elements are also directly related to the jnanendriyas and karmendriyas, through which they express themselves. The five sense organs are ear, skin, eye, tongue and nose. The ear relates to shabda, sound and the ether element; skin to sparsha, touch and the air element; eyes to rupa, sight and the fire element; tongue to rasa, taste and the water element; and nose to gandha, smell and the earth element. The five organs of action also relate to the five sense organs and the five elements. They are the mouth, hands, feet, urinogenital/reproductive organs and anus. The mouth corresponds to the ether element and sound (shabda). The hands relate to the air element (sparsha) and touch. The feet relate to the fire element (rupa) and sight. The urinogenital/reproductive organs relate to taste and the water element (rasa), and the anus relates to smell and the earth element (gandha).

All of these sense organs are responsible for our relative experiences and bring consciousness into form. Each of the organs, elements, tanmatras and sense organs has unique characteristics that make up the temporal world.

## The Five Elements

*bhuta maintmanay kali*
*porikalaintumanay*
*bodhamaki nintray kali*
*poriyai vinci nintray*

You became the five elements, Kali,
and you became the five senses.
You became awareness, Kali,
and you became the spirit.

*~ Yadumaki Nintray,*
*Bhajanamritam 2010 Supplement*

Consciousness takes form as the five great elements through which we know creation. From these, all of the many objects of the external world are composed. The mahabhutas are experienced in the subtle (non-physical) realm. From and within space/ether emanates air (thinness, lightness, airiness), then fire (energy), then water (flow, fluidity), then earth (solidity, form).

In daily life, it is helpful to be aware of the elements and what a vital part they play in sustaining creation. Awareness leads us to gratitude, which in turn leads us to love and patience. When we live a life of gratitude we are at peace with ourselves and nature. Amma gives great importance to the five elements and the vital role that they play.

Amma says, "There is no inert matter in the creation of God. Without earth, we cannot live. Earth is the substratum of our life. So we are taught by the Eternal Truth (Sanatana Dharma) to worship Mother Earth. By worshipping Mother Earth, we can avoid ecological degradation. Similarly, water is worshipped as God because we cannot live without water. Also, *agni* (fire)is worshipped. We need heat to live. Both extremes of heat and cold would make it impossible to live. So we need a right balance of all the natural resources. The same is true of air. This is why all the five great elements are worshipped in Hinduism. In Sanatana Dharma we are taught to visualize unity in diversity."

The five elements (pancha mahabhutas) form the basis of all things that are a part of creation. To balance them in a way that is unique for every human is the basic principle of Ayurveda.

## Ether or Space

Space is where we live, and this is the place where everything happens; it is the container of creation. It can also be called the stage where *lila* (the divine play) unfolds. The cells of our bodies also contain space. Ether is the subtlest of all the elements. Ether manifests as pure ideas and inspiration, and allows the connectivity and exchange between all things. It manifests as self-expression, holding space for creation to birth itself. It is expansive, subtle, light, clear, infinite and eternal. Ether comes from consciousness and the mind, and later returns to consciousness. When ether moves from its original, unmanifest state it becomes air.

## Air

Air is transparent and lofty, and causes activity within space. The biological functions that originate from sensations are considered to be functions of air. Likewise, the movements of thought and desire, which are functions of the mind, are also considered to be a function of air. Air is light, mobile, clear, dry, rough, inconsistent and like the changing wind. Air is the subtle movement responsible for directional force; it is in constant flux, everchanging. Air is the power of propulsion and, when it moves fast enough, causes friction and creates light or fire.

## Fire

Movements cause friction and thereby produce heat, which we call fire, the third element. This process changes matter from one state to another. Fire assists in the functions of the body, e.g., digestion and absorption. Fire has the qualities of being hot, sharp, liquid or fluid, penetrating, light, luminous, ascending and dispersing. The fire element also gives perception. Fire radiates heat and gives direction (internal and external) through sight and insight. When fire condenses, it becomes water.

## Water

Water represents the liquid state and is necessary for the survival of all living beings. Our body is composed primarily of water. Bodily fluids, including blood, saliva and hormones, help our body to transport energy and remove waste products. Water is fluid, heavy, wet, lubricating, cooling, softening, cohesive and stable. It is part of the impulse that nurtures and gives birth to life and is related to the reproductive organs and the conception process. Water is also womb-like in its nurturing qualities; it gives birth to new creative ideas and processes. When water coagulates, it becomes earth.

## Earth

Earth represents the solid state. The solid and stable structures of the human body are created from the earth element. It feeds and provides sustenance for all living things, and therefore creates a sense of permanence and security. Earth has the qualities of being thick, dense, hard, solid, heavy and stable.

Each element contains one-tenth of the previous element. Ether is the self-sustaining substratum in which creation takes place. Ether is in air. Air and ether are in fire. Fire, air and ether are in water. And all of the elements exist in earth.

The *doshas* (bodily constitutions) arise from the five elements. The concept of the doshas was evolved by the rishis of Ayurveda to differentiate between sentient and non-sentient beings. The *sarira* (human body) is made up of the pancha mahabhutas. Life blossoms only when the Atma, indriyas and manas unify within the human frame. Doshas are the biological units of the living body, and are responsible for all its functions.

There are three doshas – *vata, pitta* and *kapha* – each of which is made of a combination of the mahabhutas. *Vayu* (wind) and *akash* (space) form vata, agni forms pitta, and *jala* (water) and *prithvi* (earth) form kapha dosha.

The word dosha is derived from the word *dusa,* which means "to vitiate." In the balanced state of equilibrium the doshas support and nourish the body, and when vitiated they produce disease. The doshas play an important role in the pathogenesis, diagnosis and treatment of diseases. (The doshas will be discussed in detail later in this book.)

The principles of Sankhya philosophy are the basis and substratum of Ayurveda. The path of Ayurveda and yoga is a means of awakening. When awareness of the Self dawns in our consciousness, we are eternally free. The scriptures say that the whole universe dwells inside the Self. All the principles of Sankhya are part and parcel of the one Self. As we incorporate the principles of Ayurveda into our lives, may we awaken fully on the journey from darkness to light, from death to immortality.

| Element / Dosha | Tanmatra | Karmendriya | Jnanendriya |
|---|---|---|---|
| Ether / Vata | Sound (Shabda) | Speech, Mouth | Hearing (ears) |
| Air / Vata | Touch (Sparsha) | Grasping, Hands | Touch (hands) |
| Fire / Pitta | Form (Rupa) | Walking, Feet | Vision/Sight (eyes) |
| Water / Kapha | Taste (Rasa) | Procreation, Urogenital/ Reproductive organs | Taste (tongue) |
| Earth / Kapha | Smell (Gandha) | Elimination/ Excretion, Anus | Smell (nose) |

*A human being is part of the whole, called by us Universe.*

*~ Albert Einstein*

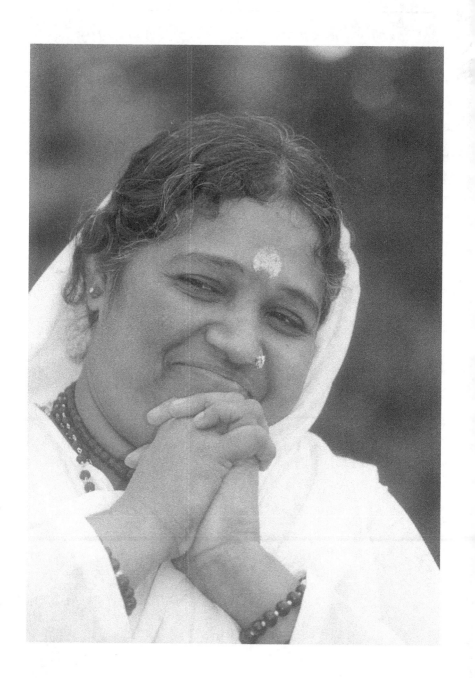

# Chapter 2

# Yoga

*Spirituality can be experienced only in stillness and silence.
If you think you will jump in the sea only after the waves
subside, you will never be able to enter the water. Don't
think you can pray and communicate with God only when
your mind is pure. Don't delay starting spiritual practice.*

*- Amma*

The purpose and goal of yoga (union) is to unite with our true Self. Through the constant practice of various methods, we train the mind to be still and listen to the sound of the inner Self. Amma describes the various yogic paths in this way: "Though there are many paths, there are four predominant paths: Bhakti Yoga (yoga of devotion), Karma Yoga (yoga of action), Jnana Yoga (yoga of knowledge) and Raja Yoga (yoga of controlling the mind and senses). The purpose of all yoga is control of the mind, which means control of the thoughts. Whatever the path may be, attainment of the goal is possible only if the *vasanas* (habits and tendencies) are attenuated. It cannot be said which path is best because each one is great and unique in its own way."

Amma always reminds us: "All paths lead to the same goal, and all paths incorporate love and devotion as essential to the practice." Amma further elaborates on the purpose of yoga, "The aim of all yogas is *samatva bhava* (the attitude of equal vision). What is known as yoga is *samatva*. There is no God beyond that, whatever the path may be. That state should be attained."

Yoga is a path of discipline, imposing restrictions on diet, sleep, company, behavior, speech and thought. It should be practiced only under the careful supervision of a master. Yoga is a path to control the mind and attain perfection. It heightens the power of concentration, arrests the wanderings and vagaries of the mind and helps us to attain the super-conscious state or *nirvikalpa samadhi*. Yoga destroys the body's restlessness, removes impurities and steadies the mind. The ultimate goal of yoga is to teach how the individual soul can attain complete union with the Self, or *Paramatman* (Supreme Being). This union of the individual soul (jiva) with the Supreme Purusha is greatly accelerated by controlling the *vrittis* (fluctuations) of the mind.

Yoga is an ancient spiritual science. The goal of yoga, like Ayurveda, is Self-realization. It serves as a roadmap for making one's life full with meaning and joy. Yoga, like Ayurveda, finds its origins in the Sankhya Philosophy. The yoga founded by the great sage Patanjali is a branch of the Sankhya philosophy. *The Patanjali Yoga Sutras* is the main text for all branches of yoga. The *Yoga Sutras* consists of four chapters forming the oldest yoga scriptures. The first chapter, *Samadhi Pada*, addresses the nature and aim of samadhi (the state of super-consciousness in which absolute Oneness is experienced along with all-knowledge and bliss). The second chapter, *Sadhana Pada*, explains the methods to attain samadhi. The third chapter, *Vibhuti Pada*, gives a description of supernatural powers or *siddhis* that can be attained through yoga practices.

Yoga, like Ayurveda, is an art, a science and a philosophy. It expounds on all aspects of life, including the physical, mental, emotional and spiritual. Both ayurvedic and yogic systems traditionally use herbs, meditation and *pranayama* (breathing exercises), as well as diet and lifestyle regimes. The main principles of both are to live a happy, peaceful and dharmic life. Yoga provides a wonderful guideline of how to achieve this balance.

Although numerous systems of yoga exist, classical yoga is grouped into one of the four main types (bhakti, karma, jnana and raja) and all other yogas fall within these categories. Other yogas such as Hatha Yoga, Mantra Yoga, Laya Yoga and Tantra Yoga are all included in one of the four main branches. Patanjali's yoga is Raja or Ashtanga Yoga (the yoga of eight limbs). This Ashtanga Yoga deals with the discipline of the mind and soul. Hatha Yoga consists of methods of bodily control and regulations of breath. Raja Yoga is the culmination of Hatha Yoga. A progressive sadhana in Hatha Yoga leads to the attainment of Raja Yoga. Thus, Hatha Yoga serves as a ladder to the stage or summit of Raja Yoga.

## Bhakti Yoga

Bhakti Yoga is the yoga of devotion. It is often said that Bhakti Yoga is the highest of all yogas, and all other yogas are manifestations of bhakti, for there is no higher path than the path of love. This yoga is union through pure selfless love from the heart. A bhakti *yogi* believes that whenever he thinks of God or the *Guru*, God thinks even more of him. A relationship between a *bhakta* and God/Guru can never be described in words.

Amma says, "Crying to God for five minutes is equal to one hour of meditation. If tears do not come by themselves, try to cry by thinking, 'Why am I not able to cry?' Try to develop devotion. That is the easiest way."

There are as many types of bhakti as the heart can fathom. Bhakti focuses on opening the spiritual heart, like a lotus blossoming in the morning sunlight. Singing and praying to God are the most common methods, as they help one to transcend the mind and enter into the secret cave of the heart. Amma says, "Try to sing to God with overflowing love and devotion. Let the heart melt in prayer. Unfortunate indeed are those who think that crying to God is a weakness. As the wax melts, the flame of the candle burns brighter. Through crying to God, one gains strength. It washes away the impurities of the mind. It makes the mind easily absorbed in the remembrance of God."

Bhakti Yoga also uses the constant repetition of mantras, the names of God, in ritual worship that can also be classified as tantra yoga. Prayer and meditation are common practices that help the heart melt in divine, unconditional love. In the *Srimad Bhagavatam*, one of the classical Bhakti Yoga texts, there is a nine-fold definition of the path of bhakti.

### 1. *Shravana:* listening to *satsang* or scriptures

Amma reminds us, "Scriptures were written by the sages from their own experience. We should make the scriptural truths our own."

### 2. *Kirtan and Bhajans:* devotional singing

Kirtan is singing the names of God. Bhajans are lyrical songs, often with narrative and a story, whereas kirtan is the repetitive '*Namavali*' or repetition of the names of deities. The goal of singing to God is for the heart to take over and the mind to lose its attachments. How bhajans and kirtan are sung is very important. Amma suggests, "Children, sing from the depth of your hearts. Let the heart melt in prayer. The joy of singing God's name is unique. These bhajans help us to pour out all our hearts' accumulated dirt. Leave aside all shyness and open your hearts to God."

### 3. *Smarana:* constant remembrance of God, which includes the repetition of mantras

Amma explains the benefit of this practice: "Mental purity will come through constant chanting of the divine name. This is the simplest way. You are trying to cross the ocean of transmigration, the cycle of birth, death and rebirth *(samsara)*. The mantra is the oar of the boat; it is the instrument you use to cross the samsara of your restless mind, with its unending thought waves. The mantra can also be compared to a ladder that you climb to reach the heights of God-realization."

### 4. *Seva:* selfless service

Amma repeatedly stresses this point to us: "Selfless service and repeating your mantra is enough to attain the goal. If these are lacking, however much penance you do, you will not be able to attain the goal. If you do spiritual practices without performing selfless actions, it will be like building a house without any doors, or a house that doesn't have a path to approach it. Be courageous. Do not be idle. Love and beauty are within you. Try to express that love and beauty through your actions and you will definitely touch the very source of bliss."

## 5. *Archana:* daily worship

This practice includes the chanting of scriptures. At Amma's Amritapuri Ashram in India, archana includes the daily chanting of the *Sri Lalita Sahasranama,* the Thousand Names of the Divine Mother.

Amma explains, "The archana brings prosperity to the family and peace to the world. It will remove the effects of past mistakes. We will get the strength to understand the Truth and live accordingly. We will get a long life and wealth. The whole atmosphere gets purified. If we chant the *Sri Lalita Sahasranama,* the energy in every nerve of our body will be awakened. *Devi* (the Divine Mother) will always protect those who chant the *Sri Lalita Sahasranama* everyday with devotion. They will never face a shortage of food or basic necessities, and will also grow spiritually."

## 6. *Vandana:* praise of God, prayer

We may have many different purposes for prayer, but Amma says, "Pray for a contented mind in all circumstances. Prayer becomes genuine only when you pray for a peaceful, contented mind, no matter what you receive."

## 7. *Dasa:* to become or adopt the attitude of a servant of God

Not many people like to think of themselves as servants, and yet Amma assures us: "What the world needs are servants, not leaders. Everyone's wish is to become a leader. We have enough leaders who are not real leaders. Let us become real servants instead. That is the only way to become a real leader."

8. *Sakhya:* friendship with God

Amma describes how this step is the key to the fullness of love: "Love is of two kinds. Love toward the world and its objects is love of a lower nature. Love toward God is devotion, love of the highest kind, and that is pure love. There is love within everyone but it manifests fully only when it is directed toward God." Eventually, you can make God your best friend.

9. *Atma Nivedana:* surrender or dedication to God

Complete surrender is one of the hardest processes for a human to go through, due to identification with the ego. It requires having total faith in God. Amma describes the nature of surrender as follows: "When you surrender to a higher consciousness, you give up all your claims; you release your grip from everything that you've been holding on to. Whether you gain or lose, it doesn't matter now. You don't want to be something any longer. You long to be nothing, absolutely nothing, so you dive into the River of Existence."

This is the nine-fold path of Bhakti Yoga. Following any of these practices wholeheartedly allows the heart to melt and true love to blossom.

## Karma Yoga

Karma means "action," and Karma Yoga is the path or yoga of selfless acts of service. The main text on Karma Yoga is the *Bhagavad Gita*, the Song of God. This text describes Karma Yoga as the main path of yoga. Without real love (bhakti), no real selfless action can take place. Bhakti and Karma Yoga are part and parcel of one another. Karma Yoga must be rooted in bhakti, because for any action to be successful, love is needed.

For a karma yogi, the activities of life are God's grace, granted to us so that we may be allowed to serve Him/Her. The karma yogi doesn't feel that the world is maya (an illusion), nor does he experience the ego during the peaks of success or the valleys of failure. A real karma yogi is detached while carrying out his duties on earth. Karma Yoga is beautifully described by Sri Krishna in the *Bhagavad Gita*: "Worshipping Him with proper actions, one attains Self-realization." One key to Karma Yoga is the performance of right action and service for its own sake, without attachments to the fruits of the actions. A karma yogi offers all of the fruits of his actions to God.

Amma tells us, "Children, you must do your work with sincerity. Whether you consider it significant or insignificant, whether you like it or not, you should do your work with interest and love. When you work in this way, when love begins to flow into all that you do, your work becomes sadhana (spiritual practice)."

When one acts selflessly, it becomes seva and the heart begins to melt. When an action is performed with real selflessness is becomes an offering to the world, because most actions are done for personal benefit. There is really no difference between Bhakti Yoga and Karma Yoga. They are one and the same, just like purusha and prakriti, Shiva and Shakti. Karma Yoga is the fragrance of love, the manifestation of pure bhakti. Amma explains: "Only action performed with an attitude of selflessness can help you to go deeper into meditation. Real meditation will happen only when you have become truly selfless, because it is selflessness that removes thoughts and takes you deep into the silence." Karma Yoga is also practiced as a means to achieve bhakti. In the beginning, due to many previous wounds, our hearts may not be open. The more we serve without personal desire for reward or the result of our action, the more our hearts become purified and we can open to real bhakti. It is for this reason that Amma often says, "Selfless service is the soap that purifies."

## Jnana Yoga

Jnana Yoga is the path of knowledge and wisdom. A jnana yogi seeks to understand the transcendental truth. He wants to transcend the mystery of birth and death, and realize the purpose of life. Vedantic texts often describe a jnana yogi as one who chants the ancient mantra *neti neti,* meaning "not this, not this," to distinguish between the real and unreal, or the permanent and impermanent. He uses *viveka* (mindful discrimination) to move from *avidya* (ignorance) to *vidya* (supreme knowledge). A real jnana yogi knows that the world perceived by the senses is not real, but an illusion created by the projections of thoughts and the mind. Jnana Yoga is described in the Upanishadic statement: "In the method of reintegration through knowledge, the mind is everbound to the ultimate goal of existence, which is liberation. This method leads to all attainments and is ever auspicious."

Amma explains: "Bhakti is not different from jnana. Real devotion is actually wisdom. Medicine should be applied to a cut only after the wound has been cleaned with a disinfectant. Otherwise, it could get infected and become a serious wound. Likewise, having destroyed the ego through devotion, wisdom should be established. Apply the medicine of jnana after cleansing the mind with the disinfectant of bhakti. Only then will there be true wisdom." Meditation, sadhana, Karma Yoga, Bhakti Yoga and self-inquiry are some of the various methods used in Jnana Yoga.

One who is established in jnana always engages in karma and Bhakti Yoga. All enlightened masters practice all three. Even though they are beyond any such practices, they manifest these yogas as an example for humanity. In the highest sense, jnana is Self-knowledge or Self-realization, the wisdom of the highest truth. The knowledge of the Self dawns in consciousness when all the dirt has been washed away through Karma Yoga and Bhakti Yoga. In the *Atmabodha Upanishad,* Sri Shankacharya has given a clear analogy about the nature of divine knowledge: "Just as fire is the direct cause of cooking, without knowledge no emancipation can be had. Compared with all other forms of discipline, knowledge of the Self is the one direct means to liberation."

## Raja Yoga

Raja yoga, also known as Ashtanga Yoga, is the founding principle of yoga that guides the seeker toward the goal of Self-realization. Also contained within Raja Yoga is the foundation of Ayurveda. Raja means "king" or "royal." This path of yoga outlines a method for moksha, which is liberation, knowledge of the Self, and freedom from all bondages. These methods are clearly described in Patanjali's *Yoga Sutras*, the foremost authoritative text on yoga.

The eight limbs of yoga as described in the *Yoga Sutras* are:
1. *Yamas* (restraint)
2. *Niyamas* (observances)
3. *Asana* (posture)
4. *Pranayama* (control of breath)
5. *Pratyahara* (withdrawal of the senses)
6. *Dharana* (concentration)
7. *Dhyana* (meditation)
8. *Samadhi* (the super-conscious state)

## Yamas

Yamas are external observances of righteous behavior. These codes of conduct for living a dharmic life are our way to purify ourselves by developing the power of self-observation.

The five yamas maintain harmony within ourselves and our environment. These guidelines apply, whether we live in the world, an ashram or a Himalayan cave. They prepare the aspirant for the real practice of yoga. The yogic student should practice non-violence, truthfulness, continence, non-stealing and non-acceptance of gifts that are conducive to luxurious living. Purity, contentment, austerity, sacred study and surrender to God should also be part of his or her practice. The most important of these is *ahimsa* (non-violence). All other virtues are rooted in ahimsa. Non-violence is abstinence from malicious intent toward all living beings – in thought, word or action – at all times. It is not merely non-violence, but also includes non-hatred.

### 1. *Ahimsa* non-violence, non-harmfulness

Ahimsa means "being devoid of violence, or committing no violence in any way." It includes not hurting another sentient being by thought, word or deed. This principle extends to all living things in creation including plants, animals and minerals. Our negative emotions harm us as well as others. Martin Luther King, Jr. once said: "Non-violence is the answer to the crucial political and moral questions of our time; the need for us to overcome oppression and violence without resorting to oppression and violence. We must evolve for all human conflict a method, which rejects revenge, aggression and retaliation. The foundation of such a method is love."

With love comes tolerance and forgiveness. Practicing real ahimsa is to sincerely forgive the trespasses committed by others. There is a profound Buddhist principle that states: "When someone whom I have benefitted, or in whom I have placed great trust and hope, harms me or treats me in hurtful ways without reason, may I see that person as my precious teacher." Ahimsa is not just the practice of non-violence, it is the action of pro-peacekeeping and prayer for the welfare of all sentient beings, including Mother Nature.

### 2. *Satya* truthfulness, non-lying

Embodying this principle begins with being honest with ourselves. The principles of satya should expand into every aspect of our lives. When we don't tell the truth, we communicate to the universe that we don't trust or that we lack faith. While it is important to speak the truth, it is also essential to avoid unnecessary conflicts. If speaking the truth could harm someone, then it is better to remain silent. We must first observe the principle of ahimsa.

## 3. *Brahmacharya* "*to find God, to walk with God*"

The literal translation of *brahma* is "Veda" and *charya* means "vow to study the Vedas," which traditionally includes living in a *gurukula* (home of a Guru or traditional school) and observing celibacy.

In yogic terms, *brahmacharya* refers to right use of sexual energy. For a *sadhak* (spiritual aspirant) it often means celibacy. For a house-holder it means to avoid sexual misconduct and to follow certain disciplines, rules, timetables and dietary restrictions. Detailed information on these codes of conduct can be found in the ayurvedic text *Astanga Hridayam*. One of the main purposes of this practice is to prevent the loss of *ojas* (subtle spiritual energy) gained from sadhana. When ojas is depleted the body and mind become susceptible to external negative vibrations. These vibrations can distract us from the spiritual path and the real goal of Self-realization. When ojas is lost, our aura, *koshas* (our subtle bodies), and physical, mental and spiritual immunity decrease. Wrong use of sexual energy can cause deep psychological imbalances. Preservation of sexual energy leads to increased healing and spiritual energy.

A whole system of herbal and dietary considerations accompanies brahmacharya, whether one is a sadhak or a householder. Unused or transmuted sexual energy can be channelled into creative energy for the upliftment of the world. It is often said that the sexual energy is the lowest part of the higher self. While it has its place for a householder, it must be used correctly for any spiritual benefit to be obtained.

Amma repeatedly says, "Children, you should use your discrimination while enjoying worldly pleasures. Through constant discrimination, you will reach a mental state where you can give up everything. Relatives, riches, sensual pleasures and the like can only give temporary happiness. They are all non-eternal. It is not external objects that give us happiness. There are many people who have all the material pleasures, but are still unhappy and discontent. Many commit suicide even while living in air-conditioned rooms. If the air-conditioned room were the source of their happiness, then why would these people commit suicide in it? So, even if we have everything, if there is no mental peace we cannot lead a happy life. If you go on craving for worldly pleasures, happiness cannot be gained. Understand that objects are ephemeral. Search for the eternal, the real source of happiness – the Self. Be satisfied with what you have. Renounce greed, selfishness and jealousy. If you can do this, in due course you will reach the state where all desires end."

### 4. *Asteya* non-stealing

The meaning of this principle is not to take what doesn't belong to us, including both material and non-material things. Praise and blame can be considered in this category. Taking credit for something we didn't do or blaming and defaming someone for something are also ways of stealing. Even wasting food can be considered theft. Amma explains: "Things meant for human sustenance can be used. If, for instance, you need only two potatoes, take just two and not three. Suppose two potatoes are sufficient to cook a dish; if you still take a third one, you are acting indiscriminately. You are committing an *adharmic* (unrighteous) act. This wastefulness can also be considered stealing. As you don't need to use the third potato, you are wasting it. You really need only two; the third one is extra. You could give it to someone else, perhaps to your neighbor who does not have anything to eat. Thus by taking that extra potato, you are denying him food. You are stealing his food and committing an unrighteous act."

### 5. *Aparigraha* non-possessiveness, non-coveting, non-greediness

This principle comes from the awareness that nothing really belongs to us. We come into this world empty-handed and we shall leave the same way. While we are here, we should use only the things we truly need, without taking any excess. Excess is the reason for all the poverty in this world. People often take more than they need, especially food. Imagine a world where humans take only what they need. If everyone takes excessively, there will never be enough. But if everyone in the world uses only what they need and gives the rest away, no one will ever go without.

Even to think that our accomplishments are due to our own efforts alone is to be possessive. Both self-effort and God's grace are required for any action to be successful. Amma explains the true nature of the situation: "The real dirt is the attitude, 'I am the doer,' and that is hard to wash away. All powers are God's powers. A plant shouldn't say, 'Look at my flower! How beautiful it is!'"

Amma also tells us: "Constant watchfulness makes you so pure that, at last, you yourself become the very embodiment of purity – and that is your true being. Once you reach this highest state, your every intention, word and action becomes pure. The burden of impurity is no longer there. The light of purity is all that exists. You then behold everything as pure consciousness. This means that you see everything as equal. External appearances are no longer significant, for you have developed the ability to penetrate deeply and to see through everything. Matter, which is ever-changing, loses its importance. Within everything you see only the immutable Atman (Self)."

## Niyamas

*Niyamas* are the internal attitudes, observances or principles of dharma that allow one to open up to higher consciousness. These are the basic formulas for living an ayurvedic or yogic lifestyle. The five niyamas define aspects for our inner development and our progress along the spiritual path. If we apply these niyamas properly, they will help us to grow strong – physically, emotionally and spiritually – like the fertilizer, water, sunlight and air that nourish a plant.

1. *Sauca* cleanliness or purity

This term refers to internal as well as external purity. Externally it refers to our way of living. The cleanliness of one's home, one's diet, clothes, appearance and other external manifestations are a reflection of the internal state. Purity of the heart and mind is the most important aspect of sauca. Yogic practices, such as bhakti, karma and jnana, help us to attain inner purity. A pure mind is full of love and compassion; it is free from anger, hatred, jealousy and other negative emotions. When we have clean hands (free from unrighteous action) and a pure heart, we are able to access our true inner wisdom.

Amma further points out: "Going to an ashram or a temple is fine, but our main aim should be to purify our mind. Countless visits to holy places won't do us any good if we cannot remove the selfishness within us and our hatred toward others."

## 2. *Santosha* contentment

Our goal is to have equal-mindedness in all circumstances and in all situations of life. When we have true *santosha*, we maintain our equanimity no matter what arises. This composure leads to inner peace and happiness. In order to maintain equanimity, Amma advises: "Try to stand back as a witness of the thoughts in your mind, like someone standing on the bank of a river, watching the water flow."

## 3. *Tapas* to purify by fire

In the yogic sense, *tapas* refers to self-discipline. It is the desire for the goal. If we want to succeed in any endeavor we must make an effort. Tapas is the effort we put forth on the spiritual path. It is as much the spiritual practices we perform, such as meditation, fasting and observing silence, as the consciousness and love we put into each action we perform. Sometimes this can appear to be a struggle. However, if we want the highest truth, Self-realization, we must pay the highest price, our ego. If we are intent on the goal then the tapas we perform becomes a great joy.

Amma explains: "A real *tapasvi* (one who practices austerities) wishes to serve others through self-sacrifice, just like a candle gives light to others while it melts and burns down. Their aim is to give happiness to others while forgetting their own struggles. This is what they pray for. This attitude awakens the love for God within them.

Mother is waiting for such individuals. Liberation will come searching for them and will wait on them like a servant maid. Liberation will come flying to them like leaves in the wake of a whirlwind. Others, whose minds are not as expansive, will not attain realization no matter how long they may be doing tapas."

### 4. *Svadhyaya* Self-study

This refers to the study of the Self through meditation, self-inquiry (*atmavichara*), and the study of scriptures, such as the Vedas. These practices are meant to increase good qualities and bring us closer to our divine nature. All yoga practices are intended for this purpose alone: self-examination resulting in the realization of the real Self. Amma says, "When we know that the juice is inside the fruit, we peel the fruit and throw the peel away. With this attitude, a sadhak will look for the essence of everything."

### 5. *Ishvara Pranidhana* surrender to the Divine Will, devotion to God

The purpose of surrender is to eliminate the ego. Only through surrender to a perfect master will we ourselves become perfect. This surrender is the dissolution of the small limited self, and the birth of the infinite Self. Amma speaks of the many benefits of surrender: "Amma can say, from Her own experience, that if you surrender totally to God, He will make sure that you don't lack anything. Surrender removes all fear and tension. Surrender leads one to peace and bliss. Where there is surrender, there is no fear, and vice versa. Where there is surrender there is love and compassion, whereas fear results in hatred and enmity. But in order to surrender, one needs a lot of courage, the courage to give up one's self. It demands a daring attitude to sacrifice one's ego. To surrender is to welcome and accept everything, without the least feeling of sorrow or disappointment. Surrender makes you silent. Surrender destroys the ego and helps you to experience your nothingness and God's omniscience. Once you know that you are nothing, that you are totally ignorant, then you have nothing to say. You have only unconditional and undivided faith; you can only bow down in utmost humility. When you surrender to a higher consciousness, you give up all your claims; you release your grip from everything that you've been holding on to. Whether you gain or lose, it doesn't matter now. You don't want to be something any longer. You long to be nothing, absolutely nothing. So you dive into the River of Existence."

The act of surrendering the ego can be terrifying, because it means that you dissolve the personality into the unknown. That unknown is, in fact, where truth and unconditional love reside. Through the act of surrender, truth and love blossom in the heart of the seeker. This is the essence of Bhakti Yoga.

When you are "in love" with someone, your thoughts are always on that person. You surrender to the experience of love. You are totally in the moment. The lover is only thinking of the beloved. He or she is not thinking of the future, but is totally in the present. Surrendering the ego to the Divine is actually the most beautiful and fulfilling of all love affairs. The Guru guides the disciple through the stages of intoxicating love to the point of merging with the beloved forever. Whereas worldly love eventually comes to a painful end, divine Love increases exponentially through eternity. As Amma says, "Real surrender and faith is Self-realization."

## Asana

Asana is a steady, comfortable posture. Being able to maintain an asana (seat or posture) is of great physical importance to concentration. When we obtain mastery over the asana, we are free from the disturbance of the pairs of opposites. Asanas are physical yoga postures that are also an integral part of Ayurveda. They allow for strength of body, mind and spirit. They are used as a way of keeping the body strong and healthy. Diet, herbs and seasonal cleansing are often part of a traditional hatha yoga practice. When adopted as part of one's personal sadhana, the practice of asana can greatly assist in meditation and the attainment of inner peace. Amma says,

"Try to stand back as a witness to the thoughts in your mind, like someone standing on the bank of a river, watching the water flow." A consistent yoga practice gives one the inner and outer strength to slowly become the witness. In hatha yoga practice, the mind and breath become one, and an inner awareness and stillness eventually dawn in the consciousness of the practitioner.

## Pranayama

Pranayama is the practice of controlling our "life force" or *prana*. In hatha yoga, pranayama includes specific breathing exercises that assist in maintaining the health of the body and achieving deep inner awareness through stilling the mind. Pranayama leads to inner peace, tranquility, steadiness of mind and good health. Asana and pranayama usually go hand in hand. A simple form of pranayama is the repetition of mantras along with the inhalation and exhalation. For example, one can practice the *So-Hum* meditation technique. Silently repeat *So* while breathing in and *Hum* while breathing out. Focus internally on the vibration of the sound. As we repeat this type of pranayama, the breath and the sound vibration unite as one to take the yogi into deep states of meditation. With movement, the breath of the yogi unifies and the stillness of consciousness dawns. It should be noted that Amma advises that complex pranayama exercises should only be practiced under the guidance of a competent master.

## Pratyahara

Pratyahara is introversion, or the withdrawal of the senses from their objects of attachment. One takes the awareness from external objects to the internal. When our sense faculties become detached from "things," the mind enters into a deeper stillness. By controlling sensory input, one can attain inner calm and peace.

Amma declares, "The thoughts of the mind are like the waves of the ocean. One cannot stop the waves by force. But when the ocean is deep, the waves subside. Similarly, try to concentrate the mind on one thought, instead of trying to stop all thoughts by force. The ocean of the mind will become deeper and it will become quiet. Even if there are small waves on the surface, it will be peaceful." Regular withdrawal of the senses, e.g. through weekly fasting and silence, greatly helps to calm the mind, and one's attachments to the outer world start to diminish. There is a saying in the scriptures that if we cannot control the tongue (speech and food), then it is not possible to control the mind. Fasting and observing silence once a week or every other week is a very useful tool to make the waves of the mind subside.

## Dharana, Dhyana and Samadhi

*Jyotirmayam anantam – shantidhamam*
*Ananda sagarantam*
*Sachidanandasandram – jnanaghanam*
*Ninde lokam mahesi*

O Goddess of the universe! Your abode is eternal light,
Abode of Peace and Ocean of Bliss.
It is full of sat-chit-ananda and dense with knowledge.

*~ Kali Mahesvariye*
*Bhajanamritam 2010 Supplement*

Dharana is the effort to fix the mind steadily upon a single object or point of reference. In Bhakti Yoga one focuses on the form of one's beloved God or Goddess. One may also focus on the sound of a mantra or the form of a *yantra* (geometrical design correlated with a deity, mantra or planetary vibration). Dhyana is the continuous and unbroken focus of the mind upon the object. This is the state of meditation. It isn't actually a practice. Samadhi is the merging of the mind upon the object with such intensity of concentration that the individual and the object become one. The mind is wholly merged in and identified with the object upon which it is fixed. This merging is the true state of yoga (union).

Patanjali declares that dharana, dhyana and samadhi are the last three aspects of Raja Yoga. They are collectively termed *samyama* (control of the mind and its fluctuations). All three aspects should be considered together, for dharana, dhyana and samadhi are progressively advanced stages of concentration. They form a continual process toward gaining mental concentration and are thus three parts of a whole. In truth, they are not separate. For as one advances along the path, there is no dividing line between these stages. When one progresses in dharana, one automatically enters the dhyana stage; likewise, as one progresses in dhyana, one automatically enters the samadhi stage. The three stages gradually merge into each other like a river flowing back into the ocean.

## Dharana

Dharana is concentration and contemplation. Dharana literally means "immovable concentration of the mind." The principle idea is to hold the concentration or focus of attention in one direction. The concentration should not be forced. It is one-pointed focus that brings the mind inward. Immersed contemplation and inner reflection will create the right inner environment, so that the focus on a single object becomes more intensified. These meditative techniques encourage one particular focus of the mind. The more the focus intensifies, the more the other preoccupations of the mind cease to exist.

Dharana often uses mantras or yantras to concentrate the mind. Inner points of reference such as the *chakras* may also be used in dharana. If mantras are too subtle, one can try gazing at a candle flame to help focus the mind. Meditation on one's *ishta devata* (beloved form of God) may also be used. Any method that brings the mind to one-pointedness is considered a dharana practice. Amma adds, "By concentrating on a form, sound or light, we learn to constantly be in that state of inner aloneness and to be joyful in any situation."

# Dhyana

Dhyana, the seventh limb of yoga, means profound spiritual meditation or worship. It is the state of perfect awareness or contemplation. It involves concentration upon a point of focus with the intention of knowing the truth. As we enter into real meditation we differentiate between the perceiver, the means of perception, and the objects perceived – between words, their meanings and ideas. Dhyana is a state of undifferentiated awareness. One must apprehend both subject and object clearly in order to perceive their similarities.

During the practice of dharana, the mind becomes single-pointed. During dhyana, it becomes completely identified and immersed in the object of attention. This is why dharana precedes dhyana. The mind is like a wild monkey jumping from branch to branch. The monkey must be stopped for meditation to occur. Dharana becomes the method of making the mind still and focused. Dhyana is the result of prolonged dharana.

In effect, the practices we call dharana encompass the techniques that many call meditation. Dhyana is the experience of meditation; it is what happens when the mind becomes still and aware. Even so, there are numerous "meditation" techniques that bring the mind to one-pointedness and eventually, through practice, to stillness. The power of true meditation is very great. Real meditation is simply the mind's natural state of awareness or being.

# Samadhi

Samadhi is complete immersion into the Self. Samadhi means "to place firmly," "to bring together" or "to merge." Patanjali refers to this in the *Yoga Sutras* as *Svarupa Avasthanam* (establishment in one's true Self). In samadhi, our personal, separate identity completely dissolves. At the moment of samadhi external awarenss ceases to exist. This doesn't mean that we are physically dead. It simply means that we experience the whole universe as the one Self. We become one with the Divine. The conscious mind merges back into the source from which it was born. The absolute and eternal freedom of an individual soul is beyond all techniques and stages, and beyond all time and place. Once free, the soul does not return to *samsara* (the cycle of birth , death and rebirth).

Samadhi is the ultimate goal. All paths, practices and methods culminate in samadhi. The rishis say that in the state of perfect samadhi, the soul experiences the complete light of Absolute Reality. Such an enlightened being maintains an individual personality in order to function in the world and guide all sentient beings to the goal. However, those who have merged in samadhi are completely free of all attachment to the created personality.

Samadhi is the only eternally true reality; everything else is constantly changing and can never bring everlasting peace or happiness. The scriptures say that once it is attained, staying in samadhi is effortless. Amma is constantly in this state. She is in the absolute state, but in appearance comes down to our level to lift us up to Her level.

*Mahasamadhi* is when a *mahatma* (great soul), consciously leaves the body for the final time during that incarnation. In mahasamadhi all prana (life force) is consciously withdrawn and the body is rendered dead. The soul merges into the Supreme Being (Paramatman) forever.

For the attainment of samadhi, or union with the Divine, the practice of yamas and niyamas is absolutely necessary. Along with constant practice and self-effort, divine grace is indispensable. One may practice for years or lifetimes with little progress. It is really the divine grace of the Guru or God that is the determining factor. In any case, the aspirant must practice the yamas and observe niyamas side by side. It is virtually impossible to attain perfection

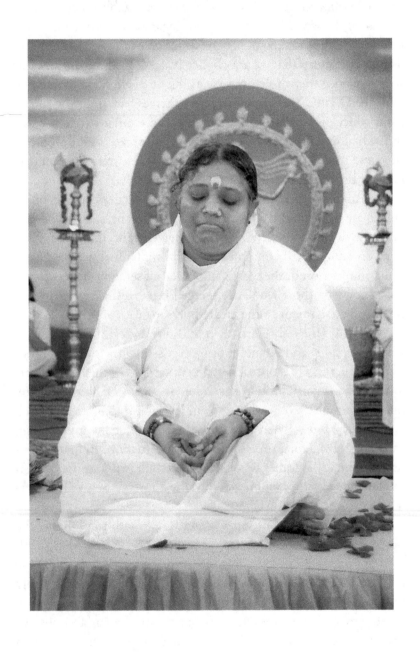

in meditation and samadhi without these observances. One cannot have concentration of mind without removing the negativities hidden deep within. Without concentration of mind, meditation and samadhi cannot be attained.

Amma describes the search for the samadhi experience in this analogy: "A musk deer searches for the source of the fragrance of musk, but it won't find it, because the fragrance comes from within itself. Bliss is not to be found outside of us; it exists within us. While God may not be visible to you now, He is always there, guiding and controlling you, holding the reins of your life. To begin with, God allows you long reins, and you don't notice that He is actually in charge. But remember, everything is in God's hands. You are not aware of it, but as you proceed through life, God is gradually shortening the reins. Finally, one day you realize that you cannot move another inch. At that point, when you are utterly helpless, you will feel God tugging at the reins as He begins to pull you back toward Him. You may at first put up a struggle, but you will soon find that the pull is of an unworldly power, and you have no choice but to surrender to His pull. It is at this point that you begin your journey back to God, the source of your existence. This journey has to happen. You will inevitably find that you can't do anything other than move toward God."

If we find it difficult to have faith or to surrender, we can pray to God to help us develop these qualities. Having the humility to pray for this guidance aids in overcoming the ego. The Guru is our lighthouse through the dark night of the soul. He/She is the ocean liner that transports us across the ocean of suffering to the shores of eternal peace. By grace alone, may we have the strength to offer ourselves at the feet of a perfect master such as Amma.

The ultimate goal of yoga and Ayurveda is spiritual communion with the Self. Carl Jung talked about this when he said, "Your vision will become clear only when you look into your heart. Who looks outside, dreams. Who looks inside, awakens." There is a saying, "Promote spiritual literacy, journey inward." All the great masters of all traditions are pointing in only one direction – toward the Self, toward the One. Self-realization comes from seeking and journeying to the inner mountain peaks and to the depths of the soul's valleys. A beautiful Hopi proverb states, "We are the ones we've been waiting for." The wait is over. We can start the journey home by sitting down and being still and taking time to listen to the voice within, the voice of God.

# Chapter 3

# The Four Goals of Life

*Our body is perishable. Only the soul is permanent.*
*This is a rented body. We will be asked to leave at any time.*
*Before that, we should look for a place in a permanent abode.*
*Then, when we leave the body, we will move to that permanent*
*abode, the eternal house of God.*
*No one brings anything into this world,*
*nor does anyone take anything with him when he leaves.*

*- Amma*

Knowing that we are in "rented" bodies, we sense that there must be some higher purpose or goal for us than to simply enjoy the material comforts and pleasures of a temporary existence. Ayurveda and yoga state that there are four goals or desires in life that are considered legitimate or worthwhile. These are referred to as the *purusharthas*, and are considered applicable to every human being. These universal, basic desires are at the heart of all other desires.

The four goals or desires identified in the *shastras* (Vedic scriptures) are *kama, artha, dharma* and *moksha*. All beings pursue one or all of these goals. Once a goal has been identified, we must contemplate the right means and then work to attain it. The goal should be clear, cherished and sought with intensity and awareness. The degree to which we are seeking any of these four goals determines the balance and harmony we keep in life and the success we will achieve. The first three are catalysts for the fourth and ultimate goal of *moksha* (Self-realization).

## The Four Goals of Life

1. *Kama* (desire): Kama means satisfying legitimate desires with the assistance of one's possessions (artha).
2. *Artha* (wealth): Artha means the accumulation of wealth or possessions while fulfilling one's duties (dharma).
3. *Dharma* (career/life path): In addition to one's career or work, dharma means the fulfillment of one's duties to society. Ideally, one's career and societal duties are in alignment with one another.
4. *Moksha* (liberation): Moksha is Self-realization and the realization that there is more to life than duties, possessions and desires (dharma, artha, kama).

# Kama

Translated literally as "desire," kama is the achievement of one's personal aspirations. All ambitions and desires, including lust, are considered kama; however, on a deeper level, kama represents the innate urge to attain one's aspiration.

For most creatures, enjoyment is the essence of their existence. Everyone wants to be happy and free from suffering. However, in the world today, most people seek happiness from external things. Real, lasting, unfluctuating happiness comes only from deep within one's Self, and not from external objects. External objects do serve valid purposes, but one should understand their proper place in life.

For example, many people in the world today crave sexual satisfaction; this desire guides many of their decisions and actions. Eventually, one must realize that the body and the world will inevitably perish – the true source of happiness lies within. This doesn't mean we shouldn't enjoy the objects of the world; it simply means that we need to understand their transient nature and let go of our attachment to those things. It is the attachment to external objects that is the cause of our suffering. Amma wants us to remember: "Nothing in this material world is everlasting. Everything can go at anytime.

Therefore, live in this world with the alertness of a bird perched on a dry twig. The bird knows that the twig can break at any time."

## Artha

Artha means wealth or prosperity. It refers to the accumulation of wealth. We need a certain amount of wealth to live our lives. Our basic necessities include clothing, food, shelter and medicine when we are sick. Money represents a means of attaining resources. It facilitates the fulfillment of our desires and duties, and helps brings about a sense of security. Wealth essentially allows us to function comfortably in life.

One's attitude toward money and work should be properly considered. If we are selfless and share what blessings we have with others, then there will always be enough for the whole world. If we hoard wealth, then people will go without and suffer. The universe is compassionate. Mother Earth is compassionate. She will always provide for her children if her bounty is not abused.

The sage Sri Adi Shankaracharya wrote in the *Vivekachudamani* (The Crest Jewel of Discrimination), "There is no hope of immortality by means of riches – such indeed is the declaration of the Vedas. Hence it is clear that works cannot be the cause of liberation."

If we are fortunate enough to have accumulated some wealth and we regularly donate a portion of our earnings to charitable causes that alleviate suffering, then we are performing a form of selfless service (Karma Yoga). Amma says, "There is a difference between buying medicine to relieve your own pain and going out to get medicine for someone else. The latter shows a loving heart."

The poverty of countries such as India is astounding. People suffer because they can't even afford a ten-rupee painkiller to alleviate a headache. Some people even die because they can't afford a three-dollar antibiotic. If we use a portion of our income to help such people, our lives will become blessed. When we serve selflessly, we start to feel the presence of the Divine blossoming within our hearts.

# Dharma

*Dharayati iti dharma* means "that which sustains all." Dharma refers to right conduct and a righteous way of living in the world. Dharma can simply refer to our career or vocation. But it can also refer to how we live in the world. Following the path of right conduct and living a life of harmony and love is the real dharma. In its highest sense, dharma means the ultimate way or the natural law or way of things. Just as it is the dharma of the sun to shine and the dharma of the planets to revolve around the sun, humans have a dharma to follow. When followed carefully and with awareness, dharma will carry us across the ocean of samsara. To follow one's dharma is to surrender to the cosmic flow and natural law of the universe. The true role of spirituality is to reveal to each individual their unique dharma. However, at present, the involvement of the ego often relegates dharma to dogma and ritual. Dharma is much more than religion. It transcends all castes, limited viewpoints and philosophies. It is a way of life that enables peaceful co-existence with others, and is conducive to the attainment of all our worldly and spiritual goals.

Amma gives a clear example of this in Her address, *Compassion: The Only Way to Peace*: "From approximately 5000 years ago until the rule of the great Indian king Chandragupta Maurya, founder of the Maurya Dynasty, truth and dharma played a central role in all wars fought in India. Even back then, defeating and, if need be, destroying the enemy was a part of war. However, there were clear rules that had to be followed on the battlefield and during combat. For example, foot soldiers were only allowed to fight with foot soldiers and horsemen could only fight with horsemen. Warriors riding elephants or in chariots could only fight with similarly mounted opponents. The same rules applied to those fighting with maces, swords, spears and bow and arrows. A soldier was not allowed to attack injured or unarmed soldiers, nor would he harm women, children, the elderly or the sick. Battles

70

began at dawn with the blowing of a conch and ended exactly at sunset, with the soldiers of both sides forgetting their mutual enmity and dining together as one. Battle would then resume the next morning at sunrise. There were even incidents of victorious kings happily returning the entire kingdom and the riches they had won to the king they had defeated or his rightful heir. Such was the great tradition of dharmic wars, in which the enemy was considered with respect and kindness, both on and off the battle-field. The sentiments and the culture of the citizens of the enemy kingdom were also respected. Such was the courageous outlook of the people living then."

The way each of us manifests dharma is unique. Mark Twain demonstrated his knowledge of the positive effects of dharma when he wrote, "Always do right. This will gratify some and astonish the rest." Everyone has unique talents for a specific reason. Amma says, "You cannot simply adopt any path that you feel like. Each one will have a path, which they followed in the previous birth. Only if that path is followed will one progress in one's practice."

If we put forth self-effort, God's grace will soon follow. Part of this effort involves looking within and finding our own path, our dharma. It is our responsibility to ourselves, to the world and to all of creation to allow our talents to be manifested in the world. The world is God's beautiful creation and each person has a role to play in it. Playing our role in the world's perfection is the pinnacle of dharma, and in order to do so, we must not act blindly or apatheti-cally. When each of us follows our individual and universal dharma, truth and righteousness will be restored to the world.

## Moksha

Moksha means "freedom from the bonds of ignorance." The jiva can merge with Atman while living in the world. Moksha is complete freedom from the cycles of birth, death and rebirth; it is Self-realization. It is the freedom from all limitations of the mind, from limitations of time and space, and from the dependence on artha and kama. Moksha is the realization of our Self as Brahman. This alone is Enlightenment. Anyone can reach this goal. Amma says, "It is possible to reach your spiritual goal while leading a family life, provided you remain detached, like a fish in muddy water. Perform your duties toward your family as your duty toward God. In addition to your husband or wife, you should have a friend – and that should be God."

The first three purusharthas – goals of life – are outer goals, whereas the desire for moksha is an inner goal and the true purpose of life. Through knowledge of the impermanent, the desire for the permanent awakens. Eventually the desire for name, fame and wealth falls away. One does not have to give these things up; one only has to dissolve the attachment to and identification with them. This natural dissolution of old attachments is the first step toward renunciation of the materially-focused life in order to reach the goal of moksha. Allowing these attachments and false identifications to fall away is real knowledge. Knowing that nothing is ours and all will pass in time awakens the discerning mind to the temporality of existence.

Amma knows the nature of each of our minds in relation to renunciation. She eloquently explains, "The word *renunciation* scares some people. Their attitude is that if contentment can come only through giving up, then it is better not to be content. They wonder how they can lead a contented life without wealth, without a beautiful house, a nice car, a wife or husband, without all the conveniences and comforts of life. Without all these, life would be impossible; it would be hell, they think. But do you know anyone whose possessions make them really happy and content? People who look for happiness in life's many conveniences and comforts are the most miserable ones. The more wealth and comforts one has, the more worries and problems one will have. The more one desires, the more one will feel discontent, because desires are endless. The chain of greed and selfishness continues to lengthen. It is an endless chain."

When considering the four goals of life, dharma should always come first. We must try to establish our lives in righteousness. Our actions should be motivated by love and compassion instead of selfishness. Then, the proper use of artha and kama will manifest of their own accord. Through life experience, dispassion will arise and the mind will turn inward. True, lasting happiness will come from this inward awareness of the Self. Ayurveda says that if we can follow these principles, then we can live harmonious, disease-free, healthful lives. Also, if we sincerely follow these guidelines, then we will assist in the restoration of harmony in the world. Sri Adi Shankaracharya said, "What greater fool is there than the one who, having obtained a rare human body, neglects to achieve the real end of this life?"

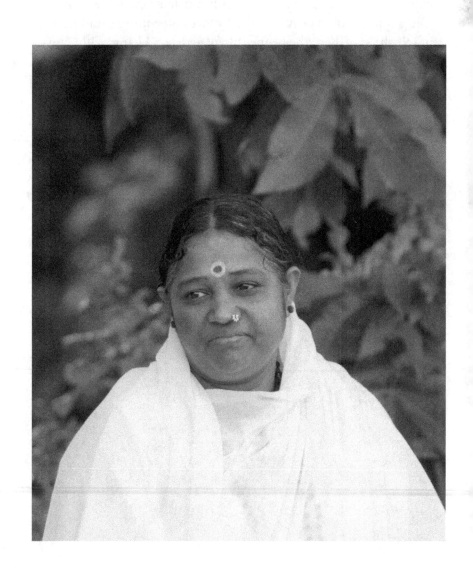

# Chapter 4

# The Doshas

*In the cave of the body is eternally set the one unborn.*
*The earth is His body.*
*Moving within the earth, the earth knows Him not.*
*The water is His body.*
*Moving within the water, the water knows Him not.*
*The fire is His body.*
*Moving within the fire, the fire knows Him not.*
*The air is His body.*
*Moving within the air, the air knows Him not.*
*The ether is His body.*
*Moving within the ether, the ether knows Him not.*
*The mind is His body.*
*Moving within the mind, the mind knows Him not.*
*The intellect is His body.*
*Moving within the intellect, the intellect knows Him not.*
*The ego is His body.*
*Moving within the ego, the ego knows Him not.*
*The mind-stuff is His body.*
*Moving within the mind-stuff, the mind-stuff knows Him not.*
*The unmanifest is His body.*
*Moving within the unmanifest, the unmanifest knows Him not.*
*The imperishable is His body.*
*Moving within the imperishable, the imperishable knows Him not.*
*Death is His body.*
*Moving within death, death knows Him not.*

*He, then, is the inner Self of all beings,*
*sinless, heaven-born, luminous, the Supreme Purusha.*

*~ Adhyatma Upanishad, verse 1.1*

The most fundamental and characteristic principle of Ayurveda is that of *tridosha,* or the three humors. All matter is composed of the five elements (*panchamahabhutas*) that exhibit the properties of earth (*prithvi*), water (*jala*), fire (*tejas*), wind (*vayu*) and space (*akasha*). All of creation is a dance or a play of these five elements. The structural aspect of our body is made up of these five elements, but the functional aspect of the body is governed by three doshas. Ether and air constitute vata; fire, pitta; and water and earth, kapha. They govern psychobiological changes in the body and physio-pathological changes. Vata, pitta and kapha are present in every cell, tissue and organ.

Doshas are to be seen as all-pervasive, subtle manifestations. Vata regulates movement and governs the nervous system. Pitta is the principle of biotransformation and governs the metabolic processes in the body. Kapha is the principle of cohesion and functions through the body fluids. In each individual, the three doshas manifest in different combinations and thereby determine the physiologic constitution (prakriti) of an individual. Vata, pitta and kapha manifest differently in each human being according to the predominance of their gunas.

The word dosha actually means "vitiated" or "out of balance." Imbalances occur due to factors such as improper diet, seasonal changes, physical or mental stress, etc. Imbalances occur to protect the body from physiological harm. In harmononious conditions, the doshas sustain a balance within us. The doshas are responsible for biological, psychological and physio-pathological processes in our body, mind and consciousness. They can maintain homeostasis or wreak havoc in our lives when they are disturbed.

Each individual in creation is a unique blend of the three doshas. From the three doshas come the seven constitutional types. There are three mono dosha types – vata, pitta and kapha. There are three dual-dosha types – vata-pitta, vata-kapha and pitta-kapha. Some people are *tridoshic*, meaning that they have an equal balance of all three (vata-pitta-kapha). When the tridoshas are balanced, the individual experiences health on all levels, mental, physical and spiritual.

When the following characteristics are in place, the doshas are said to be in balance, and a harmonious state of health is achieved.

- Happiness – a sense of well-being
- Emotions – evenly balanced emotional states
- Mental Functions – good memory, comprehension, intelligence and reasoning ability
- Senses – proper functioning of eyes, ears, nose, taste and touch
- Energy – abundant mental and physical energy
- Digestion – easy digestion of food and drink
- Elimination – normal elimination of wastes: sweat, urine, feces and others
- Physical Body – healthy bodily tissues, organs and systems.

There are generally two types of imbalances – natural and unnatural. Natural imbalances are due to time and age. Vata, pitta and kapha increase and become predominant during different periods of one's life, during seasonal changes and at certain times of the day. For example, vata is predominant during the latter part of one's life, during the rainy season and during late afternoon, as well as during the last part of night and the last part of digestion. Pitta is predominant during middle age, during the fall season, at midday, at midnight and during the middle part of digestion. Kapha is predominant during childhood, during the spring season, in late morning, at the first part of evening and during the early part of digestion. These natural imbalances can be rectified through lifestyle adjustments. Unnatural imbalances of the doshas can be caused by inappropriate diet or lifestyle, physical, mental or emotional trauma, viruses, parasites, etc. While some of these factors are beyond our control, the way we live, the foods we eat and our actions are within our control. By following the correct lifestyle regime for our personal dosha, we can minimize unnatural disturbances.

To learn to balance the doshas, one must first understand what causes each dosha to increase. According to the principles in Ayurveda, "Like increases like." For example, if you are cold and you eat ice cream, you will become colder. Herein lies one of the true beauties of Ayurveda: its principles are so simple, basic and natural.

*Om trikutayai namah*
I bow to Her who is in three parts.
~ *Sri Lalita Sahasranama, verse 588*

## Vata

Vata is the energy of movement or prana that is part of everything in creation. Vata contains the ether and air elements, space and movement. It is located in the colon, thighs, hips, ears, bones and the organs of hearing and touch. Its primary site is the colon. It governs assimilation and elimination. It is the impulse of expression, creativity and propulsion. It gives life to all things. Vata is responsible for breathing, movement, flexibility and all biological processes. It governs the nervous system as well as our sensory and mental functions. Vata is dry, light, cold, mobile, active, clear, astringent and dispersing. The rainy season is governed by vata. Vata times of day are mid to late morning and afternoon. When in balance, a vata person has strong healing capabilities with robust energy and good health.

On a physical level, vata-predominant individuals have thin, light, flexible bodies, often with protruding veins, tendons and bones. They may also have small, recessed and dry eyes. Their teeth are large and protruding with thin, small, dark or chapped lips. They will have erratic appetite and thirst, which is one reason why their digestive systems are easily disturbed.

On an emotional and mental level vatas are easily excited and act without considering what they are doing. They are very alert and aware but easily forget. They are quick and unsteady in thought, word and actions. Often they are considered unreliable and indecisive. They tend to be fearful and lack courage due to high levels of anxiety.

A balanced vata is filled with light and love, has expansive consciousness and sees the universal principle in all things. Additional indications of balanced vata are mental alertness and an abundance of creative energy, good elimination of waste matters from the body, sound sleep, a strong immune system, enthusiasm, emotional balance and orderly functioning of the body's systems. Signs of imbalanced vata are worry, fatigue, low stamina, nervousness, poor concentration, anxiety, fearfulness, mental agitation, impatience, spaciness, shyness, insecurity, restlessness, difficulty in making decisions, underweight, difficulty gaining weight, insomnia, waking up during the night, an aching and painful body, swollen, stiff and painful joints, sensitivity to cold, nail biting, rough, dry and flaky skin, fainting, dizziness, heart palpitations, chapped lips, constipation, intestinal bloating, gas, belching, hiccups, dry eyes and a sore throat. These can be alleviated by following vata lifestyle regimes, which will be discussed in depth throughout this book. Vata dosha is divided further into five types according to its location and the different functions it performs.

## Useful Tips to Balance Vata Dosha

### To Balance Vata

- Use *abhyanga* (ayurvedic oil massage).
- Stay warm in cold, windy weather.
- Consume predominately warm, cooked foods (less raw food).
- Go to bed early and have adequate rest and sleep.
- Favor warm, oily, heavy food with sweet, sour and salty tastes.

## Caution

- Avoid light, dry, cold, pungent, bitter and astringent foods.
- Avoid raw foods, juices and fasting.
- Avoid stimulants, smoking and alcohol.
- Refrain from excessive aerobic activity.

# Pitta

Pitta is fiery and transformative. It gives light and energy. Pitta is the seat of our digestive fire. The word pitta comes from the root *tapa,* which means heat. This dosha is responsible for digestion and metabolism. Pitta is located in the small intestine, stomach, sweat and sebaceous glands, blood, lymph and eyes. Pitta rules over blood and nourishment. Pitta is hot, slightly wet, light, subtle, mobile, sharp, soft, smooth and clear. It is governed by tejas, which brings forth the inner light of consciousness. Pitta is responsible for all transformation in our body and mind. It gives one the perception to comprehend reality and understand the true nature of things.

Pitta-predominant people can be very sensitive and react easily without much provocation. They tend toward anger and rage when disturbed. They have the ability to be great leaders and have intellectual capabilities. A pitta person has a medium build with good muscle tone and a bright complexion. Their eyes are piercing and their lips are soft and smiling. Often due to excessive heat in the body or mind, they tend to bald early in life. They have a strong appetite for food and life, which sometimes drives them to excess. Pittas do best in cool, calm environments that balance their internal fire.

When a person exhibits strong powers of digestion, vitality, goal-setting inclinations, good problem-solving skills, keen powers of intelligence, decisiveness, boldness, courage and a bright complexion, pitta is balanced.

Pitta is imbalanced when there is excessive body heat, digestive problems, hostility or anger, a tendency to be overly controlling and impatient, exertion of excessive effort to achieve goals, vision difficulties, a tendency to make errors in judgment due to mental confusion, passion or emotions that distort one's power of intellectual discernment.

## Useful Tips to Balance Pitta Dosha

### *To Balance Pitta*
- Keep cool. Avoid hot temperatures and hot food.
- Favor cooling, heavy, dry, sweet, bitter and astringent foods.
- Keep all activities in moderation.
- Keep regular mealtimes, especially lunchtime.

### *Caution*
- Avoid sesame and mustard oils, fish, buttermilk, mutton, acidic fruits, alcohol, meat and fatty, oily foods.
- Restrict pungent, sour, salty, warm, oily and light foods.
- Avoid overworking.
- Avoid excessive or prolonged fasting.

## Kapha

Kapha is governed by water and earth. It binds things together and solidifies creation. Kapha is also called *slesma* (slimy/sticky). One of its main functions is to provide nutrition to bodily tissues. Kapha is nourishment and support. It is located in the chest, throat, head, pancreas, sides, stomach, fat, nose and tongue. Kapha creates bodily tissues and holds the bones and muscles together. Kapha, like Mother Earth, is abundant and giving. Kapha-predominant types are motherly, patient and compassionate. They have energy to endure through long and arduous tasks. They tend to be slow learners but once they have learned something, they never forget. They are pure and gentle, yet firm.

Kapha is heavy, slow, cold, oily, wet/liquid, slimy, dense, soft, static, sticky, cloudy and gross. Kapha bodily frames are large with wide eyes, large lips and bones, thick skin and strong teeth. Their hair is full and often curvy or very wavy. They have a consistent appetite with slow to sluggish digestion. They have deep faith in God and love for humanity. Kapha types are abundant with health, fertility and longevity. However, when out of balance, kaphas are "couch potatoes." Kaphas tend to be overweight and can become obese. They can become dull and lifeless, immobile and lazy. Their minds become dull and move into slumps of depression and non-responsiveness, becoming almost catatonic. When kapha is harmonized it has excellent strength, knowledge, peace, contentment, love and longevity. In India, kapha is often considered to be the most desirable constitution. (Whereas in the West, vata is preferred as is reflected in most of the advertising, modeling and diet programs forced on the masses.)

Kapha is balanced when there is physical strength, a strong immune system, serenity, mental resolve, rational thinking, and ability to conserve and use personal resources, endurance, adaptability, love and compassion.

Imbalances in kapha are indicated by sluggish thinking, grogginess, apathy, loss of desire, depression, sadness, sentimentality, slow comprehension, slow reaction, procrastination, lethargy, clinginess, greedy, possessiveness, materialism, sleeping too much, exhaustion in the morning, drowsiness during the day, weight gain, obesity, congestion in the chest or throat, mucus and congestion of the sinuses, nausea, diabetes, hay fever, pale, cool, and clammy skin, edema, bloatedness, sluggish digestion, high cholesterol, aching joints or heavy limbs. These kapha excesses can be diminished by following kapha lifestyle regimes.

## Useful Tips to Balance Kapha Dosha

### To Balance Kapha

- Exercise regularly. Begin with *surya namaskar* (sun salutations) to warm up the body, which should be followed by vigorous activity.
- Prefer warm temperatures. Stay warm and dry in cold, damp weather.
- Eat fresh fruits, vegetables and legumes.
- Favor pungent, bitter, astringent, light, dry and warm foods.

### Caution

- Reduce heavy, oily, cold, sweet, sour and salty foods.
- Avoid heavy meals.
- Sleep promotes kapha, hence avoid excessive sleep.
- All frozen desserts are to be avoided.

Determining one's dosha and following the appropriate lifestyle modifications is essential for living a harmonious, disease-free life. Dietary and lifestyle regimes vary depending on the unique balance of the individual.

## Qualities of Nature

The three doshas are the gross manifestation of the three gunas. The three doshas are governed by the twenty attributes or qualities of nature (prakriti), which manifest as ten pairs of opposites and are the dual forces of the universe.

### The Ten Pairs of Opposites

- cold (*shita*) and hot (*ushna*)
- oily or wet (*snigha*) and dry (*ruksha*)
- heavy (*guru*) and light (*laghu*)
- gross (*sthula*) and subtle (*sukshma*)

- dense (*sandra*) and liquid (*drava*)
- stable (*sthira*) and mobile (*chala*)
- slow or dull (*mandha*) and sharp (*tikshna*)
- soft (*mridu*) and hard (*kathina*)
- slimy or smooth (*slakshna*) and rough (*khara*)
- clear (*vishada*) and cloudy (*pichilla*)

## The Twenty Attributes and the Doshas

**Hot** relates to pitta and the fire element. It increases pitta while decreasing vata and kapha.

**Cold** relates to kapha and vata and increases both, while decreasing pitta.

**Dry** is one of the primary attribute of vata. Dryness greatly increases vata, yet greatly decreases kapha and mildly decreases pitta.

**Wet** is the primary attribute of kapha dosha and the water element. It decreases vata and mildly increases pitta.

**Heavy** correlates to the earth and water element, thus it increases kapha. It moderately decreases both vata and pitta.

**Light** is of the fire, space and air elements, so it greatly increases vata, moderately increases pitta, and decreases kapha.

**Gross** is similar to heavy, as it relates to earth and water. It increases kapha and decreases vata and pitta.

**Subtle** is similar to light. It increases vata and pitta while decreasing kapha.

**Dense** relates to earth. It increases kapha and decreases vata and pitta.

**Liquid** or **flowing** corresponds to water and fire. It increases pitta and decreases vata and kapha.

**Mobile** relates primarily to air, but also to fire. It greatly increases vata and moderately, pitta. It decreases kapha.

**Stable**, sometimes called **static** or **slow**, relates to water and earth elements. It increases kapha and decreases vata and pitta.

**Dull** corresponds to earth and water. It increases kapha and decreases vata and pitta.

**Sharp** relates to fire, space/ether and air. It increases pitta and vata while decreasing kapha.

**Soft** corresponds to water. It increases kapha while decreasing pitta and vata.

**Hard** relates to the earth and air elements. It increases vata while decreasing pitta and kapha.

**Smooth** is similar to soft. It relates primarily to water. It greatly increases kapha and mildly increases pitta. It decreases vata.

**Rough** is of the earth and air elements. It increases vata and decreases pitta and kapha.

**Clear** or **Light** corresponds to fire, ether and air. It increases vata and pitta while decreasing kapha.

**Dark** or **Cloudy** is of the earth and water elements. It increases kapha and decreases pitta and vata.

Other qualities such as masculine and feminine are also present in the doshas. Pitta is more masculine while kapha is feminine. Vata is neutral. The balance of the masculine and feminine energies within oneself depends on the prakriti. It is ideal to have equal amounts of both masculine and feminine energies.

## Ojas, Tejas, Prana

*The mind alone is the cause of bondage and liberation.*
*The mind that is attached to the objects of the senses*
*leads them to bondage.*
*Freed from the objects of attachment,*
*it leads them to liberation.*

*~ Satyayaniya Upanishad, verse 1.1*

The doshas are composed of the five elements. Ojas, tejas and prana are the very subtle forms of the doshas. These three are the positive, life-giving aspects of the doshas. Prana is our vital life force and is the healing energy of vata. Tejas is our inner light and is the healing energy of pitta. Ojas is the ultimate energy reserve of the body that manifests from kapha. In Ayurveda, one wants to reduce excess in the doshas to prevent disease, while developing more prana, tejas and ojas for good health. A person with strong, healthy prana has vitality, breath, circulation, movement and adaptability. Someone endowed with good tejas has radiance, luster in the eyes, clarity, insight, courage, compassion and fearlessness. A person with strong ojas has strong immunity, endurance, calmness and contentment.

Like the doshas and gunas, it is necessary that these elements are in alignment with each other and within our consciousness, giving us physical, psychological and spiritual stamina.

Ojas in its pure form relates to kapha and the water element. Tejas in its subtle form relates to pitta and the fire element. Prana in its subtle form relates to vata and the ether element. They are often compared to the principles of *yin, yang* and *chi* of the Chinese medical system. Ojas is the yin, tejas the yang and prana the chi. When ojas, tejas and prana are functioning harmoniously, the mind enters a state of waking stillness and we experience peace deep within. As with the doshas, when our life force is out of balance, we feel disturbed and our health diminishes. If we maintain balance, our life becomes peaceful, happy and free from disease.

## Ojas

*Om prema-rupayai namah*

I bow to Her who is Pure Love.
~ *Sri Lalita Sahasranama, verse 730*

The most crucial factor in wellness is ojas, the higher aspect of kapha dosha. Ojas is the essential root power, our basic energy. Ojas is the subtle energy of the water element and thus relates to kapha dosha. It is the accumulated vital reserve, the basis of physical and mental energy. Ojas is the internalized essence of digested food, water, air, impressions and thoughts. On an inner level it is responsible for nourishing and developing all higher facilities. Ojas is our core vitality. It is the basic capacity of the immune system to defend us against external pathogens. Ojas provides endurance, resistance and strength to ward off disease. It affords not only physical immunity, but emotional and mental immunity as well. It is a superfine substance that gives strength to the bodily tissues, organs and processes. Ojas is the motherly qualities of nurturance and love. Without ojas, we are lifeless. Ojas is the pure vibration of love and compassion in the heart. When one is filled with love, the gross and subtle immune system is very strong and disease cannot penetrate into the body. Ojas is the product of pure thoughts and actions as well as the intake of pure foods and impressions. It gives us mental strength, contentment, purity, patience, calmness, adaptability and excellent mental faculties. Ojas is also the auric field that, when strong, emits a beautiful, serene glow of golden light. This field protects us from external negative influences.

Ojas is increased and maintained through proper diet (sattvic, vegetarian or vegan diet), tonic herbs, sensory control (including celibacy or proper use of sexual energy) and Bhakti Yoga (including seva).

Foods that increase ojas are whole grains, fruits and vegetables (especially root vegetables), nuts and seeds, pure quality dairy (not pasteurized or homogenized) and pure water and air. Dates, almonds and ghee are especially beneficial ojas-increasing foods and can be taken together as a tonic.

# Tejas

*Om parasmai jyotishe namah*

I bow to Her who is the Supreme Light.
*~ Sri Lalita Sahasranama, verse 806*

Tejas is our inner light and the subtle energy of the fire element, pitta. It is the radiant mental vitality through which we digest air, impressions and thoughts. On an inner level, it opens up higher perceptual abilities. Tejas is the fire of the intellect, knowledge and reason. It gives the power of proper discrimination such as knowing the eternal from the non-eternal and right from wrong. Tejas is the power of sadhana or spiritual practices such as self-discipline, scriptural study and mantra japa. Tejas is necessary for Jnana Yoga, the yoga of knowledge. It bestows clarity of mind and speech as well as courage and faith. It gives the power to know the Self and the endurance to persist on the path toward the One. Practices like *atma-vicharya* (Self-inquiry) increase the intensity of tejas within the mind and heart.

Like ojas, tejas is a vital part of our immunity. Tejas is the immune system's ability to burn and destroy toxins. When activated, it generates fever to destroy pathogens that assault the body. Tejas is our ability to attack and overcome acute diseases, which are generally infectious in nature. As fire, it is the power of digestion and the transformation of our food, thoughts, emotions and actions. Someone with strong tejas will have bright, penetrating eyes, lustrous skin and an attractive personality.

Tejas can be increased and maintained by performing tapas (purification through the heat or spiritual practices), such as controlling the tongue (fasting and observing silence). It is often said that if we cannot control the tongue we will never be able to control the mind. Chanting of mantras is an excellent way to harness the pure quality of the tongue and the mind. Studying scriptures is also very beneficial. One must do spiritual practices under the guidance of a competent guide so as to protect tejas from becoming too high. If tejas becomes too high, it can deplete ojas and harm the nervous system.

# Prana

*Om prana-datryai namah*

I bow to Her who is the giver of life.
~ *Sri Lalita Sahasranama, verse 832*

Prana is our vital life force and the subtle energy of the air element, vata. As the divine force and guiding intelligence behind all psycho-physical functions, it is responsible for the coordination of the breath, senses and mind. On an inner level, it awakens and balances all higher states of consciousness. Prana governs all aspects of our life, physical and spiritual. Prana is our ability of coordination and speech. Prana is the essence of sound and governs all mantras. It is the breath that gives life; it literally breathes life into all of creation. It is our creative impulse and desire for evolution. It is the pull of the unmanifest calling us home. Prana unifies Shiva and Shakti (purusha and prakriti). It is the Kundalini Shakti lying dormant at the base of the spine waiting to merge with Her beloved in the crown of our head at the lotus of infinite brilliant light, the Self.

Prana is the vitalized activation of the immune system's natural functions to project and develop our life force. It manifests when we are fighting off chronic diseases. It is the adaptability of the immune system and sustains all long-term healing processes. With sufficient prana, tejas and ojas, no disease can harm us.

Prana is increased through practices like meditation, pranayama, hatha yoga and the chanting of mantras, especially aum. Prana is the unifying factor between ojas and tejas. Once ojas is present, tejas is born. Prana develops from the union of ojas and tejas. Ojas and tejas could not sustain themselves without prana.

Prana, tejas and ojas are the divine manifestations of the three doshas. According to Ayurveda, when the doshas are too high or too low, they cause disease. But prana, tejas and ojas, unlike the doshas, promote health, creativity and well-being and provide support for deeper sadhana. Prana, tejas and ojas do not cause disease. They are the radiant manifestations in our life. We only have disease if they are imbalanced or lacking. As with all things in creation, conditions of excess and deficiency can arise when prana, tejas and ojas are out of balance.

Prana in excess creates a loss of mental control, sense and motor function. Its predominant manifestation is a lack of grounding or centering within one's own self. Deficient prana causes mental dullness or a lack of mental energy, enthusiasm and creativity. Tejas in excess causes the mind to become very critical and discriminating. Emotional outbursts of anger, irritation and rage may follow. There will often be headaches, fever and burning sensations in the head or eyes. When tejas is weak there will be a passiveness, a lack of proper discrimination and an inability to learn from life. Motivating factors fall away from life and result in a lack of courage and ambition. Ojas in excess may cause sluggishness of the mental faculties. An imbalanced self-contentment may lead to lack of desire to progress on one's spiritual path. An excess of ojas may manifest as high cholesterol or high kapha. A deficiency of ojas is very common due to excess use of stimulants, sex, external input and an unwholesome drive toward overindulgence. Weak ojas appears as a lack of concentration, poor memory, poor self-esteem, lack of faith and devotion, poor or no motivation, nervous exhaustion and immune weakness.

Prana, tejas and ojas may be increased through not only spiritual practices, but also positive impressions such as positive life experiences, right diet, walks in nature, warm baths and the use of colors, gemstones, crystals and essential oils. Spending time in nature increases prana most effectively. Sitting, walking or doing spiritual practices near fresh bodies of water or in a secluded forest will increase prana, tejas and ojas tremendously, because nature is the true healer.

## Diet, Doshas and Gunas

Both Ayurveda and yoga emphasize "right diet" as the foundation of all healing therapies. Food is the first and most important form of medicine. A famous ayurvedic saying expounds, "If right diet is followed, no medicines are necessary. If wrong diet is followed, no medicines can help." Ayurveda and yoga recommend a sattvic diet (pure food, following ahimsa), as it brings balance to the physical, mental, emotional and spiritual body.

However, there are references to the consumption of meat for medicinal purposes in the original ayurvedic texts. In ancient times everything had a medicinal benefit. If an animal was used for the cure of a disease, it was not considered *himsa* (violence). For example, there was extensive use of goat soup for healing numerous diseases, especially tuberculosis. However, it is strongly encouraged to follow a purely vegetarian diet, unless meat is prescribed by a qualified Ayurveda practitioner. In the present day, eating animals has numerous health, environmental, political and socio-economic consequences. Scientific research shows that animal meat, fat, proteins and cholesterol promote cancer, heart disease, diabetes, obesity and numerous other diseases. A vegetarian diet follows the principles of ahimsa and sattva, avoiding any products that involve the killing of animals. In most scenarios, eating the flesh of an animal violates the principles of ahimsa. Additionally, eating pure, organic food supports good health. Non-organic food is produced using violent and destructive farming practices that harm the earth, our Mother.

Most humans cannot readily break down animal tissues into the proper nutrients for human tissues. Instead of digesting and transforming meat into the appropriate human tissue, the animal energies are preserved and substituted for our human tissues. Thus, eating animals increases the animalistic tendencies in our bodies and brings the traits of the animal to live within us, promoting anger, lust, fear and other negative emotions. Dead animals produce a heavy or tamasic type of tissue that clogs the body's energetic channels *(nadis)*, making the mind dull and lethargic. Not only violence and crime but also religious intolerance have proven to be more common among those who eat meat. On an economic level, the grain used to produce meat to serve one family could easily serve at least five families. The entire economic and environmental status of the world would change if most people resolved to become vegetarians.

# Chapter 5

# The Subdoshas

*Fire is his head, his eyes are the moon and the sun;*
*The regions of space are his ears, his voice the revealed Veda,*
*The wind is his breath,*
*his heart is the entire universe,*
*The earth is his footstool,*
*Truly he is the inner soul of all.*

*~ Mundaka Upanishad, 2.1.4*

The subdoshas are the natural elemental intelligences of vata, pitta and kapha functioning within our bodies. Each subdosha is connected to one of the five elements and has a specific function. The five forms of vata, known as the five pranas, are the most important because they are involved in all other processes.

## Subdosha Chart

| Element | Vata | Pitta | Kapha |
|---------|------|-------|-------|
| Ether | Prana | Sadhaka | Tarpaka |
| Air | Udana | Alochaka | Bodhaka |
| Fire | Samana | Pachaka | Kledaka |
| Water | Vyana | Bhrajaka | Sleshaka |
| Earth | Apana | Ranjaka | Avalambaka |

## Vata and the Subdoshas

*mamaivamso jivaloke
jivabhutah sanatanah
manah sastanindriyani
prakrtishtani karsati*

The eternal life force in each body is a particle of My own
being. Due to the conditioned life, they are struggling
very hard with the six senses, which include the mind.

*~ Bhagavad Gita, 15.7*

Vata has numerous functions in the body and in consciousness. Of
the various functions, five are the most important; from these five,
all other functions are possible.

### The five main functions of Vata

- *Purana* (to fill space)
- *Udvahana* (to move upward)
- *Viveka* (to separate, isolate, split)
- *Dharana* (to hold together, to hold the flow)
- *Praspandanam* (to pulsate, to throb).

### Function of Vata

- Physical movements
- Maintenance of life
- Communication
- Mind, movement of thoughts, sensory organs, perception
- Emotions
- Nerve impulses
- Respiration
- Heart function
- Circulation
- Ingestion
- Peristalsis

- Enzyme secretion
- Absorption, assimilation
- Elimination of urine, feces, sweat
- Menstruation
- Childbirth
- Cellular respiration and division
- Touch
- Clarity
- Orgasm
- Creativity
- Joy

## Vata Subdoshas and Their Functions

• *Prana*: The seat of prana is the head, chest, throat, tongue, mouth and nose. It controls functions such as salivation, eructation (belching), sneezing, respiration and deglutition (swallowing). It governs the senses, creative thinking, reasoning and enthusiasm.

• *Udana*: The seat of *udana vata* is the umbilicus, chest and throat. It also provides enthusiasm, vitality and complexion to human beings. It governs quality of voice, memory and movements of thought.

• *Samana*: The functions of *samana vata* are very similar to *agni* (digestive fire/digestive juices). It regulates the secretion of gastric juice, retains the food in the stomach or intestines for the proper amount of time, and then assists in its absorption. It governs movement of food through the digestive tract.

• *Vyana*: *Vyana vata* is seated all over the body and is responsible for the pulsation of the heart and blood circulation. It controls the movement of eyes and limbs, and governs perspiration and the sense of touch.

• *Apana*: The seat of *apana vata* includes the testes, bladder, umbilical region, thigh and groin. It controls the functions of elimination of semen, urine and feces. The movements related to the delivery of a fetus are also governed by apana vata.

# Prana

Prana vata functions in the head, neck, chest region. Prana governs inhalation and perception through the senses and the mind. It is located in the brain, head, throat, heart and respiratory organs. Thinking, creativity, learning new information and inhalation are examples of prana-vata-governed activities. It is also the connection to higher functions.

Prana vata imbalances result in respiratory disorders, cognitive problems, tension headaches, worry, anxiety, neurological disorders and insomnia. Just as vata is known to lead the other doshas, prana vata is said to lead the other subdoshas of vata, which is why it is the most important subdosha to keep balanced. In balance, it makes one alert, clear-headed, exhilarated and lively. With healthy prana vata, we are drawn toward that which is harmonious and which brings us greater health and well-being. When prana vata is out of balance, we misuse the senses and internalize that which will cause disease.

The inward movement of prana is responsible for the intake of impressions and sensory impulses. It is also responsible for our intake of food, water and air. On the deepest cosmic level it governs the mind, heart and consciousness. It vitalizes them by giving energy, coordination and adaptability.

Prana vata is responsible for perception and movement of all kinds. Located in the brain, prana vata enables the body to hear, touch, see and smell. It is first pure awareness, then becomes perception, sensation, the ability to feel, then thought and finally emotion. The more erratically prana moves, the more agitated the mind becomes. When prana is disturbed in our body we experience respiratory difficulties, mental problems and neurological disorders. In harmony, prana gives the body strength for longevity, power of breath, creativity and acute awareness of the mind and senses. It carries positive, healing energy. When prana is in balance we are open to the Divine and experience the cosmic oneness of creation.

## Udana

Udana vata functions in the throat and chest region. It governs speech, self-expression, effort, enthusiasm, strength and vitality. Sneezing, singing and exhalation are examples of udana vata-regulated activities. Udana vata is the upward movement of vata. Seated in the diaphragm, it moves through the lungs, bronchi, trachea and throat.

Whereas prana is the inhalation, udana is the exhalation. In the process of exhalation, udana is responsible for sound. It is responsible for the complexion of our skin, made possible by the process of respiration of the skin. An udana vata imbalance may create disorders such as faulty speech, stuttering and muttering as well as diseases of the throat (dry cough), ears (earaches), nose (bleeding) and neck (tonsillitis). Udana vata is also responsible for general fatigue.

Udana is responsible for memory. It enters the brain and stimulates memory. If imbalanced, it can block our memory; when deranged, it may stunt our creativity. Without the proper flow of udana we feel no direction in life. When balanced, we have clear, creative ideas and inspiration to manifest our goals and aspirations. Udana gives us lightness of body, the power to chant mantras or sing bhajans, and ultimately, the power to transcend ordinary consciousness at the time of physical death.

## Samana

Samana vata works in the stomach and small intestine. It governs the flow of food through the digestive tract and is responsible for peristaltic movement of the digestive system. A balancing force that activates agni (digestive fire), samana vata stimulates the secretion of hydrochloric acid. It balances the upper and lower parts of the body. Located in the small intestine, it is the power of the digestive system. Samana stimulates hunger in the body by sending messages to prana in the brain to take in food. It rules over appetite, digestion, absorption and assimilation. When it is out of balance, there is a lack of appetite and nervous indigestion. Samana vata also governs over the liver, spleen, pancreas, stomach and part of the large intestine. Imbalance of samana vata is responsible for too slow or too rapid digestion, gas, diarrhea, nervous stomach, inadequate assimilation of nutrients and emaciated tissue formation. When weak or out of balance, one may also experience irregular and weak digestion, improper formation of the *dhatus* (tissues), anorexia and lymphatic stagnation.

When samana is functioning properly, impressions are properly absorbed. Balanced samana vata brings peace, balance, harmony, subtlety, concentration, one-pointedness and equilibrium within us and our environment.

## Vyana

Vyana vata radiates from the heart to the entire body through the circulatory system and the skin. Vyana vata is the circulatory movement that maintains cardiac activity, the beating and rhythm of the heart, the circulation of the blood and lymph, the nutrition and oxygenation of the cells and organs, and locomotion. Sweating and the sense of touch are examples of vyana vata activity. Vyana vata is also responsible for the movement of the joints and skeletal muscles. It governs our breathing process, senses, emotions, thoughts and consciousness.

When vyana is disturbed it blocks oxygen flow and shuts off blood from the heart and brain. This blockage results in heart attacks, seizures, strokes, aneurisms, heart disease, paralysis, edema and other heart and circulatory diseases such as high blood pressure and arrhythmia (irregular heartbeat). In addition, vyana blockage results in numerous nervous disorders as well as other disease processes.

Vyana is the free-flowing manifestation of our inspirations and goals. When it is harmonized, we feel a sense of expansion, adaptability, freedom, openness to Divine Consciousness and free-flowing prana.

## Apana

Apana vata works in the colon and pelvic area and governs such functions as menstruation and the elimination of wastes. Located between the navel and the anus, apana vata governs all downward impulses (such as urination, elimination, menstruation and sexual discharges). It is situated in the colon, rectum, urinary tract, cecum, pelvic cavity, kidneys and the reproductive organs. It is responsible for flatulence and the act of conception. Deficiency in apana vata prevents successful conception. Impairment of apana vata leads to constipation or diarrhea, retention of urine, delayed or lack of menstruation, or excessive and painful menstruation. It also creates sexual dysfunction, lower back pain, swollen prostate and muscle spasms. As it nourishes the bones, apana is responsible for osteoporosis and other bone disorders. When apana is harmonized, there is strong immune function and the feelings of stability, calmness, groundedness and well-being prevail.

## Pitta and the Five Subdoshas

*aham vaisvanaro bhutva*
*praninam dehamasritah*
*pranapanasamayuktah*
*pacamyannam caturvidham*

Taking the form of fire lodged in the body of all creatures
and united with their exhalations and inhalations,
it is I who consume the four kinds of food.
*~ Bhagavad Gita, 15.14*

The five forms of pitta are known as the five *agnis*, or fires. As fire gives warmth, light and transformation, so do the five agnis transform inside us. Pitta governs bodily metabolism, digestion, absorption, and assimilation. It maintains body temperature, appetite, thirst, taste, color, luster of eyes, hair, skin, body. It maintains intelligence, understanding, comprehension, knowledge, courage, ambition, transformation and visual-mental perception. The five forms of pitta are *sadhaka, alochaka, pachaka, bhrajaka* and *ranjaka*.

## Pitta Subdoshas and Their Functions

• **Sadhaka**: *Sadhaka pitta* is seated in the heart *(hrdayam)* and is responsible for intelligence and the ego. It is due to sadhaka pitta that all the functions of the mind and body are coordinated. It controls desire, motivation, decisiveness and spirituality.

• **Alochaka**: *Alochaka pitta* is located in the eyes and governs all functioning of the eyes.

• **Pachaka**: *Pachaka pitta* is located in the stomach and intestinal region, also known as *grahani*. Its main function is digestion; it also augments the pitta situated elsewhere in the body. It governs digestion, assimilation and metabolism for healthy nutrients and tissues.

• **Bhrajaka**: The seat of *bhrajaka pitta* is the skin; it is responsible for pigmentation and the healthy glow of the skin.

• **Ranjaka**: The seat of *ranjaka pitta* is the liver and spleen. Its main function is to convert plasma *(rasa)* into blood *(rakta)*. It is responsible for healthy, toxin-free blood.

## Sadhaka

Sadhaka pitta is located both in the grey matter of the brain and in the cardiac plexus or heart chakra. It is responsible for mental digestion, mental energy and the power of discrimination. Sadhaka pitta governs emotional balance, contentment, intelligence and memory. It gives the energy to achieve and realize. It is the primal force behind the desire for liberation and gives the energy to do sadhana. In the heart, sadhaka pitta gives the power of love and compassion, governing feeling and emotion. As it eventually unifies with the higher self, it is ultimately transformed into unconditional love. In the brain, sadhaka pitta produces neurotransmitters. For these reasons, when sadhaka pitta is deficient one may experience sadness, depression and low self-esteem. There may be chemical imbalances in the brain. Other imbalances in sadhaka pitta are linked to heart disease, memory loss, emotional disturbance (sadness, anger, heartache) and indecisiveness. When harmonious, sadhaka pitta gives the power to perceive the true nature of reality. With proper perception, one can see the unity in all creation and can truly say that the heart and the divine mind are functioning in harmony.

## Alochaka

Alochaka pitta functions in the eye region and governs vision and perception. Alochaka pitta governs good or bad vision, depending on if it is in balance or out of balance. It also connects the eyes with emotions. An imbalance in alochaka pitta creates bloodshot eyes, vision problems and eye diseases of all kinds. In balance, it creates bright, clear, healthy eyes that emanate a warm, content gaze. It governs intake of external stimulus through the eyes as well as the ability to look and see within one's own self.

When alochaka pitta is strong, the eyes are filled with a spark of light; hence it is often said that the eyes are the window to the soul. The brighter the inner light, the clearer the eyes are, and they radiate that light. Alochaka pitta is also the higher power of perception, the ability to perceive things as they are.

As our perception becomes clear, we begin to see the world and creation as the beautiful manifestation of God. William Blake said, "When the doors of perception are cleansed, things will appear as they truly are, infinite." The illusion of maya disappears like a mirage in the desert when we come close to it. We perceive truth everywhere.

# Pachaka

Pachaka pitta is located in the duodenum/lower stomach and small intestine. It regulates the transformation and digestion of food that is broken down into nutrients and waste. Producing digestive enzymes, pachaka pitta is the power to digest, absorb and assimilate nutrients. On the mental and emotional level, it is our ability to digest life's experiences. In the body, it digests starch, glucose and fructose – all of the sweets. Pachaka pitta is often associated with *jathara agni*, the fire of the stomach. This agni is the internal central fire in which all food is "cooked." When there is an excess in pachaka pitta one may experience inflammation, gastritis, ulcers, hyperacidity, indigestion, anorexia, hypoglycemia and dyspepsia. Deficient pachaka pitta may cause poor absorption and assimilation of food and nutrients, low body heat and weak agni. Pachaka pitta supports all the other forms of agni. It balances the fires of the body and regulates metabolism. When in balance, pachaka pitta affords strong mental faculties, great inner wisdom and clarity, and a strong spiritual or humanitarian inclination.

# Bhrajaka

Bhrajaka pitta is located in the skin. It regulates the biochemical processes that occur therein and governs the luster, complexion, temperature and pigmentation of the skin.

Bhrajaka pitta is the fire that warms the body and gives a bright complexion. It is the power of circulation. It is also the warmth we feel and are able to give to the world. It fuels the senses of touch, pain, temperature and stereognosis. It assists in digesting or assimilating oils and other medicines like pastes that are applied to the skin. An imbalance of bhrajaka pitta is responsible for skin disorders such as rashes, acne, boils, skin cancers, eczema, psoriasis, dermatitis and loss of sense of touch, tingling and numbness.

Emotionally, bhrajaka rules the feelings of anger, irritability and impatience. If you look at someone who is angry, you may notice that their skin is very red or they may appear "hotheaded." This is due to a combination of bhrajaka pitta and prana imbalances. Likewise, you may have noticed that when you see someone who is scared, filled with fear and anxiety, they may appear white, or "as pale as a ghost." When bhrajaka pitta and prana are balanced, a gentle glow and warmth of the body, mind and aura manifest. One who has this balance radiates vitality and happiness.

## Ranjaka

Ranjaka pitta resides in the liver, gall bladder and spleen; it is responsible for blood composition and the distribution of nutrients to cells and tissues throughout the blood. It governs the formation of red blood cells and gives color to blood and stools. Ranjaka pitta is the fire that imparts color to the body. Situated in the liver, gall bladder, spleen and stomach, it produces bile and liver enzymes. Its home is the blood, and when imbalanced, it aggravates the liver. The liver gives color to the skin, hair and eyes. Ranjaka pitta is responsible for the creation of red blood cells in the bone marrow from blood plasma. Ranjaka in the spleen is responsible for destroying unfriendly bacteria and parasites. It also produces white blood cells and strengthens blood and the immune system. When deviated, ranjaka pitta causes hepatitis, jaundice, anemia, chronic fatigue syndrome, mononucleosis, gallstones, high cholesterol, fatty deposits in the liver or liver degeneration, anger and hostility. Toxins in the body from impure food, air, water, alcohol or cigarettes are a primary cause of pitta imbalances, acting through ranjaka pitta.

## Kapha and the Five Subdoshas

*gamavisya ca bhutani*
*dharayamyahamojasa*
*pusnami causadhih sarvah*
*somo bhutva rasatmakah.*

Permeating the soil,
it is I who supports all creatures by My vital power.
Becoming the nectarous moon, I nourish all of the plants.
*~ Bhagavad Gita 15.13*

Kapha, being of earth and water, acts like glue by binding things together. Kapha governs lubrication, nourishment, support and stability, groundedness, growth, stamina, energy, repair and regeneration, gaseous exchange in the lungs, gastric secretion, water electrolyte balance, fat regulation, strength, sleep, memory retention, contentment, forgiveness, compassion, taste perception and olfactory perception. The five forms of kapha are tarpaka, bodhaka, kledaka, sleshaka and avalambaka.

## Kapha Subdoshas and Their Functions

• *Tarpaka*: *Tarpaka kapha* is seated in the head. It nurtures the mental faculties and is responsible for moisturizing the nose, mouth, eyes and brain.
• *Bodhaka*: *Bodhaka kapha* is seated on the tongue. It governs the sense of taste, which is essential for good digestion.
• *Kledaka*: *Kledaka kapha* is seated in the stomach. It is slimy (*picchila*) in quality, sweet in taste and has the task of moistening the ingested food. It also protects the digestive organs from being hurt by the digestive juices. It controls moisture of the stomach and intestinal mucosal lining.
• *Sleshaka*: *Sleshaka kapha* is seated in the joints. Its function is to lubricate the joints and keep skin soft and supple.

• *Avalambaka*: *Avalambaka kapha* is located in the chest cavity where it gives nutrition to the heart. It protects the heart, gives strong heart muscles and promotes healthy lungs.

## Tarpaka

Tarpaka kapha, located in the head, sinuses and cerebrospinal fluid, provides lubrication to nerve and brain tissue and nourishment to the sense and motor organs. It also provides calmness, happiness and stability. Tarpaka kapha is responsible for the nourishment of the mind. The word *tarpaka* means "contentment" and is also translated as "to nourish, to retain, to record." Tarpaka kapha is the cerebrospinal fluid that surrounds the brain and spinal cord. It protects the myelin sheath and, when deficient, can cause multiple sclerosis. Additionally, it forms the predominance of the white matter of the brain, and serves as a repository that stores or records past experiences and memories. It is located in the heart and gives peace and satisfaction.

Tarpaka kapha governs stability, happiness, joy, bliss and memory. In terms of memory, it is responsible for our past-life impressions and has an effect on our subtle or astral bodies known as the koshas. It also governs our awareness and attention while working on the conscious and subconscious levels. It keeps the nose, mouth and eyes moist, protecting these sense organs. It maintains the spinal fluid that is essential for the central nervous system. Imbalance of tarpaka kapha is responsible for sinus congestion, hay fever, sinus headache, impaired sense of smell and general dullness of the senses. When tarpaka kapha is deficient one often sees symptoms such as memory loss, confusion, Alzheimer's, stroke paralysis, brain tumors, multiple sclerosis, discontentment, malaise, nervousness and insomnia.

## Bodhaka

Bodhaka kapha is located in the tongue and throat and governs taste. It also governs the lubrication of food and facilitates swallowing. Bodhaka kapha is responsible for perception of taste. Bodhaka means "to make known." Kaphas relate to the world primarily through taste, along with smell. Kaphas who have abused the sense of taste often develop the problem of compulsive eating. If one eats too much or too often, the taste buds lose their sensitivity. Bodhaka kapha may also be desensitized by overuse of only a few of the six tastes such as eating primarily sweet and salty foods. When taste diminishes, the body becomes much more vulnerable to other kapha problems such as obesity, food allergies, congestion of mucous membranes and diabetes.

Bodhaka kapha is responsible for the production of saliva and is responsible for the first part of digestion. It stimulates the salivary glands and makes digestive enzymes. Since the taste buds are located on the tongue, out-of-balance bodhaka kapha leads to an inability to taste food or smell properly. If bodhaka kapha is low, the salivary glands do not secrete sufficient saliva, leaving the palate too dry to taste food. Harmonized bodhaka kapha produces plentiful saliva that helps to absorb our food and nourish *rasa dhatu* (plasma).

## Kledaka

Kledaka kapha functions in the gastric area. Located in the upper part of the stomach, it moistens and liquefies ingested food in the initial stages of digestion. Its principal function is the lubrication of ingested food for easier digestion.

Kledaka kapha is that which moistens or softens. It is soft, oily, liquid and slimy by nature. It is located in the stomach and digestive tract as the mucous lining. It liquefies our food and starts the digestive process. When there is improper liquefication of our food, excess phlegm accumulates and irregular stomach secretions occur.

_daka in the stomach can result in irritation and lead gastritis. This deficiency can also cause nausea, vomiting and severe stomachaches. Like other aspects of kapha subdoshas, when kledaka is harmonized, it brings contentment, affection and a feeling of being nourished. When out of balance, it leads to feelings of anxiety, insecurity, loneliness, grief, sadness and depression. Other physical ailments caused by kledaka kapha are obesity, overeating, hyperglycemia, diabetes and high cholesterol.

## Sleshaka

Sleshaka kapha is located in the joints and provides lubrication to keep the joints smooth and flexible. It is thick, sticky, fluid, oily and slimy, manifesting as the synovial fluid that facilitates easy movement. When impaired, arthritic conditions arise that can be accompanied by mild to severe joint pain and congestion or swelling. Imbalance of sleshaka kapha also contributes to loose, watery or painful joints, various joint diseases and sciatica. Deficient sleshaka kapha indicates excessive vata and results in the bones becoming brittle and dry. The most common sleshaka diseases are degenerative and rheumatoid arthritis. When sleshaka is balanced there is good prana and a strong, clear and conscious mind. It gives strength, endurance and determination.

## Avalambaka

Avalambaka kapha resides in the heart, chest, lungs and lower back. It governs the lubrication of the heart and lung tissue, which slows down wear and tear. It also provides strength to the back, chest and heart. Avalambaka kapha is that which supports. It is the transport system that carries prana to every cell, tissue and organ in the body. The physical stamina of kapha comes from these areas, so the kapha physique usually exhibits a powerful chest and shoulders.

In balance, avalambaka kapha provides strong muscles and a well-protected heart. Its liquid quality forms the pericardial fluid that surrounds the heart. It is the source of prana in the heart and lungs. It is also located in the lining of the lungs, trachea, bronchi and the bronchioles. Avalambaka kapha is also responsible for the gaseous exchange that takes place in the alveoli. It assures the removal of carbon dioxide and absorption of oxygen. When avalambaka is out of balance, one may experience respiratory problems, an accumulation of mucous and phlegm, lethargy, lower back pain, heart diseases and lung congestion accompanied by swollen glands. Avalambaka kapha governs plasma, the body's main water constituent. Avalambaka kapha also governs lung disorders such as bronchitis, asthma, pneumonia, wheezing, emphysema and bronchial collapse. If out of balance, one may suffer from persistent back pain in the area behind the chest and heart, and may experience deep sadness and prolonged grief. When functioning harmoniously, avalambaka is responsible for love, compassion, receptivity and caring.

The subdoshas of each of the three main doshas have direct correlations with each other and together govern all of the processes in our bodies. Prana vata, sadhaka pitta and tarpaka kapha are responsible for brain, heart and nervous system functioning. Udana vata, alochaka pitta and bodhaka kapha are responsible for functions in the head and govern sensory activity, such as perception, aspiration and will. Samana vata, pachaka pitta and kledaka kapha govern the digestive processes. Vyana vata, bhrajaka pitta and sleshaka kapha govern movement of the limbs, and the health of skin. Apana vata, ranjaka pitta and avalambaka kapha are the support for the other subdoshas.

For optimal health, the goal is to balance and harmonize the subdoshas, or the subtle levels, with the other overall doshas, or the gross levels. When all of these aspects are in harmony we attain a deep sense of inner peace and contentment.

## ubdosha Charts

| dosha | | Balanced | Imbalanced |
|---|---|---|---|
| *Prana* | Heart | Breathing and swallowing | Hiccups, bronchitis, asthma, cold, hoarseness of voice |
| *Udana* | Throat | Speech and voice | Diseases of eye, ear, nose and throat |
| *Samana* | Stomach and small intestine | Helps action of digestive enzymes, assimilation of end products of food and separation into their various tissue elements | Indigestion, diarrhea, defective assimilation |
| *Vyana* | Heart | Maintains circulation | Impairment of circulation, fever |
| *Apana* | Colon and pelvis | Elimination of stool, urine, semen, fetal and menstrual blood | Urinary and bladder diseases, diabetes, diseases of anus and testicles |

### Pitta

| Subdosha | Site | Balanced | Imbalanced |
|---|---|---|---|
| *Sadhaka* | Heart | Memory and other mental functions | Psychic disturbances, cardiac diseases |
| *Alochaka* | Eyes | Vision | Impairment of vision |
| *Pachaka* | Stomach and small intestine | Digestion | Indigestion, anorexia |
| *Bhrajaka* | Skin | Color and luster of the skin | Leucoderma, other skin diseases |

| *Ranjaka* | Liver, spleen and stomach | Blood function | Anemia, jau~~n~~ hepatitis |

## Kapha

| Subdosha | Site | Balanced | Imbalanced |
|----------|------|----------|------------|
| *Tarpaka* | Brain | Nourishes the sense organs | Loss of memory, impairment of sense organs |
| *Bodhaka* | Tongue | Perception of taste | Impairment of digestion |
| *Kledaka* | Stomach | Moistens food, which helps digestion | Impairment of digestion |
| *Sleshaka* | Joints | Lubrication of joints | Pain in joints, impairment of joints |
| *Avalambaka* | Heart | Energy in limbs | Laziness |

# Chapter 6

# Ayurvedic Anatomy

*The five sheaths of the Self are those of food, the vital air, the mind, the intellect and bliss. Because the Self is enveloped in them, it forgets its real nature and becomes subject to transmigration. The gross body, which is the product of the quintuplicate elements, is known as the food sheath. That portion of the subtle body which is composed of the five vital airs and the five organs of action, and which is the effect of the rajas aspect of prakriti, is called the vital sheath. The doubting mind and the five sensory organs, which are the effect of sattva, make up the mind sheath. The determining intellect and the sensory organs make up the intellect sheath. The impure sattva which is in the causal body, along with joy and other vrittis (mental modifications), is called the bliss sheath. Due to identification with the different sheaths, the Self assumes their respective natures. By differentiating the Self from the five sheaths through the method of distinguishing between the variable and the invariable, one can draw out one's own Self from the five sheaths and attain the supreme Brahman.*

*~ Sri Panchadasi, verse 33-37*

## The Dhatus

There are seven *dhatus*, or layers of tissue, in the human body. The word dhatu literally means "to hold together," "to firm" or "to construct." Dhatus are the layers of bodily tissue that support and hold the body together, giving it form. The nutrients we receive from our digested food create the dhatus. Each tissue is governed by one of the three elements, and each dhatu is developed from the preceding tissue layer, beginning with *rasa* (plasma). If the plasma is not healthy, then all the other layers are affected. Each dhatu produces a secondary tissue known as its *upadhatu,* as well as a type of *mala* (waste material).

Dhatus are the sites in the body where diseases manifest. Each dhatu can be in excess, deficient or balanced in relation to the rest of the body. When one dhatu is diseased or impaired it affects the next dhatu and subsequently the next, as each receives its nutrients from the preceding one.

The seven dhatus in order of production are *rasa* (plasma), *rakta* (blood), *mamsa* (muscle), *meda* (fat), *asthi* (bone), *majja* (marrow and nerves), and *shukra/artava* (male/female reproductive fluid). Each dhatu is formed from the previous dhatu. Rasa becomes rakta, rakta becomes mamsa, mamsa becomes meda, meda becomes asthi, asthi becomes majja, and majja becomes shukra and artava. The formation of ojas is the final product of the nutritional process of the dhatus.

Each of the dhatus has two main aspects: *sthayi* (stable) and *asthayi*(unstable). As the dhatus develop, several processes occur. First, the formative parts of the dhatu turn into a stable form through the dhatu agni (the agni or digestive process of each tissue). Through this process the upadhatus are formed. Then mala (waste material) is formed through a process similar to the digestion of food. In the final stage, the purified form of the formative tissue is made for the next dhatu.

# The Seven Dhatus, Upadhatus, Malas and Their Functions

1. *Rasa dhatu* (plasma tissue): Rasa derives from digested food, and then nourishes each and every tissue and cell of the body; it is analogous to plasma. The upadhatus for rasa are breast milk and menstrual blood. The mala of rasa dhatu is phlegm.

2. *Rakta dhatu* (blood tissue): Rakta is viewed as the basis of life and is analogous to the circulating blood cells. It nourishes the body tissues and provides physical strength and color to the body. The upadhatus for rakta are the blood vessels, skin and tendons. The mala of rakta dhatu is bile.

3. *Mamsa dhatu* (muscle tissue): Mamsa is muscle tissue, and its main function is to provide physical strength and support for the meda dhatu. The upadhatus for mamsa are the ligaments and skin. The malas of mamsa dhatu are the waste materials of the outer bodily cavities like the ears and nose, for example earwax and nasal crust.

4. *Meda dhatu* (fat tissue): Meda consists of adipose (fat) tissue providing support to asthi dhatu. Meda lubricates the body. The upadhatu for meda is omentum, the peritoneal fat of the abdomen. The mala for meda dhatu is sweat.

5. *Asthi dhatu* (bone tissue): Asthi is comprised of bone tissue, including cartilage. Its main function is to give support to the majja and mamsa dhatus. The upadhatu of asthi is the teeth. The malas for asthi dhatu are the nails and hair.

6. *Majja dhatu* (marrow and nerve tissue): Majja denotes the bone marrow tissue, nervous system and brain. Its main function is to lubricate the body. It is a very soft, jelly-like substance that fills the bone cavity. The upadhatu for majja is the sclerotic fluid in the eyes. The malas of majja dhatu are tears and other secretions of the eyes.

7. *Shukra and artava dhatu* (semen and reproductive tissue): The main purpose of the reproductive tissue is to aid in reproduction and to strengthen the body. The upadhatu for shukra and artava

dhatus is ojas. The mala for shukra and artava dhatus is smegma, the waste secreted from the genitals.

## Rasa

Rasa, or plasma, contains all of the digested nutrients and gives nourishment to all the dhatus, organs and bodily systems. The word rasa means "juice" or "sap." Rasa is kapha by nature and contains all five elements and the three gunas. Its main sites in the body are the heart, blood vessels, lymph fluid, skin and the mucous membranes. Rasa gives the feeling of fullness. It is responsible for the hydration of the bodily tissues.

When plasma is in its excess state, there will be excessive saliva and phlegm, blocked channels, decrease or loss of hunger, lymphatic congestion and nausea. When rasa is deficient the skin will be rough to the touch and the lips will be dry and chapped; both are signs of dehydration. The body and mind may be tired and weary with a hypersensitivity toward loud or sudden noises. There may be heart tremors or palpitations and a general feeling of exhaustion, premature aging, wrinkled skin due to dryness and emaciation.

Some causes of rasa imbalances are heavy food, cold food and drinks, tamasic food, overeating, oily and fried foods, excessive sugar and salt intake, bad food-combining, excessive thoughts, worries and fears, bacteria, worms, parasites and excessive *ama* (toxins).

When rasa is in harmony, there will be a good complexion, healthy, flowing hair, glowing skin, good stamina and strength, and joyful feelings. Plasma is built by drinking plenty of water, juices and other healthful liquids. Pure, organic, non-homogenized dairy products also build rasa by strengthening ojas.

# Rakta

Rakta, or blood, is fed by healthy rasa. Rakta is composed of the fire and water elements and has generally a pitta-dominant nature. The word *rakta* means "that which is red." Healthy blood is our vital life force. It oxygenates our cells. When the blood is strong, our lives are full and healthy and there is a deep feeling of love and abundance.

Excess rakta leads to skin disorders, abscesses, enlarged liver and spleen, burning, redness and/or bleeding of the skin, eyes and urine. All inflammatory conditions are due to pitta and rakta.

Deficient rakta results in anemia, paleness of skin, low blood pressure, craving of cold and sour food, dryness of the head, collapsing blood vessels and rough or cracked skin.

Rakta imbalances are caused by eating food that is too hot, spicy food, too much sugar and salt, sour foods, oily and fried food, bad food-combining, drug use (including alcohol and tobacco), blood loss, iron and vitamin B-12 deficiencies, radiation (including from cell phones), anger, hatred, jealousy, repressed emotions, bacteria, worms, parasites, and any liver or spleen disease.

When rakta is healthy there will be good skin tone throughout the body. The eyes will have a glow and the skin will be warm to the touch. There will be strong vitality and a passion for life. Rakta is strengthened by iron-rich foods like seaweed, black sesame seeds, molasses, jaggery, dark grapes and root vegetables like beets, carrots and burdock.

# Mamsa

Mamsa is muscle. Mamsa strengthens our body and gives us the capacity for work and action. Mamsa is mostly composed of the earth element and holds the body together. Mamsa is predominantly kapha with a small amount of pitta. Mamsa is responsible for the movement of urine, lymph, sweat and blood. Whenour muscles move, our blood moves, which gives us strength, ambition and courage.

When there is too moch mamsa there will be swelling and tumors of the muscles, heaviness and swelling of the glands, obesity, an enlarged liver, anger and aggression. In women this can result in uterine fibroids or miscarriages, and there may even be infertility.

When the mamsa is deficient there will be emaciation, fatigue, loose limbs, a lack of coordination, fear, anxiety, insecurity and general depression and unhappiness.

Causes of mamsa deficiency are an excessive or deficient intake of protein, consumption of meat and too much dairy, bad food-combining, lack of exercise, sleeping during the day, poor quality of sleep, physical trauma, emotional or mental stress, liver disorders, tuberculosis or typhoid fever.

The muscles of the body make up half of the body's weight. When mamsa is balanced there will be good muscle tone, good physical strength for the individual constitution, flexibility, adaptability in movement, a good build of shoulders, neck and thighs, and a feeling of courage and security. Mamsa is strengthened by whole grains, beans, nuts, and seeds containing protein, especially hemp seed. It is also nourished by all other foods containing easily digestible forms of protein and amino acids.

## Meda

Meda, or fat, is fed by mamsa. Meda is oily and lubricates all of the dhatus. It is the adipose tissue or the loose connective tissue that includes fat, phospholipids, cholesterol and other types of lipids. Meda means "that which is oily." The Sanskrit word for "oily" is *sneha*, which also means "love." Meda is soft, comforting and of a motherly nature. It warms and protects. When there is a lack of love from another human being, people often turn to food for comfort and this excess intake can lead to obesity. Obesity is a serious problem in the western world today.

When there is an excess of meda, there will be obesity, fatigue, a lack of mobility, swelling and inflammation such as arthritis, asthma, sexual debility, incontinence, hypertension, high blood pressure, high cholesterol, gallstones, blockages of the bile duct, diabetes, a short life span, and a sagging belly, breasts and thighs. Emotional imbalances may occur as well, which in turn can create food cravings.

When there are deficient amounts of fat, there will also be fatigue, as well as cracking joints and tendons, enlargement of the spleen, emaciation of limbs and abdomen, brittle nails and teeth, and weakness of hair and bones. There will also be emotional imbalances including fear, doubt and lack of self-love.

Causes of meda disorders include too much sugar, carbohydrates, salt, dairy, meat, oily and fried food, poor quality fats, poor food-combining, emotional eating, stress, unresolved emotions, lack of or too much exercise (depending on the dosha dominance), use of drugs (i.e., alcohol, marijuana, tobacco and amphetamines) and typhoid fever.

When meda is in equilibrium, there will be an adequate amount of fat per body type, the tissues, hair, eyes and feces will have sufficient lubrication and the speech will be harmonious. Emotionally, one will be content, sharing love, affection, joy and humor as a result of the balance one has in all areas of life. Meda is increased by fats such as ghee, butter, sesame oil and dairy products.

## Asthi

Asthi is bone. It is fed by the meda dhatu, and gives structure to the body and to our lives. It is made up mostly of the earth element and is ruled by kapha dosha. It is partially air and contains marrow, which is composed of vata. As bones are responsible for movement, asthi upholds the tissues and makes them firm. The word *asthi* comes from the word *stha*, which means "to stand or endure."

When there is an excess of asthi dhatu there may be extra bones, bone spurs, extra teeth, an excessively large body frame, painful joints, fear, anxiety and weak endurance. There will be a tendency toward arthritis and bone cancer.

When asthi is deficient there will be weariness, weakness, pain and looseness in the joints, loss of hair, teeth and nails, poor bone and teeth formation, receding gums and ringing of the ears.

Disturbances in asthi dhatu are due to poor diet, mineral deficiency, lack of protein, poor physical posture, excessive exercise, physical trauma, psychological factors such as loneliness and insecurity, a weak thyroid, menopause and hormone replacement therapy.

When asthi is balanced, there will be a tall frame with large, prominent and strong joints. There will be flexibility, straight, large, strong, white teeth and possibly long hands and feet. Emotionally, there will be concern for others, patience, acceptance, dependability, stability and consistency. Asthi is strengthened by foods high in minerals (especially calcium, magnesium, iron and zinc). Foods that support the formation of asthi are sesame seeds, sunflower seeds, raw and organic dairy products, hemp seeds and seaweeds.

## Majja

Majja is the bone marrow and nerve tissue, and is contained within the empty spaces of the body such as the nerve channels, bones and brain cavity. It sends nerve impulses and governs the sense of pain and of pressure. Majja is also responsible for the production of red blood cells, hemoglobin, and synovial fluids, and assists in lubricating the eyes, feces and skin. Majja is that which fills; when we are full there is a feeling of contentment and sufficiency.

Excess majja creates a feeling of heaviness in the eyes, limbs and joints, as well as non-healing wounds.

Deficient majja leads to weakness, porosity of bones, pain in the small joints, dizziness, spotting in the vision, darkness around the eyes, sexual debility and a deep feeling of emptiness and fear. Many neurological conditions are associated with a weakness or deficiency of majja, such as multiple sclerosis, Parkinson's, epilepsy, ADHD, Bell's palsy, paranoia and schizophrenia.

Majja disturbances are caused by poor diet, poor food-combining, physical trauma, emotional and physical stress, conflict, excessive stimulus, lack of sleep, disturbing dreams, high fevers, bacterial or viral infections, heavy-metal toxicity, radiation, drug and alcohol abuse and over-stimulation of the nervous system.

When majja is harmonized, the eyes are large and clear with good vision, joints are strong, senses are sharp, speech is clear and powerful, the pain threshold is high and the intellect is sharp, clear, sensitive and responsive. In this healthy state, the memory is also strong and feelings of receptivity and compassion are prevalent. Majja is supported by the intake of ghee, hemp seeds and other seeds, and nuts (especially raw almonds, soaked and peeled).

## Shukra and Artava

Shukra and artava are the male and female reproductive tissues. Shukra is the masculine tissue and artava is the feminine tissue. They contain elements of all the dhatus. Shukra and artava are ojas in its pure form and have the capacity to create new life. These tissues have the nature of water and are both pitta and kapha. Shukra, the male reproductive tissue, means "seed" or "luminous." Kapha's cool and passive qualities best describe shukra. Artava, the female reproductive tissue, is hot and active and is therefore pitta by nature. The female egg contains prana, apana, vyana, the twenty attributes, the five elements, the three doshas, the seven dhatus and the three gunas.

When the reproductive tissue is in excess there will be excessive sexual desire or lust, anger, excessive reproductive fluid, an enlarged prostate, stones in the semen, and ovarian or uterine cysts.

When shukra and artava are weak or deficient there will be a lack of vigor, a lack of sexual desire, impotency, sterility, dryness of the mouth, fatigue, lower back pain, difficult or painful ejaculation, a lack of lubricating sexual fluids in women and inability for orgasm or intimacy. Emotionally, there will be repression, fear, anxiety and a feeling of lack of love.

Causes of disturbance in the reproductive tissues are poor food-combining, wrong use and timing of sex, overindulgence of sexual activity, frequent or multiple orgasms, sex during menses, sex while under the influence of intoxicants, violent sex, wrong positions during sex, physical or surgical trauma, sexual diseases, genetic predisposition, tantric practices without proper guidance, as well as emotional distress, worry and anxiety.

Reproductive tissues that are balanced in relation to the body are evidenced by luster in the eyes, strong hair, well-formed reproductive organs, an attractive body, charisma, and the capacity to love, empathize and be compassionate. Shukra and artava are increased by pure dairy products like milk and ghee, raw sugar, almonds and seeds.

## Ojas and the Dhatus

Ojas is the product of all of the dhatus. It is produced by shukra or artava dhatu and is the end product of the nutritional process. If there is disturbance in the formation of the dhatus, ojas will be weak. It is considered to be the eighth dhatu. Ojas is the vital energy of the body that gives vigor, stamina and will power.

Ojas is lost when we have emotional imbalances like anger, worry, sorrow, stress and negative thoughts. It is also depleted by the use of drugs, unnatural sexual activity, environmental pollutants, devitalized foods and an adharmic lifestyle, all of which weaken the mind and drain our life force. When ojas is low, it creates susceptibility to infections, nervous disorders, chronic and degenerative diseases, immune weakness, Epstein Barr virus, HIV, AIDS, hepatitis, sexually transmitted diseases and premature aging. All forms of physical, emotional and mental indigestion weaken and destroy ojas. Positive emotions like tolerance, forgiveness, patience, compassion and love increase ojas and enliven our entire lives.

## The Three Malas

Mala is our body waste. The word *mala* means "bad" or "tainted." The three malas are the three types of waste materials in the body: feces, urine and sweat. Just like the organs and dhatus, the malas can have four types of imbalances: excess, deficiency, damage and increase/decrease.

## Feces

An excess or build up of feces (*purisha*) can cause abdominal pain, abdominal cramping, constipation, heaviness and painful excretion. Results of deficiency include gas, dehydration of the intestines, abdominal distention, as well as lower back pain, palpitations, generalized body pain and prolapse of the colon. Deficiency is usually due to dryness caused by high vata. Feces can be damaged by excessive or wrong use of colonics or purgatives, eating the wrong foods for your dosha, wrong food-combining, excess movement or travel, stimulants, drugs, antibiotics, parasites and wrong use of sex. Feces can be increased with the use of laxatives like triphala and chitrak, as well as bran, whole grains, root vegetables and dark, leafy greens. Feces can be decreased by fasting, the use of purgatives and consuming light food or fruit juice.

## Urine

Urine (*mutra*) in excess can cause pain, cramping or pressure in the bladder, frequent urination, or the feeling of having to urinate again immediately after urinating. When urine is deficient there may be difficulty when urinating, scanty urination, discoloration, blood in the urine and thirst. The urinary system is damaged by excessive use of diuretic herbs, drugs, food, alcohol and sex, as well as emotional disturbances like sudden shock or trauma to the body. Urine is increased by the intake of liquids and is decreased by fasting from liquids or by strong heat such as a sauna or sweat lodge.

## Sweat

An excess of sweat (*svedha dhatu*) causes profuse perspiration, bad body odor and skin eruptions like eczema, psoriasis, boils and fungal invasions. When sweat is deficient, there will be stiffness and dryness of the hair on the skin, dry or wrinkled skin, dandruff and other surface deficiencies. Svedha is damaged by excessive use of diuretics, saunas, sweat lodges, hot tubs, exercise (according to body type) and dry foods. It can also be damaged by a lack of salt in one's diet. Extreme or inadequate exercising (according to one's dosha) will also damage sweat production. Sweat can be increased by drinking sour fruit juice with salt and by exposure to heat like saunas, hot tubs and sweat lodges. It is decreased by exposure to cold and a decrease in water intake.

## The Organs

In ayurvedic anatomy, the doshas are produced and accumulated in the organs of the digestive tract. When these organs are healthy, the doshas and dhatus are also healthy. Each organ relates to our emotions. When the organs are not healthy, our emotions become imbalanced. Likewise, when we are emotionally out of balance, the health of our organs is affected.

There are six solid organs and six hollow organs, matched in corresponding pairs. These pairs are lungs (solid) and large intestine (hollow), liver (solid) and gall bladder (hollow), pericardium (solid) and tridosha or triple heater (hollow), heart (solid) and small intestine (hollow), spleen/pancreas (solid) and stomach (hollow), and kidney (solid) and bladder (hollow).

## The Lungs and Large Intestine

The lungs are responsible for the respiration process. The lungs like moisture and thus contain kapha; they rule breath and prana, and thus also contain vata. The large intestine is the counterpart of the lungs, and it is vata by nature. Air or gases accumulate in the large intestine. The lungs and large intestine also govern the emotions of sadness, grief and loss. Chronic sadness creates disharmony in the lungs and weakens their functioning. If we eat when we are emotionally upset, we experience indigestion. As the large intestine also governs prana, we may disturb all of the dhatus if we eat too quickly or eat the wrong types of food. This disharmony leads to insufficient energy in the whole body, which in turn creates further levels of disharmony.

The large intestine is where nutrients are absorbed and malas are then processed for expulsion. Their function correlates directly to being able to "let go" of that which does not support optimum health. If one is emotionally stuck and is holding onto the past, there will be blockages in the large intestine and constipation or hemorrhoids may result. When we are happy and flowing in our life and have a balanced emotional state, we breathe deeply and experience clarity, lightness and peace of mind; our body reflects this balance and functions with ease.

## The Liver and Gall Bladder

The liver relates to the digestive and circulatory systems and is pitta by nature. It helps to metabolize sugar and fat and also cleanses the blood and body of ama (toxins). The liver stores repressed or negative feelings like anger, hatred and jealousy. When the liver is balanced, it is the organ of individual will power, creativity and expression. The liver governs the eyes, muscles, tendons, fingernails and some aspects of the throat. It also controls the menstrual cycle and plays a major role in the reproductive process. For women, maintaining a healthy liver supports painless menstrual cycles, strong fertility and balanced moods. For men, especially the athletic type (pitta), a calm and healthy liver will prevent torn muscles, an injured back, tinnitus and headaches.

The gall bladder is both pitta and kapha by nature. It is kapha as it stores bile and pitta as it works in conjunction with the liver to cleanse the body. When there is excess kapha in the liver there may be gallstones and obesity, as the bile necessary to break down fats is hindered.

## The Pericardium and the Triple Heater (Tridosha)

The pericardium and the triple heater (also known as the tridosha) are considered very important in both Chinese medicine and Ayurveda. The pericardium is the protective covering of the physical heart, and also of the emotional heart. Sadhaka pitta governs the pericardium. It assists in transforming our emotions into love. Unprocessed emotions become stagnant and create numerous diseases. Emotional stress is one of the biggest factors in heart disease and depression. When the pericardium and triple heater are functioning harmoniously, we experience joy and happiness in our lives; we experience the beauty of creation.

Tridosha refers to both the process of water metabolism and the *srotas* (channels) of metabolism. It also works on the psychological level as it governs the balance of prana, tejas and ojas. While it is not a specific organ, it assists prana in its movements and has a direct correlation to the circulatory and nervous systems.

## The Heart and Small Intestine

The heart is both pitta and kapha by nature. Its activity emulates pitta, and its solidity (being made of the earth element) expresses kapha. Physically, it governs the pumping and circulation of blood. It can also be considered vata as it is a major site for prana distribution through the control of the blood flow. The heart governs the health of the blood vessels. It rules love, compassion and other emotions. When there is an excess of energy in the heart, we experience over-excitement (different from an ordinary sense of happiness). When people are overexcited, their body temperatures rise quickly and their hearts beat faster and are stressed. Heart fire results in agitation, insomnia, palpitations and undue exertion of pressure on the other organs. This also disturbs the internal harmony of the masculine and feminine energies. It is ideal to maintain a balance of emotion. When we process our experiences in a healthy, balanced way, we feel contentment. When we do not fully process our life experiences, we may be suppressing a range of emotions. These repressed emotions affect both the physical and emotional aspects of the heart.

The small intestine is primarily pitta by nature. It is the seat of agni (digestive fire), and is responsible for the absorption of nutrients and overall nutrition of the blood. The small intestine governs how much we absorb and to what extent we experience a sense of union with our life experiences.

## The Stomach, Spleen and Pancreas

The stomach is a solid kapha organ. Undigested food within it creates excess phlegm in other parts of the body. The stomach works directly with the spleen and pancreas to form digestive enzymes that break down food and assist in the absorption of nutrients. The spleen also behaves as a kapha organ, and governs sugar metabolism and the transportation of blood. It governs the health of muscles. Due to its connection to blood and muscle nutrition, the spleen can also be associated with pitta and our natural immunity. The primary emotion that correlates to the stomach, spleen and pancreas is worry. Worry comes from too much mental and intellectual stimulation. When we think too much or worry, we run the risk of upsetting our peace of mind and internal harmony. The organ most affected is the spleen, leading to loss of spleen energy, indigestion and loss of appetite.

Any type of mental or emotional stress can intensify worry and result in fatigue, lethargy and inability to concentrate and think clearly. When the digestive system is affected, it fails to nourish the other organs and results in organ malfunction. If the problem is not rectified early, it can cause permanent damage. Many times, worry and other emotions that go along with the stomach, spleen and pancreas come from early childhood traumas and the feeling of not being nurtured by the world. Trauma and a lack of nurturing is more of a societal problem than an individual problem. However, we can assist the healing of the world by creating our own personal well-being.

## The Kidneys and Bladder

The kidneys and bladder are both vata and kapha by nature. They control water metabolism and are connected to the bones, marrow and reproductive organs. The kidneys separate water from waste products to produce urine. Because the kidneys and bladder dry the body by eliminating water, they have vata traits. The primary emotion related to the kidneys and bladder is fear. To some degree, fear is a normal and adaptive human emotion. However, when fear is chronic, it leads to disharmony in the kidneys. In cases of extreme fear, the kidneys lose their ability to hold energy. This loss of energy may result in enuresis (incontinence), which is quite common in children when they encounter fear. Deficient kidney energy creates a whole series of problems in the balance of body fluid. It affects the bones and marrow and hinders the well-being of the brain. Again, fear is a societal dilemma and seems to be at an all-time high level. Mainstream media presents an onslaught of images that create fear in the minds of the masses. Watching television and reading about violent events deplete the kidneys while increasing negative emotions. If we want to live happy, wholesome lives, we must overcome fear and focus on the light of consciousness. Avoiding negative mental images makes this much easier.

## The Organs and the Dhatus

The organs and dhatus have direct relationships with each other. Plasma correlates to the lungs and heart. Blood correlates to the heart, liver and spleen. Muscle correlates to the liver and spleen/pancreas. Fat is associated with the kidneys, liver and pancreas. Bone relates to the colon and kidneys. Marrow is governed by the brain and the colon. Reproductive tissue is ruled by the kidneys and the reproductive organs (testes and ovaries). The organs and tissues have extremely interdependent relationships with each other. When one of the organs or tissues is out of balance, it is likely that its counterpart will be imbalanced as well.

## The Srotas

*Srotas*, meaning channels or pores, are present throughout the visible body as well as at the subtle level of the cells, molecules, atoms and subatomic particles. It is through these channels that nutrients and other vital substances are transported in and out of our bodies, to the tissues and organs. Srotas act like a vast network of rivers and canals, with many small rivers merging into larger rivers and finally meeting at their home in the ocean. They serve as the pathways for the nutrients, waste products and doshas during the process of metabolism, and enable the products to reach their destination. They transport the dhatus while undergoing transformation. Srotas are physical structures and specific in their functions. Each srota has a *mula* (root), a *marga* (the passage or pathway it travels) and a *mukha* (an opening or mouth). While the basic sites of srotas with different functions are fixed, their openings are innumerable.

When the srotas are flowing properly we experience good health. When they are blocked, we become stagnant and excess materials accumulate, creating disease. The srotas have four improper ways of flowing: in excess, deficiently, blocked and flowing through the wrong channel. The same factors that derange or damage the organs and the tissues also disturb the channels through which they flow.

Along with a combined knowledge of dosha imbalances, the dhatus, the state of the agni and other specific diagnostic methods, assessment of the srotas is one of the ways in which diseases can be distinguished. By knowing which srotas are affected, and the nature and extent of their disturbance, one can gather much information about the disease process.

There are a total of fourteen main srotas in the body, plus additional srotas in women. The fourteen main channels are:

1. *Pranavaha Srotas*: carry prana, which is our breath and life force
2. *Annavaha Srotas*: carrying food
3. *Ambuvaha Srotas*: carrying water
4. *Rasavaha Srotas*: supplying and carrying plasma
5. *Raktavaha Srotas*: supplying and carrying blood
6. *Mamsavaha Srotas*: supplying the muscles with nutrients
7. *Medavaha Srotas*: supplying the body with fat (adipose tissue)
8. *Asthivaha Srotas*: supplying the bones with nutrients
9. *Majjavaha Srotas*: nourishing the marrow and nerve tissues
10. *Shukravaha/Artavavaha Srotas*: Shukravaha srotas supply the male reproductive system, including the testes, prostate and semen. Artavavaha srotas supply the female reproductive system, including the ovaries, areola of the nipples and fallopian tubes.
11. *Svedavaha Srotas*: carrying sweat
12. *Purishavaha Srotas*: carrying feces
13. *Mutravaha Srotas*: carrying urine
14. *Manovaha Srotas*: carrying thoughts

The additional srotas in woman are:

15. *Rajahvaha Srotas*: While similar to artavavaha, it is specifically connected to the fundus (large upper end) of the uterus, endometrium, cervical canal and vaginal passage.

16. *Stanyavaha Srotas*: the lactation system (channels that carry breast milk)

Below is an explanation of each of the srotas.

1. **Pranavaha Srotas:** The pranavaha srotas carry our life force and run through the entirety of the respiratory system. The mula (root) is the left chamber of the heart where oxygenated blood from the lungs and gastrointestinal tract are received. The marga (passage) is the respiratory system, which includes the whole bronchial system and the alveoli. The mukha (opening) is the nose. The prana is absorbed through the lungs and the colon.

The pranavaha srotas also connect to and work with the pranamaya kosha. Pranavaha srotas are disturbed mostly by vata-type activities such as smoking, exposure to polluted air, loud noise, sudden jolting, excessive exercise and sex. They are further damaged by malnutrition, the suppression of natural urges (e.g. going to the toilet, sneezing, and ejaculation), excessive dryness and other vata-provoking activities.

Symptoms of excess flow are rapid breathing and hyperventilation. Symptoms of deficient flow are slow or shallow breathing and shortness of breath. If there is a blockage, there will be difficulty in breathing accompanied by coughing, wheezing or asthma. There may also be hiatal hernias. If energy is flowing out of the wrong channel, the lungs could be perforated.

2. **Annavaha Srotas:** The annavaha srotas are the channels responsible for carrying our food. The mula (root) is the esophagus and the greater curvature of the stomach. The marga (passage) is the gastrointestinal tract, starting with the lips and ending at the ileocecal valve. The mukha (mouth/opening) is the ileocecal valve. These srotas are the main channels in the body. Annavaha srotas are disturbed by improper eating habits, such as eating at the wrong

time, overeating, eating tamasic foods, eating the wrong types of food for one's dosha and emotional eating.

Excess flow results in an excessive appetite, hyperacidity and possibly diarrhea. A deficient flow results in a suppressed appetite as well as hypoacidity, anorexia and constipation. Blockage to the flow may result in intestinal obstruction and the formation of tumors. If the flow is not exiting through the correct channel, there may be vomiting and perforations of the stomach or intestines, or perforated ulcers.

3. **Ambuvaha Srotas:** The ambuvaha srotas are the channels that carry water and other fluids throughout the body, including the cerebrospinal fluid, saliva, and the gastric mucosal and pancreatic secretions. This is the fluid-absorbing aspect of digestion. These srotas govern the assimilation of water and foods that contain water. They are deranged by overexposure to heat, the presence of ama (toxins) in the body, emotions like fear and sadness, consumption of alcohol and excess dryness.

Excess flow results in excessive thirst, a sharp taste in the mouth and hypoglycemia. Deficient flow results in a lack of taste in the mouth, nausea and hyperglycemia. Blocked flow may result in diabetes or other serious problems of the pancreas such as cancer. If the flow exits through the wrong channel, there may be vomiting and anorexia.

4. **Rasavaha Srotas:** These are the channels of the lymph (rasa) dhatu that carry the plasma. They are connected to the lymphatic and circulatory systems. The mula (root) is the right chamber of the heart and the blood vessels. The marga (passage) is the network of blood vessels and the lymphatic system. The mukha (opening) is the arteriole-venous junction in the capillaries, which form the primary web or network of channels through the body. Rasavaha srotas are deranged by overeating, eating foods that are heavy, cold and mucous-forming, and by emotional eating.

Excess leads to edema, as well as swelling of the glands and lymph nodes. Deficiency may lead to dehydration and emaciation. Blocked flow may result in overly swollen glands, major lymphatic obstructions and lymphatic cancer. If the flow exits through the wrong channel, there may be bleeding as well as the coughing up of blood.

5. **Raktavaha Srotas:** These channels carry the blood and relate to the circulatory system. The mula (root) is the liver and spleen. The marga (passage) is the circulatory system and the mukha (opening/mouth) is through the skin. Raktavaha srotas are deranged by consuming excess stimulants, foods and beverages that are too hot and oily, and by too much exposure to thesun or heat.

Excess flow may result in a rapid pulse, heart palpitations and hypertension. A deficient flow may result in a slow pulse with hypotension and varicose veins. If the flow is blocked, there may be arrhythmia, an enlarged liver or spleen, clotting of the blood, tumors or heart attacks. If the direction of the flow is incorrect, there may be different types of bleeding disorders.

6. **Mamsavaha Srotas:** These channels supply the muscle tissue with nutrients. The mula (root) is formed by the ligaments and skin where the muscle tissues are attached. The marga (passage) is through all the muscles of the body. The mukha (opening) is through the skin. Mamsavaha srotas are deranged by foods that are too heavy, gross, oily and liquid. Sleeping directly after eating or sleeping during the day also has a damaging effect on mamsavaha srotas.

If there is an excess of the flow, there may be hyperactivity of the muscles and tremors may occur. If the flow is deficient, there may be under activity of the muscles that can cause loss or lack of muscle tone and spasms. If the flow is blocked, there can be chronic inflammation in the muscles, as well as tumors. Wrong flow may result in muscles that are more easily torn.

7. **Medavaha Srotas:** These channels supply fat tissue with nutrients. The mula (root) is formed by abdominal fat, the kidneys and the adrenals. The marga (passage) is the subcutaneous fat tissue and the mukha (opening) is the sebaceous glands. Medavaha srotas are deranged by stagnation and la ack of proper exercise. Additionally, sleeping during the day or right after eating can aggravate these

srotas. Consuming foods that are fatty and oily and drinking alcohol also deranges the medavaha srotas.

Excess flow may lead to edema and obesity. Deficient flow may cause emaciation with dryness of the skin. When the flow is blocked, there may be tumors in the adipose tissue. Wrong flow may lead to the tearing of fat tissue.

8. **Asthivaha Srotas:** These channels nourish the bones and skeletal system. The mula (root) is the adipose tissue and hips/pelvic girdle/sacrum, which contain the largest bones of the skeletal system. The marga (passage) is the skeletal system and the mukha (opening) is through the nails and the hair. Asthivaha srotas are deranged by physical work or exercise that jolts, shocks or strains the bones. Eating foods that increase vata (dry, light, etc.) will cause aggravation as well.

When there is excess flow, there will be excess bone tissue. Likewise, if there is deficient flow, there will be weak bones, deficient bone tissue and osteoporosis. When the flow is blocked there may be bone spurs, calcification of the bones and cancer. Wrong flow also occurs when a bone is broken.

9. **Majjavaha Srotas:** Majjavaha srotas supply the nerve tissue and bone marrow with nutrients. The mula (root) is formed by the joints and bones, and secondarily by the brain and spinal cord. The marga (passage) is the entire nervous system (central, sympathetic and parasympathetic). The mukha (opening) is synaptic space. As the entire nervous system connects to the brain and spinal cord, it contains connections to the motor and sensory nerves. Majjavaha srotas are deranged by any traumatic experience, either physical or emotional. Violent sensory input, like horror movies or the evening news, can disturb the nervous system. Additionally, improper food-combining or eating in a disturbed atmosphere will aggravate the nerves.

Excess flow leads to hypersensitivity, pain, insomnia, tremors and an overly heightened sense of perception. If the flow is deficient, there will be hyposensitivity, numbness (physical and emotional), dullness, lethargy and a clouded sense of perception. If the flow is blocked, there can be convulsions, multiple sclerosis and one may even enter into a coma. Wrong flow will result in nerve tissue damage.

10. **Shukravaha and Artavavaha Srotas:** Shukravaha srotas are the channels through which nutrients are transported to the male reproductive system. The mula (root) is formed by the testes and the nipples. The marga (passage) is formed by the prostate gland, urethra, epididymus and the urogenital tract. The mukha (opening) is the opening of the urethra. These srotas are also connected to the secretions that occur during sexual activities. Shukravaha srotas can be deranged by the suppression of natural sexual urges, excessive sexual indulgence/activities, sexual activities at the wrong time of day, promiscuity and reproductive surgeries.

Excess flow results in spermatorrhea, involuntary nocturnal emissions, premature ejaculation and leucorrhea. Deficient flow results in a difficulty to attain an erection, as well as delayed ejaculation. A blocked flow may result in an inability to ejaculate, testicular swelling, prostate stones and tumors. If the flow is incorrect, the sperm may enter into the bladder.

The mula (root) of artavavaha srotas is formed by the ovaries and areola; the marga (passage) is formed by the fallopian tubes, uterus, cervical canal and vagina; and the mukha (opening) is the labia. The artavavaha srotas have some responsibility for menstruation and also nourish the reproductive tissue, or the ova. It governs the production of hormones and other sexual secretions. Artavavaha srotas are deranged by activities similar to those that aggravate the rajahvaha and shukravaha srotas. Additionally, excessive or deficient sexual activity, lack of nutrition, and emotions like anger, grief, sadness, worry and fear all affect the reproductive system. The symptoms are the same for both the rajahvaha and artavavaha srotas.

11. **Svedavaha Srotas:** These are the channels that carry sweat, the sebaceous glands. The mula (root) is formed by the sweat glands. The marga (passage) is through the sweat ducts. The mukha (opening) is the pores of the skin and the sweat glands underneath the skin.

These srotas are intrinsically connected to the adipose (fat) tissue. The more fat the body has, the more the body sweats. Svedavaha srotas are deranged by excessive exercise, overexposure to the sun or heat, eating foods that are too hot or too cold and imbalanced emotions.

If there is excess flow, profuse sweating will occur. If there is a deficient flow, there will be a temporary lack of sweating. Blockages can lead to the complete inability to sweat. If the flow is through the wrong channel, the sweat will enter into the lymphatic system (rasa) dhatu.

12. **Purishavaha Srotas:** These are the channels that carry feces. The mula (root) is formed by the cecum, rectum and the colon. The marga (passage) is through the large intestine. The mukha (opening) is the anus. Purishavaha srotas are deranged by the suppression of the urge to defecate, overeating, eating tamasic foods, eating when a previous meal has not been completely digested and weak agni (digestive fire).

Excess flow leads to diarrhea; if the flow is deficient, there will be constipation. When the flow is blocked, there will be obstructions to the colon and there may be diverticulitis or tumors. Incorrect flow may lead to perforations in the colon.

13. **Mutravaha Srotas:** These channels carry the urine, and include the entire urinary system. The mula (root) is the kidneys. The marga (passage) is through the ureters, urethra and the bladder. The mukha (opening) is through the opening of the urethra. Mutravaha srotas are deranged by inordinate intake of food or liquid, excessive sex, suppression of the natural urge to urinate, and by diseases or traumas. Additionally, excess travel can aggravate these channels.

Excessive flow can lead to excessive or frequent urination. Likewise, if the flow is deficient, there will be scant (deficient) urination. If the flow is blocked, there will be painful and difficult urination, and there may be stones in the urinary tract. If the flow exits through the incorrect channel, the bladder can burst.

14. **Manovaha Srotas:** These are the channels of the mind that carry thoughts. They are not only physical channels, but subtle

channels as well, and are critical in the development of a balanced mind. These channels are located in the nerve tissue and are part of our emotional process. The mula (root) is formed by the heart or cardiac plexus and the ten sensory pathways (subtle channels that carry input to the five senses). The marga (passage) is the whole body. The mukha (opening) is the sense organs, the ears, skin, eyes, tongue and nose, as well as the *marma* points (energy points, similar to acupuncture points). The manovaha srotas make up the subtle body and are part of the manomaya kosha. The mind is directly connected to the parts of the nervous system and physical body that are responsible for the sensory and motor systems. When in its higher state of awareness, the mind transcends physical body consciousness. Manovaha srotas are deranged by excessive emotional processes, suppression of emotions, use of drugs, alcohol or stimulants, and disturbing stimuli like loud music, violent or pornographic cinema/ images, disturbing news, etc.

Excess flow leads to mental unrest. In such cases, the mind and the senses may be hyperactive and one may worry or have a lot of anger. Deficient flow leads to dulled senses and depression, with predominant emotions of grief and sadness. Blocked flow results in blocked or suppressed emotions. If the flow is wrong, there will be major psychological problems like delirium, delusion (including delusions of grandeur) and schizophrenia.

15. **Rajahvaha Srotas:** Rajahvaha and artavavaha srotas are similar physically but have different functions. The mula (root) of rajahvaha srotas is formed by the ovaries and areola. The marga (passage) is formed by the fallopian tubes, uterus, cervical canal and the vagina. The mukha (opening) is the labia. Rajahvaha srotas carry out the process of menstruation. They are deranged by excessive repression of sexual urges, overuse of sex, sex at the wrong time of day, promiscuity and surgery on the reproductive system.

Excess flow leads to menorrhagia (excessive or prolonged menstruation). Deficient flow leads to scant or delayed menstruation. Blocked flow may lead to a lack of menstruation (amenorrhea), painful menstruation (dysmenorrhea) or tumors. Wrong flow may cause menstrual blood to enter into the urine or feces.

16. **Stanyavaha Srotas:** These are the channels that carry the breast milk for lactating women. The mula (root) is the lactation glands, which are directly connected to the marga (passage), the lactiferous ducts. The nipple is the mukha (opening). (The mukha functions only when a woman gives birth.) Stanyavaha srotas are deranged by not having children, breastfeeding for too long, and suppressing the breast milk by not feeding the baby.

Excessive flow can lead to an excess of breast milk. Likewise, if the flow is deficient there will be a lack of breast milk. If the flow is blocked then there may be no breast milk, painful and swelling breasts, mastitis, cysts, tumors or cancer. Incorrect flow may result in injury to the breasts.

# Chapter 7

# Subtle Anatomy

*In the center of the castle of the soul, our own body, there is*
*a tiny mansion in the shape of a lotus. Within can be found*
*a tiny room. This small space within one's own heart is as*
*expansive as the universe. There is a light that shines beyond*
*all things on Earth, beyond us all, beyond the stars, beyond*
*the universe. This is the light that shines in the Lotus Heart.*

*~ Chandogya Upanishad, 8:1:1-2*

## The Chakras

Chakras are powerful energy centers that affect our causal, subtle and gross bodies and everything we do. Chakras have a relationship to specific functions of the physical and emotional body. Physically, each center correlates to major nerve ganglia that branch forth from the spinal column. The first five chakras are connected to specific sense organs. They store psycho-physical energy, which then flows to all seven chakras. The breath activates this flow from one chakra to the next. In addition, the chakras also correlate to levels of consciousness, archetypal elements, developmental stages of life, colors, sounds, bodily functions and more.

Chakras relate to different energetic sites of the human body, as well as to parts of the endocrine system. Made of prana, the chakras function to take in higher vibrational frequencies from everything around us. They transform each frequency into a form of energy useful to the physical body. Each major chakra vibrates at different rates, and each will absorb energy harmonically related to its own natural frequency. The chakras absorb energy from the environment. The *nadis* (subtle energy channels) then direct this energy to the organs.

Ayurveda considers the chakras a vital part of health, healing and spiritual growth. Chakras are affected by impressions of sound, touch, smell, sight and taste. In numerous healing systems, sound, aromatherapy, crystals and gemstones, color (or light), tuning forks and other vibrational methods are utilized for chakra balancing. Such chakra therapy has become popular in western healing systems. Traditionally, mantras, yantras, yagnas and yoga asanas were also used to harmonize the chakras.

Situated along the *sushumna nadi* (the central nerve channel), the seven chakras relate to different emotions, thoughts and actions. Each chakra has a specific mantra and relates to one of the senses and organs of action.

The chakras are represented by different forms of lotus flowers; each lotus represents an awakened state of consciousness. The word chakra means "wheel." When all of the chakras are "spinning," open, bright and clean, our chakra system is balanced. When a chakra becomes blocked, damaged or muddied with residual energy, our physical and emotional health can be affected. Often these disorders occur habitually as the result of negative belief systems. The effects of our habits, feelings, beliefs, thoughts and desires can be found in our chakras. They may be utilized as a pathway for gaining a strong, clear and balanced energy system. An open state of being affords the most efficient flow of energy through the system.

This flow of energy is essential for vitality, health and growth on all levels. Ideally, all chakras contribute to the wholeness of our being. This inspires our instincts to work together with our feelings and thoughts to create positive emotional and spiritual balance.

All of our senses, perceptions, states of awareness – everything that is possible for us to experience – can be divided into seven categories. Each category can be associated with a particular chakra. In this way, each of the chakras represents not only particular parts of the physical body, but also specific parts of consciousness. Some chakras are not open enough or are underactive; to compensate, others are overactive. The chakras are constantly trying to create a harmonious balance.

## Muladhara (Root Chakra)

The first chakra, *muladhara*, is located at the base of the spine. *Mula* means "root." It has four petals and is correlated with the earth element. Its mantra is *lam* and its color is red. Muladhara is the resting place of Kundalini Shakti, the divine feminine principle. When She awakens, She rises to the *sahasrara* (crown chakra), the abode of Shiva, the divine masculine.

Muladhara chakra correlates to the organs of elimination. It governs our physical existence, our bodies and our health. It rules the nose, the sense of smell, the anus and elimination. It corresponds to the sacrum and gives the feeling of being grounded. It relates to our biological needs and comfort.

On a psychological level, it relates to fear and ignorance, or maya. In a balanced state, it gives a sense of stability and groundedness, and gives the strength to manifest our visions. Muladhara also relates to survival instincts, safety, connection to our body and the physical plane. Ideally, this chakra brings us health, prosperity, security and dynamic presence.

## Svadishtana (Sacral Chakra)

Located in the abdomen, lower back and sexual organs, just above the root center, the second chakra, *svadishtana*, relates to the reproductive organs. Svadishtana means "the abode of the Self." It has six petals and is of the element water. This chakra's mantra is *vam* and its color is orange. It rules the tongue, sense of taste and the reproductive organs. The second chakra relates to emotions and sexuality. It connects us to others through feeling, desire, sensation and movement. In balance, this chakra brings us fluidity and

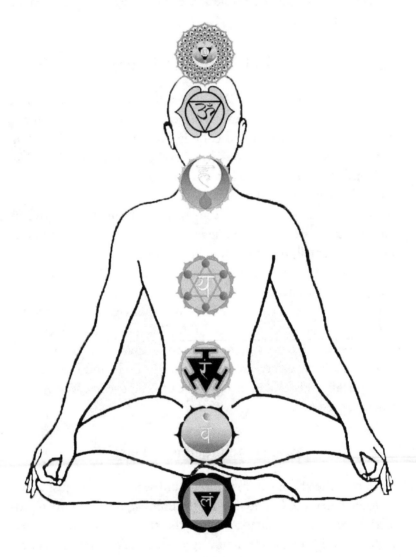

*The seven chakras*

grace, creativity, depth of feeling, sexual fulfillment and the ability to accept change.

## Manipura (Solar Plexus Chakra)

The third chakra, *manipura*, is located near the navel in the solar plexus. Manipura means "the city of gems." It has ten petals and rules the element fire. This chakra's mantra is *ram* and its color is yellow. Manipura governs the navel center and our digestive organs. It rules the eyes and sight as well as the feet and movement. It also governs agni, the fire that digests food as well as life experience. Manipura is the seat of ego and will power. In harmony, it is the power to surrender to the will of the Divine. Manipura is the fire of self-discipline. It rules personal power, autonomy and metabolism. When balanced, manipura brings us energy, effectiveness, self-confidence, spontaneity and non-dominating power.

## Anahata (Heart Chakra)

The fourth chakra, *anahata*, governs the heart. Anahata means "the unstruck sound." It has twelve petals and rules the air element. Anahata's mantra is *yam* and its color is green. This chakra rules the skin, the hands and the sense of touch; it also creates prana. It represents the two polarities of body and spirit as interconnected in perfect balance. When this chakra is in harmony, one feels unconditional love, empathy and devotion. Anahata governs the experience of interconnectedness. Through love, it integrates the opposites in the psyche: mind and body, masculine and feminine, persona and shadow, ego and unity. A healthy fourth chakra allows us to love deeply, feel compassion, and have a deep sense of peace and centeredness. To fully open the heart chakra, we need to bring the various aspects of our existence into balance.

## Vishuddha (Throat Chakra)

The fifth chakra, *vishuddha*, is located in the throat. Vishuddha means "pure." It has sixteen petals and is the color blue. Vishuddha rules the throat, ears and mouth and governs sound. Its mantra is *ham*. An imbalanced vishuddha chakra leads to blockages in communication and expression, as well as repressed feelings. When harmonized, it is a source of inspiration and expression. Vishuddha is related to communication and creativity; furthermore, when activated, we experience the world through vibrations, such as the vibration of sounds representing language.

## Ajna (Third Eye Chakra)

The sixth chakra, *ajna,* is located behind the pineal gland. It is commonly known as the "third eye." Ajna means "commanding" or "infinite power." It has two petals and is the color indigo. Ajna's mantra is *ksham,* and it governs the mind, giving the power of divine perception to see things as they truly are. Ajna governs the pineal gland. It gives the powers of discrimination, creativity, detachment, inner vision and stillness of the mind. It is related to the act of seeing, both physically and intuitively, and as such it opens our psychic faculties, capacities and our understanding of archetypes.

## Sahasrara (Crown Chakra)

The seventh chakra or crown chakra is called *sahasrara*. It has one thousand petals and its mantra is *aum*. Sahasrara is the place of Divine Consciousness and the dissolution of ego. When Shakti awakens, She rises to merge with Shiva, who is the pure consciousness that resides in the sahasrara. The seventh chakra is at the crown of the head, and is violet fading to white as it moves further away from the body. This chakra enables the connection to our higher selves and to the Divine. It is associated with wisdom and integration of our eternal self with our physical self. The sahasrara is like an umbilical cord to God. When the crown chakra is open and active, we can become a vessel for God to work through. Ultimately, this chakra helps us relate to consciousness as pure awareness. This chakra is our connection to a timeless, spaceless place of all-knowing. When developed, sahasrara brings us knowledge, wisdom, understanding, spiritual connection and bliss.

## The Nadis

Together with the chakras, the nadis – variously translated as "conduits," "nerves," "veins," "vessels" or "arteries" – constitute the subtle or yogic body. Like the Chinese meridians, the nadis are flowing channels or rivers that carry prana throughout the body. Most authorities say there are 72,000 nadis. The text *Siva-Samhita* says there are 350,000. It is agreed that there are fourteen main nadis. The main nadi system connects the seven major chakras to each other and to 72,000 other nadis. The 72,000 nadis are further divided into two main channels:
1) The invisible channels of the mind, or mental body
2) The visible channels, which include the nerves, muscles, arteries, veins, cardiovascular system, lymphatic system and the meridians in the body
Of all the nadis, the three most important and principle nadis are *shushumna, ida* and *pingala.* This nadi system is divided into three channels: one channel flows up the spinal column and the other two reside in the brain. Centrally located shushumna is the only nadi that passes through the spinal column. Shushumna is associated with the mystical Saraswati River. It is said that the Saraswati River manifests at the point of spiritual awakening. It runs up the body from just below muladhara chakra to sahasrara chakra at the crown of the head. Shushumna pierces the chakras, and is like a pole or current around which the ida and pingala nadis dance.

Ida is the left channel and is pure white, sattvic, feminine and cold. It represents the moon, and is associated with the River Ganga (Ganges). Originating in muladhara, ida culminates its journey at the left nostril.

Pingala is the right channel and is red, rajasic, masculine, hot and represents the sun. It is associated with the river Yamuna. Originating in muladhara, pingala's journey culminates at the right nostril. Ida and pingala cross and meet at each chakra. A blockage in the nadis may manifest as emotional blockage, nervous tension, repressed self-expression or emotional suffering.

## The Koshas

*The spiritual aspirant, in the quest for Self- and God-realization, passes under the guidance of the master through each of these selves in turn, finally attaining the Absolute or Brahman, which is synonymous with the highest or Bliss-Self.*

~ *Taittiriya Upanishad, 1.5.1-1.6.1*

The ancient yogis created a map to penetrate and awaken the deepest levels of our being. This inward journey is yoga. The concept of having five selves within our body first appeared in the *Taittiriya Upanishad*. Fifteen hundred years later, *Advaita Vedanta* (non-dual philosophy) refined this concept into the koshas, the five sheaths that veil the light of our True Self (*Atman*). The koshas can be compared to layers of an onion; they form a barrier that prevents us from realizing our true nature of bliss and oneness with the universe. Ayurveda and yoga are tools to peel back these layers to bring our awareness deeper into our bodies, eventually reaching the innermost core, our True Self. Experience and understanding of the koshas helps us know the depth of the human mind and, ultimately, realize dhyana, or meditation. When we can see clearly through the

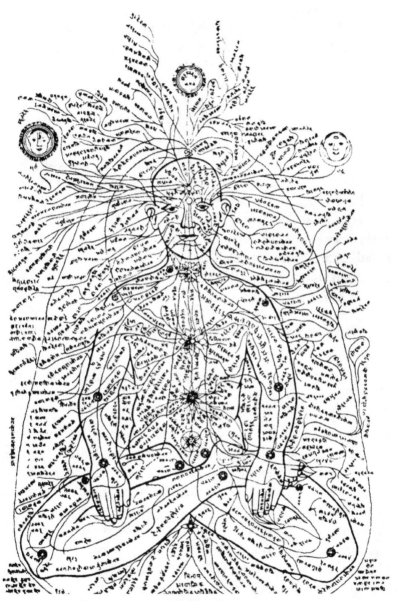

*This traditional diagram illustrates the nadis
in conjunction with the chakras.*

layers of the koshas, we may then attain a state of yoga, or oneness, with the universe.

The koshas form our most subtle body. The five koshas make up our subtle body and determine the quality of our chakras. They are vibrational by nature and affected by all impressions including those of the mind. Our *samskaras*, collected mental patterns, are stored in the koshas. They are both conscious and unconscious. The unconscious patterns are said to be our *vasanas*, or karmic impressions. These are created by strong desires, emotions, wounds, ecstatic moments, violence, jealousy and illusions. All thoughts and emotions contribute to the vibration at which our koshas resonate.

The five koshas are *annamaya kosha* (food sheath), *pranamaya kosha* (breath sheath), *manomaya kosha* (mind sheath), *vijnanamaya kosha* (knowledge or wisdom sheath) and *anandamaya kosha* (bliss sheath). Each kosha is hidden within the next, until consciousness reaches the physical, gross body. Each kosha depends on the previous for its nourishment.

## Annamaya Kosha

The first and most basic sheath is annamaya kosha. *Anna* means "food;" this sheath feeds our awareness into the other layers and sustains the other four koshas. This kosha determines the physical body, created and sustained by the intake of food. The quality of food that is ingested determines the quality of the body. It feeds the tissue, muscle, fat and bone; however, it is not only the nutritional quality of the food that is ingested. The planting, preparation and love that are put into the food are also ingested. This explains why the scriptures suggest eating food prepared by someone of a pure nature or who is chanting mantras. Although science may view the physical body as different systems that control the bodily functions, yoga ascribes that these functions are nothing but manifestations of the interaction between energy and consciousness. When annamaya kosha is strong, it promotes good health, long life and long-lasting youth. The quality of the annamaya kosha feeds the pranamaya kosha.

## Pranamaya Kosha

The second sheath is pranamaya kosha. Prana means "life force energy." This sheath contains and regulates the movement of physical and mental energies through the channels and centers of energy. It is much more subtle than the first kosha. The nadis and chakras exist within the pranamaya kosha. Prana is developed through the air we breathe and through our sensory input. What we take into our bodies and senses either feeds or depletes our prana. Pranamaya governs the five pranas and all of their functions. It also makes up our etheric or auric body. When pranamaya kosha is strong, it produces courage, valor, genius and radiance. One's personality becomes magnetic and the scope and power of personal influence increases.

## Manomaya Kosha

The third kosha is manomaya, the sheath of the mind. This sheath contains thoughts and feelings. The mental realm is composed of two qualities, manas and *buddhi*. Manas is the rational, linear, sequential and thoughtful mind. Buddhi is the quality of discrimination that comes after knowledge and after the removal or the absence of ignorance. The practices of mental concentration (pratyahara) aim at realizing the nature of our manomaya kosha. Positive thoughts create a peaceful and contented vibration, as well as a spiritual glow coming from this kosha. The manomaya kosha contains the subconscious records, the samskaras that control our daily habits.

The most powerful thought we can have is mantra. Mantra can completely transform the mind into a higher state of being and awareness. It governs our higher perception and cognition. It uplifts and awakens the Self within. When manomaya kosha is strong, it enhances the wisdom, foresightedness and intelligence of a person, and one is able to maintain balance and patience during life's ups and downs.

Annamaya, pranamaya and manomaya koshas all relate to the physical body and govern its processes. Balancing pranamaya brings harmony to manomaya. The first three koshas are distinct from one another, however, they function simultaneously and interdepently.

## Vijnanamaya Kosha

The fourth sheath is vijnanamaya kosha, the sheath of wisdom and intellect. Vijnana means "knowledge;" this sheath contains intuition, wisdom and witness consciousness. It rules our ability to perceive divine knowledge. This causal body constitutes our thought patterns. Because it is established in pure awareness, consciousness perceives knowledge from within. The aspects of *chitta* and *ahamkara* are associated with vijnanamaya kosha. Chitta is the ability to know, to become the observer of what is actually happening, to be able to live a reality and not speculate or fantasize about it. Ahamkara is the knowledge and awareness that Self exists. Vijnanamaya kosha is purified through seva, satsang, bhajans and *darshan* (keeping company with holy beings). When vijnanamaya kosha is strong, it makes one gentle, generous, open-hearted and angelic.

## Anandamaya Kosha

The fifth layer is anandamaya kosha, the sheath of bliss. *Ananda* means "bliss," found at the deepest layer of our being. This quality is not merely a feeling, but a state of being that is unchanging and has always existed, but has been buried by the other koshas. Beyond this thin sheath resides the pure consciousness of our true Self. This is the natural state of being. This original state is untainted by thoughts or fluctuations in the mind. When the anandamaya kosha is strong, one's thoughts and actions become submerged in a state of continuous bliss and undisturbed peace.

## The Chakras and Koshas

The chakras are correlated with the koshas. Muladhara chakra works together with the annamaya kosha for the instinct and purpose of survival. Svadishtana chakra relates to pranamaya kosha in the soul's process of self-identification and the instinct of procreation, or continuity. The manipura chakra relates to manomaya kosha, for they work together to achieve goals through the power of ambition and will. Anahata chakra relates to vijnanamaya kosha to achieve the perfect state of love and compassion. One who has attained true wisdom naturally loves all beings as one's own Self. Vishuddha chakra relates to vijnanamaya kosha and the ability to clearly vocalize the heart's ambition. Ajna chakra relates to the anandamaya kosha, together dwelling in the stillness of the inward-drawn consciousness. Sahasrara chakra is beyond all the koshas, as it is the Self dwelling within the Self.

# Chapter 8

# Ama and Agni

*O Agni, bring us radiant light to be our mighty aid,*
*for Thou art our visible deity!*

*~ Sama Veda, 1:1:1*

## Ama

Ama is a concept unique to Ayurveda. It is an essential causative factor of disease and the disease process. Ama begins with improperly digested or processed toxic particles that clog the body's physical channels. These channels include the intestines, lymphatic system, arteries and veins, capillaries and genitourinary tract. Ama accumulates wherever there is a weakness in the body and results in disease. There are five main causes of ama.

### Causes of Ama

#### 1. *Agni-Mandya* – Low digestive fire
Digestive fire is a vital component of the complete and proper digestion of food. When digestive fire is low, food is not properly digested and toxins are formed. Absorption becomes sluggish and the poorly digested food and/or toxins are retained in the intestines. This retention causes the toxins to ferment and putrefy in the intestines. The ama remains unabsorbed in the intestines. Incomplete digestion is the root cause of most diseases.

## 2. *Dhatu-Agni-Mandya* – Low tissue fire

*Dhatu-agni (dhatvagni)* plays an important role in the process of forming tissues from nutrient substances. When the power of the dhatvagni of a particular tissue is diminished, either in the liver or in a channel, the nourishment and construction of that tissue is incomplete and ama is produced. When toxins are present in the tissues, it is called *samadhatu,* or tissues containing ama. This type of pathology is seen in most diseases. In diabetes, fat (meda dhatu) and muscle (mamsa dhatu) tissues are formed as "sama tissues" because of the diminished agni of the fat and muscle tissues. This disturbs the normal functioning activities of these tissues. In cases of obesity, a similar type of fat tissue is produced due to weak meda dhatu agni, or fire of fat tissue.

## 3. *Mala Sanchaya* – Accumulated waste products

Agni transforms food substances into body tissues. It first produces a nutritious substance, which is then converted into tissues in the second phase of digestion. This process, referred to as secondary or tissue digestion, is the anabolic activity of tissue fire. Different tissues are produced as a result of tissue fire's action on nutrient food substances. The tissues produced are utilized for the release of energy required for every bodily activity. During this process, the tissue substances are again digested, transformed and utilized for the release of heat and energy by the tissue fire. This describes the catabolic process. During this activity of tissue disintegration, minute, subtle waste products called *kleda* are formed. Small amounts of kleda are essential for the body; the excess is excreted. If this excretion is defective or deficient, kleda accumulates in the body and results in the formation of the toxic substance ama.

## 4. *Dosha Sammurcchana* – Interaction between vitiated doshas

Every dosha has unique qualities that are antagonistic to the qualities of other doshas. For example, the dry and light qualities of vata are antagonistic to the oily and heavy qualities of kapha. Likewise, the hot quality of pitta is antagonistic to the cold quality of kapha and vata. When two or three doshas become severely vitiated and combine, specific reactions between them occur. These conditions produce opposite qualities: instead of nullifying each other, they interact and produce ama.

5. *Krimi Visha* – Bacterial toxins

When pathogenic organisms cause an infection, they release a toxic substance. Pathogenic organisms can include molds, fungus, yeast, worms, bacteria and various parasites.

## Properties of Ama

- Ama is usually in the form of an incompletely digested substance (food).
- It is non-homogenous and contains a very bad odor that is experienced when it is combined with the malas (waste material), such as sweat, urine and feces, or when it is expelled from the body in the forms of sputum, vomit or mucous.
- Ama is sticky.
- Ama produces lethargy and tamas (darkness or inertia) in the body.

## Signs and Symptoms of Ama:

- Obstruction: Obstruction can occur in any of the channels (srotas). The most commonly observed obstructions are in the liver, urinary tract, fallopian tubes, blood vessels, and the gastrointestinal and respiratory tracts.
- Weakness or deficiency in any part or organ of the body
- Obstruction of the movement of vata: Ama causes disturbance in the action of the musculature of the part or organ and in the conduction of nerve impulses. Ultimately, the activity of the affected part diminishes or stops altogether.
- Heaviness and lethargy
- The tongue will be coated with a whitish, thick or greasy film, especially upon rising in the morning.
- Metabolic and digestive disturbances such as bloating, gas, constipation, diarrhea, sticky stool, sinking stool, mucous or blood

in the stool, fever, turbid urine, skin blemishes and foul-smelling stool, breath, sweat, urine and phlegm.
- One may lack mental clarity and energy and feel weary or unenthusiastic. One may even experience depression.

## Modern Symptoms of Ama

High triglycerides, atherosclerosis, adult onset diabetes, high blood sugar levels, depression, rheumatoid factor, overgrowth of H. pylori bacteria, leukocytosis or leukocytopenia (deficient or excess white blood cells), excess antibodies, candida albicans in the gut and uterus, blood urea, gout, excess platelets, high IgE levels from allergic reactions, excess red blood cells, gallstones as a sign of excess bile, kidney stones as a sign of unmetabolized calcium and oxalates, high liver enzymes, glaucoma, bacterial infection, fever, tumors

## Effects of Ama

When ama comes in contact with the doshas, dhatus or waste products, it produces sama dosha, sama dhatus and sama mala. Ayurveda describes symptoms of these stages – sama (with ama) and *nirama* (without ama) – in the doshas, dhatus and malas for all diseases.

The underlying cause of any disease is an imbalance in one or all of the doshas. For successful treatment of a particular disease, the ayurvedic specialist must determine whether the imbalanced dosha is sama or nirama.

## Treatment of Ama

### Herbs

- **Vata-Pacifying** – asafoetida (*hingwastak churna*, very effective for clearing wind, bloating and spasms from the intestines), black pepper, castor oil, cumin, fennel, garlic, fresh ginger, linseed, nutmeg
- **Pitta-Pacifying** – aloe vera, amalaki (can be used with other cooling herbs to clear heat toxins from the system), coriander, fennel, guduchi, kalmegh, neem

- **Kapha-Pacifying** – black pepper, cumin, ginger, guggulu, punarnava, pushkarmula, trikatu (renowned for its heating properties that can literally digest toxins), tulasi, vaccha

**Specific Therapies** – vigorous exercise, fasting, panchakarma, soaking in hot water, sweating, wind and sun therapy

## Ama-Pacifying Diet

- **Tastes:** Emphasize pungent, bitter, astringent
- **Fruit:** No sweet; only sour fruits such as cranberry, grapefruit, lemon, lime, pomegranate
- **Vegetables:** Steamed sprouts, steamed vegetables; some raw is good for pitta; lots of greens, microalgae such as open-cell chlorella; no roots, sweet vegetables or mushrooms
- **Grains:** No bread or pastry; less wheat and oats; barley, kichari, millet, quinoa, rice, rye
- **Beans:** Aduki, mung
- **Nuts:** None
- **Seeds:** Hemp seeds, pumpkin seeds
- **Dairy:** None. Raw goat's milk is alright in moderation because it is slightly astringent and less kapha-forming.
- **Meat:** No eggs, shellfish, saltwater fish, fats, red meat or pork
- **Oils:** None. Ghee is acceptable in small quantities, as are mustard and linseed oils, which are drying.
- **Sweeteners:** None. Sugar (mainly white and artificial sugars) is ama-forming. Honey is okay (maximum two teaspoons per day, never cooked or mixed with anything hot).
- **Drinks:** Avoid cold drinks. Drink hot teas made of cardamom, cinnamon, fennel, ginger, tulasi, and dandelion root "coffee."
- **Note:** This provides a general idea of how to pacify ama. Variations will be present depending on dosha, dhatu, agni and season. Please consult your ayurvedic practitioner for individual needs.

# Agni

Agni is the transformative principle of fire. It is the source of light and love in the universe. Without light and love, we have no life force (prana). Without love, life is empty and meaningless. On the subtle level agni is tejas, the illuminating aspect of consciousness that governs our mental processes. It generates new ideas and inspiration, as well as the energy to manifest them. Each dosha, each dhatu, each kosha, each organ and each part of nature has its own agni. As the fire aspect of the five great elements (panchamahabhutas), it exists in our bodies as the pitta dosha. Agni is the fire inside our body.

Agni encompasses all of the changes in the body and mind, from the dense to the subtle. These changes include the digestion and absorption of food, cellular transformations, assimilation of sensory perceptions, and mental and emotional experiences. The process of agni covers the whole sequence of chemical interactions and changes in the body and mind. It governs overall body metabolism.

Of the forty agnis existing in the human body, the primary are *jatharagni* (the digestive fire of the stomach), *dhatvagnis* (the seven dhatu agnis), and the five *bhutagnis* (the liver enzymes which process the components of food into elements of bodily tissue). There are also agnis for each of the srotas (channels). Without agni, the dhatus do not receive nourishment and disease manifests.

The most important agni is the jatharagni, the gastric or digestive fire responsible for digesting food. This agni correlates hydrochloric acid in the stomach and the digestive enzymes and juices secreted into the stomach, duodenum and the small intestine. Jatharagni is the main agni present in pachaka pitta. It is responsible for the digestion and the absorption of nutrients from food.

The process of digestion is divided into three stages: digestion in the stomach, in the duodenum, and in the small and large intestines. Each stage of digestion is related to the six tastes. The taste of the first morsel of food initiates the digestive process as digestive enzymes are produced in the saliva and the upper fundus of the stomach.

The first two hours of digestion relate to kapha dosha and provide nourishment for the kapha parts of the body. Sweet taste and the water and earth elements are dominant in the first hour of digestion. The second hour of digestion is the sour stage, dominated by the fire and earth elements. Agni resides in the lesser curvature of the stomach as hydrochloric acid to further assist in the digestion of nutrients. The next two hours (third and fourth stage of digestion) relate to pitta dosha and nourish the pitta parts of the body. The third stage of digestion relates to the salty taste, and to the water and fire elements. This stage of digestion occurs in the duodenum, the beginning of the small intestine. The fourth stage relates to the pungent taste, and to the air and fire elements, and takes place in the jejunum, the second part of the small intestine. The last two hours (fifth and sixth stage of digestion) relate to vata dosha and nourish the vata parts of the body. The fifth stage of digestion relates to the bitter taste, and to the air and ether elements. Located in the ileum, this stage is responsible for absorption. The sixth and final stage is related to the astringent taste, and to the air and earth elements; it is located in the cecum of the large intestine.

Balanced agni plays a vital role in maintaining optimum health, as it is necessary to destroy ama. As agni exists in every tissue and cell in the body, it is a necessary component in maintaining nutrition and the autoimmune mechanism. By destroying *krumi* (microorganisms, foreign bacteria and toxins in the stomach and the intestines), agni helps to maintain health and interrupt the disease process.

Agni protects us from both external as well as internal disorders. A disturbance or weakness of agni implies that the basic balance of the doshas has been disturbed. Disturbed or weakened metabolism, compromised immunity and lowered immune resistance are all results of impaired agni. When agni is weakened food will not be digested properly. It will not activate the chain of nutritional formation of the seven dhatus in a proper way. Instead of creating ojas, ama will be created and will accumulate in the body, clogging body channels and manifesting disease.

Agni's functioning depends on many factors, including food, clothing and shelter. It also depends on the five senses: what we see, hear, smell, taste and touch. Negative or disturbing input may contribute to ill health. Positive and loving sensory input supports wellness

# Chapter 9

# The Ayurvedic Diet

*The ayurvedic physician begins the cure of disease
by arranging the diet that is to be followed by the patient.
The ayurvedic physicians rely so much on diet that it is
declared that all diseases can be cured by following dietetic
rules carefully along with the proper herbal supplements;
but if a patient does not attend to his diet, a
hundred good medicines will not cure him.*

~ *Charaka Samhita, 1.41*

## Dharmic Dining

The ayurvedic diet not only nourishes the body, but also restores the balance of the doshas, which is essential for maintaining health. An ayurvedic diet is based on an individual's constitution. Medicine for one person may be poison for another. Each individual has unique dietary requirements; depending on one's dosha, or constitutional type, some foods can be beneficial and others should be avoided. When choosing what to eat, one must consider the season, weather, time of day and quality of food, as well as one's mental and emotional attitudes at the time of eating.

When we ingest food, we participate in the creative process of nature. Healthful food rejuvenates the cells of the whole body, especially our stomach lining and skin. How we eat also determines how food affects our body. If we feel emotionally imbalanced when we eat, our food may disrupt the body's natural order. If we overeat or eat too quickly, the poorly digested end product predisposes us to ill health. Food intake should contribute to order and coherence in the body. It should help us to stay balanced and boost our overall immunity.

Every food contains the five elements and the three doshas in different proportions. Consumption of each food will affect our elemental doshic balance in a positive or a negative way. If a person already has an element in sufficient quantity by inheritance, he or she should be careful not to ingest too much of that element, or an imbalance may manifest. Following an ayurvedic diet is not difficult. For every food that will aggravate the doshas, there are plenty of alternative, beneficial and tasty foods. Wrong eating habits are a result of past conditioning by family, friends and society. By creating new dietary patterns, we can enhance all levels of well-being.

> *Diet has a great deal of influence on our character.*
> *Children, you should take care to eat only simple, fresh,*
> *vegetarian food [sattvic food]. The nature of the mind is*
> *determined by the subtle essence of the food we eat. Pure*
> *food creates a pure mind. Without forsaking the taste of*
> *the tongue, the taste of the heart cannot be enjoyed.*
>
> *– Amma*

## Ahimsa Ahara (Non-violent Diet)

Saving the lives of animals may save your own life. Extensive evidence shows that vegetarian and vegan diets are by far the healthiest diets. Scientific research is now proving that excessive consumption of the cholesterol and saturated fats found in animal products leads to heart disease and numerous forms of cancer. The consumption of animal products also leads to obesity, diabetes, hypertension, arthritis, gout, kidney stones and many other diseases. In addition, modern-day factory farming methods use hormones, antibiotics, chemical fertilizers and drugs to increase their output and profits. Commercial animal products contain high levels of herbicides and pesticides. When humans consume animal products, their bodies receive these poisons and become toxic.

Since the 1960s, scientists have suspected that a meat-based diet is related to the development of arteriosclerosis and heart disease. As early as 1961, a study published in the *Journal of the American Medical Association* reported, "Ninety to ninety-seven percent of heart disease can be prevented by a vegetarian diet." Since that time, several well-organized studies have scientifically shown that, after tobacco and alcohol, the consumption of meat is the greatest single cause of mortality in Europe, the United States, Australia and other affluent areas of the world.

The human body is unable to process and utilize excessive amounts of animal fat and cholesterol, which accumulate on the inner walls of the arteries and constrict the flow of blood to the heart, resulting in high blood pressure, heart disease and strokes. Research during the past twenty years also strongly suggests a link between meat-eating and cancer of the colon, rectum, breast and uterus.

An article in *The Lancet*, a UK-based medical journal, reported, "People living in the areas with a high-recorded incidence of carcinoma of the colon tend to live on diets containing large amounts of fat and animal protein; whereas those who live in areas with a low incidence live on largely vegetarian diets with little fat or animal matter." Why do meat-eaters seem more prone to these diseases? Biologists and nutritionists have discovered that the human intestinal tract is simply not suited for digesting meat. Flesh-eating animals have short intestinal tracts, only three times the length of the body, to rapidly pass decaying, toxin-producing meat out of the body. Since plant foods decay more slowly than meat, plant-eaters have intestines at least six times the length of the body. Humans have the long intestinal tract of an herbivore.

Another major concern about eating meat is that of chemical contamination. As soon as an animal is slaughtered, its flesh begins to putrefy, and after several days it turns a sickly gray-green. The meat industry masks this discoloration by adding nitrites and other preservatives to give the meat a bright red color. Research now shows that most of these preservatives are carcinogenic.

Gary and Steven Null, in their book *Poisons in Your Body*, reveal something that ought to make anyone think twice before buying another steak or ham: "The animals are kept alive and fattened by continuous administration of tranquilizers, hormones, antibiotics and 2,700 other drugs. The process starts even before birth and continues long after death. Although these drugs will still be present in the meat when you eat it, the law does not require that they be listed on the package."

Many people feel concerned that they will not meet daily requirements for protein on a diet that excludes animal products. Dr. Paavo Airola, a leading authority on nutrition and natural biology said in 1984: "The official daily recommendation for protein has gone down from the 150 grams recommended 20 years ago to only 45 grams today. Why? Because reliable worldwide research has shown that we do not need so much protein, that the actual daily need is only 35 to 45 grams. Protein consumed in excess of the daily need is not only wasted, but actually can cause harm to the body, as it strains to digest it. In order to obtain 45 grams of protein a day from your diet you do not have to eat meat; you can get it easily from a 100 percent vegetarian diet of a variety of grains, lentils, nuts, vegetables and fruits."

> *Our task must be to free ourselves, by widening our circle of compassion to embrace all living creatures and the whole of nature and its beauty. Nothing will benefit human health and increase our chances of survival for life on earth as much as the evolution to a vegetarian diet.*
>
> *– Albert Einstein*

Generally, Ayurveda encourages one to follow a pure, vegetarian diet. A yogic diet, likewise, promotes sattva (purity) and ahimsa (non-violence). Killing animals for food is not only violence to animals, but is also harmful to the environment and all of the hungry people in the world. When an animal is killed, its body releases fear hormones and other toxins, which the meat-eater later ingests and absorbs into his or her body. That negative emotional vibration then enters the person's consciousness. In addition, meat is dead; it is completely void of prana. As such, according to Ayurveda, meat creates tamas (dullness, darkness) in the mind and body.

In the ancient Indian epic *Mahabharata*, there are numerous statements against killing animals. "Who can be more cruel and selfish than he who augments his flesh by eating the flesh of innocent animals? Those who desire to possess good memory, beauty, long life with perfect health and physical, moral and spiritual strength should abstain from animal food." In addition to health and ethics concerns, the vegetarian and vegan lifestyle has a higher spiritual dimension that can help us develop our natural appreciation and love of God.

## Vegan Ayurveda

*A single commercial dairy cow produces about 120 pounds of wet manure per day, which is equivalent to the waste produced by 20–40 people. That means California's 1.4 million dairy cows produce as much waste as 28–56 million people.*

*~ US Environmental Protection Agency, Fall 2001*

Traditional Ayurveda uses dairy products as both food and medicine. Unfortunately, in the current state of the world, the commercial dairy industry is a major contributor to planetary destruction and worldwide hunger. Unless needed for personal health requirements, it is essential to seriously consider minimizing or eliminating dairy consumption.

If commercialized factory farming and the use of meat were eliminated, humanity could restore traditional methods of agriculture. In such systems, cows and goats are a vital part of the ecosystem and are honored with the love and respect they deserve. In this case, organic dairy farms could serve a vital role in preservation of the ecosystem.

The term *vegan* was coined by Donald Watson in 1944 and was defined as follows:

> Veganism is a way of eating and living, which excludes all forms of exploitation of, and cruelty to, the animal kingdom, and includes a reverence for life. It applies to the practice of living on the products of the plant kingdom to the exclusion of flesh, fish, fowl, eggs, honey, animal milk and its derivatives, and encourages the use of alternatives for all commodities derived wholly or in part from animals.

Veganism is not necessarily about personal purity or separating oneself from society, but rather about applying an awareness of compassion and justice to our often unseen and ignored relationships with animals and Mother Nature.

*Children, love can accomplish anything and everything. Love can cure diseases. Love can heal wounded hearts and transform human minds. Through love one can overcome all obstacles.*

*- Amma*

## Organic Food

*Treat the Earth well.*
*It was not given to you by your parents;*
*it was loaned to you by your children.*

*We do not inherit the Earth from our ancestors;*
*we borrow it from our children.*

~ *Native American Proverb*

Many years ago, traditional agriculture used methods that respected nature's rhythms and utilized only substances that nature provided. Since the use of chemical fertilizers, pesticides and herbicides has become widespread in farming, nature's balance has been upset, threatening the well-being not only of our external environment, but also our internal environment. Having noticed these detrimental effects, many farmers have returned to using systems of organic agriculture that increase soil fertility and restore harmony of nature. These systems include natural inputs such as compost, animal manures and biodynamic preparations, as well as appropriate crop rotations. Plants grown in well-balanced, fertile soil are strong and healthy. They resist disease and pests in the same way that healthy, happy humans resist disease.

zIn addition to being completely free from all chemicals, certified organic food is never irradiated after harvest. To become certified organic, produce must be grown in soil that is tested to be free from heavy-metal contamination. There is scientific evidence showing that the accumulation of the above-mentioned toxic substances in our bodies can lead to a wide variety of health problems, including impaired immune function, cancer, allergies, autoimmune diseases, impaired fertility and birth defects. Annually, close to five million people worldwide suffer from symptoms of pesticide poisoning. Furthermore, 10,000 people actually die each year from these poisons. Studies have shown the lifespan of conventional commercial farmers is significantly shorter than that of organic farmers.

Currently many non-organic, commercial foods are being genetically modified. Genetically modified organisms (GMOs) present a profound danger to humans as well as to the ecosystem. Many species of animals, such as the monarch butterfly and bees, are becoming endangered or extinct due to GMOs. For vegetarians, GMOs pose another problem, as they are frequently spliced from animal DNA. It is hypothesized by many experts that GMO food will eventually even alter human DNA. As GMOs are a recent creation, their long-term effects are unknown.

In India and other developing nations, western-based GMO and pesticide companies are aggressively promoting heavy use of chemicals for farming. This leads to serious depletion of the soil and contamination of the water. Many insects are developing stronger resistance to pesticides, so sometimes even huge amounts of chemicals prove ineffective in protecting crops. For this reason, many farmers have little or no yield, year after year. Having gone deeply in debt to these chemical companies, the farmers begin to feel hopeless. The horrific reality is that large numbers of Indian farmers are committing suicide by drinking their pesticides. Amma has expressed deep concern about this issue and is guiding the M.A. Math's projects to help these farmers and their families. When we choose organic, non-GMO foods, we are doing our part to try to end this tragic situation.

Certified organic food has much higher nutritional content than non-organic food, so the consumer gets more for their money. Many people also find organic food tastes better. Organic food has a stronger vital life force than commercial food. Eating organic food is a primary step toward personal and global health.

*Nature gives all of Her wealth to human beings. Just*
*as nature is dedicated to helping us, we too should be*
*dedicated to helping nature. Only then can the harmony*
*between nature and humanity be preserved.*

*- Amma*

## Food as Prayer

*Not a grain of the food we eat is made purely by our own*
*effort. What comes to us in the form of food is the toil of our*

*sisters and brothers, and the bounty of nature and God's compassion. Even if we have a million dollars, we still need food to satisfy our hunger. After all, we cannot eat dollars. So we should never eat anything without first praying with a feeling of humbleness and gratitude. Consider your food to be the Goddess Lakshmi [the Goddess of Prosperity], and receive it with devotion and reverence. Food is Brahman [the Supreme Being]. Eat the food as God's prasad [blessed gift].*

*~ Amma*

Through her life and message, Amma reminds us that we are not the body; we are the Atma (the Supreme Self). So why bother to eat healthfully? Our bodies are vehicles for transporting the soul. Just as we would not put gasoline mixed with dirt into our cars, we should consider what type of fuel we put into our soul's vehicle. At the same time, we should be careful not to take our diets so seriously that we lose a sense of gratitude for whatever foods we receive. We are blessed if we have enough food to provide energy and nutrition, as millions of people worldwide do not have this. Our thoughts and attitude during meals affect our digestion and assimilation as much as the food itself.

We have infinite potential to heal ourselves and the planet by making some simple changes to our dietary habits. Amma again and again emphasizes to us that Mother Nature is very much out of balance.

# Chapter 10

# Food as Medicine

## Ayurvedic Eating Principles

*The following are general principles that should be followed when eating. They will assure optimum digestion, assimilation and elimination. Never overeat. Half the stomach should be for food, a quarter for liquid, and the remaining portion for the movement of air. The less food you eat, the more mental control you will have. Do not sleep or meditate immediately after eating; if you do, you won't be able to digest the food properly. Always mentally repeat your mantra while you eat. This will purify the food and your mind at the same time.*

*~ Amma*

- Eat to about three-quarters of your capacity. Do not leave the table very hungry or very full.
- Avoid taking a meal until the previous meal has been digested. Allow approximately 3–6 hours between meals.
- Eat in a settled and quiet atmosphere. Do not work, read or watch TV during meal times. Avoid talking, if possible.
- Choose foods by balancing physical attributes. In general, the diet should be balanced to include all six tastes sweet, sour, salty, bitter, pungent and astringent. Follow specific recommendations according to your constitution. Each taste has a balancing effect, so including some of each minimizes cravings and balances the appetite and digestion. The general North American and European

diet tends to have too much of the sweet, sour and salty tastes, and not enough of the bitter, pungent and astringent tastes.

- Choose foods that are sattvic. Choose whole, fresh, in-season, local foods.
- Yogurt, cheese, cottage cheese and buttermilk should be avoided at night.
- Follow food-combining guidelines (listed later in this chapter).
- It is best not to cook with honey as it becomes toxic when cooked.
- Take a few minutes to sit quietly after each meal before returning to activity.
- Eat optimal times for digestion: breakfast 7–9 a.m., lunch 10–2 p.m. and dinner 4–6 p.m.
- Wash face, hands and feet before meals.
- Rinse mouth before and after eating.
- Dine in an isolated, neat and clean place. The environment should be pleasant. The eater should be in a comfortable seated position.
- Eat only food prepared in a loving way. This method of food preparation increases the vitality-giving quality of the food.
- Chew food until it is an even consistency before swallowing.
- Hard items should be consumed in the beginning of the meal, followed by soft foods and subsequently, liquids.
- Do not drink cold drinks just prior to or while eating. Also do not drink large quantities of liquids during meals, for this habit weakens digestion. A few sips of warm water are okay with meals.
- Avoid heavy substances such as rich desserts after meals.
- Consumption of excessively hot food leads to weakness. Cold and dry foods lead to delayed digestion.
- No travel, vigorous excercise or sexual intercourse within one hour after a meal, as this will impede digestion. Walking (10–20 minutes) after a meal can help digestion.
- Avoid meals when thirsty and water while hungry.
- Avoid meals immediately after exertion.
- Do not eat when there is not an appetite.

- Don't suppress the appetite, as this leads to body pain, anorexia, lassitude, vertigo and general debility.
- Don't suppress thirst, as it leads to general debility, giddiness and heart disease.

### *Eating Habits that Decrease Health*

- Overeating
- Eating when not hungry
- Emotional eating
- Drinking juice or excess water while eating
- Drinking chilled water at any time
- Eating when constipated or emotionally imbalanced
- Eating at the wrong time of day
- Eating too many heavy foods or not enough light foods
- Snacking on anything except fruit in between meals
- Eating incompatible food combinations

## Six Types of Nutritional Imbalances

1. Quantitative Deficiency: malnutrition due to insufficient food
2. Quantitative Excess:
   - Excessive amounts of any food or water
   - Food taken at the wrong time
   - Food that is not appropriate for one's constitution
3. Qualitative Deficiency: wrong food-combining, which results in malnutrition, toxic conditions and lack of essential nutrients
4. Qualitative Excess: emotional overeating; eating foods that are fried, high in fat, wrong foods for constitution
5. Ama-producing: eating foods and improper food-combinations that lead to toxemia and other digestive disorders. This includes eating foods with toxins such as pesticides, herbacides, hormones and antibiotics.
6. Prakriti-disturbing: eating foods not appropriate for one's constitution, which may lead to reduced agni, immunity and disease

These six factors lead to depletion of agni and the build up of ama.

## Sattvic Eating

*The person who always eats wholesome (sattvic) food
enjoys a regular lifestyle,
remains unattached to the objects of the senses,
gives and forgives,
loves truth and serves others without disease.*

*~ Ashtanga Hridayam*


*When food is pure, the mind is pure; this creates an
oasis for awakening and provides an awakening that
affects every level of our health [body-mind-spirit].*

*~ Chandogya Upanishad, 6.5.1-4*

Ayurveda encourages a sattvic diet. According to criteria given by the rishis, this includes:
1. Foods grown in healthy, fertile soil
2. Foods that are attractive in appearance
3. Foods that are protected from animals (insects, parasites, worms and harmful bacteria)
Modern Day Additions:
1. Foods grown without pesticides, herbicides, fungicides, chemical fertilizers, hormones, antibiotics, irradiation, GMOs, etc. This includes not harming the earth or its inhabitants (ahimsa).
2. Food should be whole, fresh, unprocessed and unrefined. It should not contain any chemical additives.
3. Animal food is dead; it is tamasic and has no life force.


Sattvic foods prevent free radicals because they are rich in antioxidants. Free radicals destroy enzymes, amino acids and block cellular function. Free radicals are electron-deficient molecules that are produced from oxygen and heated fats or oils in the body. They destroy health. Health and longevity are dependent on antioxidant-rich foods and hydration. Sattvic food contains 75-90 percent water. It is filled with prana and nourishes life.

## Food-combining Guidelines

Foods in **bold** lettering are listed first because they increase ama to such a degree that they should definitely be avoided!

| Don't Eat These Foods | With These Foods |
|---|---|
| Beans | fruit, cheese, eggs, fish, milk, meat, yogurt |
| Eggs | **milk,** fruit, beans, cheese, fish, kichari, meat, yogurt |
| Grains | fruit |
| Fruit | **any other food,** except dates or almonds |
| Honey | and **ghee** by equal weight (For example, 1 teaspoon honey with 3 teaspoons ghee is not okay.) Equal volume is okay. (For example, 1 teaspoon of each is okay.) Raw honey is considered to be *amrita* (nectar), but when cooked, it adheres to mucous membranes and clogs the gross and subtle channels, producing toxins. |
| Hot drinks | mangoes, cheese, fish, meat, starch, yogurt |
| Lemon | cucumbers, milk, tomatoes, yogurt |
| Melon | any other food, including other melons |
| Milk | **fruit,** especially **bananas,** cherries, melons, and sour fruit; bread, fish, kichari, meat. Pasteurized and homogenized dairy causes ama. Instead, Ayurveda recommends consuming raw dairy and avoiding dairy produced in factory farms that use hormones, antibiotics and steroids. |

| Nightshades (tomato, eggplant, bell pepper, potato) | cucumber, dairy products |
| --- | --- |
| Radishes | bananas, raisins, milk |
| Tapioca, yogurt | **milk**, fruit, cheese, eggs, fish, hot drinks, meat, nightshades |

## The Six Tastes

The six tastes are based on the actual taste in the mouth. Each taste has unique therapeutic properties. This applies to food, herbs and minerals. Balancing the tastes according to dosha is a key to health. Each of the tastes is governed by two of the five elements and either increases or decreases the doshas.

**1. Sweet:** made of earth and water, decreases vata and pitta and increases kapha

- Sweet fruits: figs, grapes, oranges, dates, pears
- Most legumes: beans, lentils, peas
- Most grains: wheat, rice, corn, barley, most bread
- Milk and sweet milk products: cream, ghee and butter
- Sugar and sweeteners: white, refined sugars, artificial sweeteners, jaggery, maple syrup. Honey, having a secondary taste of astringent, decreases vata and kapha and increases pitta.
- Certain cooked vegetables: starchy tubers like potato, carrot, sweet potato, beet root

**2. Sour:** made of earth and fire, decreases vata and increases pitta and kapha

- Sour milk products: yogurt, cheese, whey and sour cream
- Sour fruits: lemons, sour oranges, etc.
- Fermented substances: soy sauce, vinegar, wine, sour cabbage (kimchi) and pickles

3. **Salty:** made of water and fire, decreases vata while increasing pitta and kapha
   - Salt: sea salt, Himalayan salt, rock salt, table salt, soy sauce, tamari and any other form of salt
   - Salty food: seaweed, salty pickles, chips

4. **Pungent:** made of fire and air, decreases kapha and increases pitta and vata
   - Few vegetables: radish, onion
   - Spices: ginger, cumin, garlic, chili, mustard seeds, black pepper

5. **Bitter:** made of air and ether, decreases pitta and kapha and increases vata
   - Certain fruits: olives, grapefruits
   - Vegetables: eggplant, chicory, bitter gourd and zucchini
   - Green leafy vegetables: spinach, green cabbage, Brussels sprouts
   - Certain spices: fenugreek and turmeric

6. **Astringent:** made of air and earth, increases vata and decreases pitta and kapha
   - Sweetener: Honey decreases vata and kapha while increasing pitta due to its heating properties.
   - Nuts: walnuts, cashews and hazelnuts
   - Legumes: beans, lentils
   - Vegetables: sprouts, lettuce, rhubarb, most green leafy vegetables and most raw vegetables
   - Fruits: persimmons, berries, pomegranates, unripe fruits and, to some degree, apples

Vata is decreased by sweet, sour and salty tastes. It is also decreased by foods that are heavy, oily and hot. Vata is increased by pungent, bitter and astringent tastes, as well as foods that are light, dry and cold.

Pitta is decreased by sweet, bitter and astringent tastes and cold, heavy and oily foods. Pitta is increased by pungent, sour and salty tastes as well as foods that are hot, light and dry.

Kapha is decreased by pungent, bitter and astringent tastes in foods that are light, dry and warm. Kapha is increased by sweet, sour and salty tastes, as well as foods that are heavy, oily and cold.

# Balancing the Diet

## The Benefits of Eating According to Your Constitution
- better health, concentration and memory
- youthfulness
- more energy, endurance and strength
- a gradual decrease in existing imbalances
- prevention of imbalances
- greater ability to handle stress and anxiety
- improved sleep
- better digestion, metabolism and elimination
- healthier skin and complexion
- healthier progeny
- a stronger immune system
- weight loss or gain (depending on what is needed) and better weight management
- improved meditation and yoga practice
- a more productive and happier life

# Vata-balancing Diet

Vata season is when weather is cold, windy and dry. Depending on location, vata season usually lasts from November through February. During this time of year, the qualities of vata increase naturally. Thus, one should take lots of warm food and drinks, as well as heavier and oilier foods, during this time. Eat more of the sweet, sour and salty tastes. Avoid dry or cold food and cold drinks. Eat fewer pungent, bitter and astringent tastes overall.

To balance vata, favor foods that are oily, heavy, warm, sweet, sour and salty:

- Beverages:
  - Herbal teas: ajwain, bancha, chamomile, clove, comfrey, elderflower, eucalyptus, fennel, fenugreek, ginger (fresh), hawthorne, juniper berry, lavender, lemon grass, licorice, marshmallow, oat straw, orange peel, pennyroyal, peppermint, rosehips, saffron, sage, sarsaparilla, sassafras, spearmint
  - Juices: aloe vera juice, apple cider, apricot, berry (not cranberry), carrot, cherry, grape, lemonade, mango, orange, papaya, peach, pineapple, sour juices
  - Other: almond milk, grain beverages, miso broth, rice milk, vegetable bouillon
- Condiments: chutney (mango), dulse, gomasio, hijiki, kelp, ketchup, lemon, lime, lime pickle, mango pickle, mayonnaise, mustard, pickles, scallions, seaweed, vinegar
- Dairy: butter, ghee, whole milk (cow and goat), lassi, cheese (cow and goat), fresh homemade paneer, cottage cheese, sour cream, yogurt
- Food supplements: aloe vera juice, bee pollen, amino acids, calcium, copper, iron, magnesium, royal jelly, spirulina, blue-green algae, vitamins A, B, B$_{12}$, C, D, E, and EFAs (essential fatty acids found in cold pressed oils from hemp seed, evening primrose, black currant seed, flax seed, borage oils)
- Fruits: apples (ripe and sweet, cooked), applesauce, avocado, banana, berries, cherries, coconut, dates, figs, grapefruit, grapes, kiwi, lemon, lime, mango, melons, oranges, papaya, peaches, pineapple, plums, pomegranate, prunes (soaked), raisins, rhubarb, strawberries, tamarind
- Grains: whole amaranth, cooked oats, quinoa, seitan (wheat meat), sprouted wheat bread (Essene style), white basmati rice
- Legumes: mung beans, mung dal, tur dal, urad dal

- Nuts: almonds (soaked and peeled are best), black walnuts, brazil nuts, cashews, charole, coconut, filberts, hazelnuts, macadamia nuts, peanuts, pecans, pine nuts, pistachios, walnuts
- Oils: ghee, olive oil, sunflower oil. Use coconut, avocado and sesame oils externally only.
- Seeds: chia, flax, halva, hemp, pumpkin, sesame, sunflower
- Spices: ajwain, allspice, almond extract, anise, asafoetida (hing), basil, bay leaf, black pepper, cardamom, cayenne, cinnamon, clove, green coriander leaf, cumin, dill, fennel, fenugreek, garlic, ginger (especially fresh), marjoram, mint, mustard seeds, nutmeg, orange peel, oregano, paprika, parsley, peppermint, pippali, poppy seed, rosemary, saffron, savory, spearmint, star anise, tarragon, thyme, turmeric, vanilla, wintergreen
- Sweeteners: barley malt, fructose, fruit juice concentrates, honey, jaggery, molasses, rice syrup, stevia, raw sugar or sucanat, turbinado sugar
- Vegetables: asparagus, beets, red cabbage (cooked, in moderation), carrots, green chilies, cilantro, cucumber, daikon radish (cooked, in moderation), fennel (anise), garlic, green beans, dark leafy greens (cooked, in moderation), leeks, mustard greens, okra, olives (black), onions (cooked), parsnips, peas (cooked), sweet potato, pumpkin, radish (cooked), rutabaga, summer squash, taro root, watercress, zucchini

To balance vata, reduce foods that are dry, light, cold, spicy, bitter, astringent:
- Avoid all cold foods and drinks.
- Beans: Reduce intake of beans, all of which increase vata, except mung dal.
- Dairy: Reduce use of milk or yogurt with fruit or vegetables.
- Fruits: Avoid dry, light, or astringent fruits such as apples, berries, pears and dried fruit.
- Grains: Reduce intake of barley, corn, millet, oats, rye.
- Spices: Minimize use of chilies and red pepper.

• Vegetables: Avoid raw, frozen, canned, fried and leftover vegetables, and cruciferous vegetables

## Pitta-balancing Diet

Pitta season is hot and dry, usually lasting from July through October. Again, this will vary depending on location. During this time, favor foods and drinks that are cooling. Eat foods of sweet, bitter and astringent tastes. Include fresh, sweet fruits and vegetables that grow during the pitta season. Eat fewer pungent, sour and salty foods. Avoid yogurt, cheese, tomatoes, vinegars and hot spices, as they all greatly increase pitta.

To balance pitta, favor foods that are oily, heavy, cold, bitter, sweet and astringent:
• Beverages:
  • Herbal teas: alfalfa, bancha, barley, blackberry, borage, burdock, catnip, chamomile, chicory, comfrey, dandelion, fennel, ginger (fresh), hibiscus, hops, jasmine, kukicha, lavender, lemon balm, lemon grass, licorice, marshmallow, nettle, oat straw, passion flower, peppermint, raspberry, red clover, sarsaparilla, spearmint, strawberry, violet, wintergreen, yarrow
  • Juices: aloe vera juice, apple, apricot, berry, cherry, grape, mango, mixed vegetable, peach, pear, pomegranate, prune
  • Other: almond milk in moderation, grain beverages, rice milk
• Condiments: chutney, cilantro, sprouts
• Dairy: butter (unsalted), cow or goat cheese (soft, unsalted), ghee, whole cow and goat milk (avoid homogenized), lassi
• Food supplements: aloe vera juice, blue-green algae, barley greens, brewer's yeast, calcium, magnesium, zinc, spirulina, vitamins D, E and EFAs (essential fatty acids found in cold pressed oils from hemp seed, evening primrose, black currant seed, flax seed, borage), whey protein powder as a protein supplement

177

(isolate only, not concentrates or hydrolyzed as the protein has been denatured)

• Fruits (ripe and sweet): apples, applesauce, apricots, avocado, berries (sweet), cherries, coconut, dates, figs, grapes (red and purple), mango, melon, oranges, papayas, pear, pineapple, plums, pomegranate, prunes, raisins, watermelon

• Grains: whole amaranth and barley, cereals (dry), oat bran, oats, whole grain pasta, spelt, sprouted wheat bread (Essene style), tapioca, white basmati rice

• Legumes: adzuki beans, black beans, black-eyed peas, chickpeas (garbanzo beans), kidney beans, lentils (brown and red), lima beans, mung beans, mung dal, navy beans, peas (dried), pinto beans, split peas, white beans. NOTE: All legumes should be well-cooked.

• Nuts: almonds (soaked and peeled), coconut

• Oils: coconut oil, ghee, olive oil

• Seeds: flax, hemp, pumpkin, sunflower

• Spices: basil (fresh), black pepper (in moderation), fresh ginger (in moderation), cardamom, cinnamon, coriander, cumin, dill, fennel, mint, peppermint, spearmint, saffron, turmeric, rock salt

• Sweeteners: agave, barley malt, fruit juice, honey, maple syrup, rice syrup, stevia, raw sugar or sucanat, rock crystal sugar

• Vegetables: artichoke, asparagus, beets, bitter melon, broccoli, Brussels sprouts, cabbage, carrots, cauliflower, celery, cilantro, cucumber, dandelion greens, fennel, green beans, kale, dark leafy greens, leeks, okra, olives (black), onion (cooked), parsley, parsnip, peas, sweet potatoes, prickly pear leaves, pumpkin, rutabaga, spaghetti squash, sprouts, squash (winter and summer), taro root, wheat grass sprouts, zucchini

To balance pitta, reduce foods that are dry, light, warm, salty, spicy and sour:

• Dairy: Reduce use of cheese, cultured buttermilk, sour cream and yogurt.

- Fruits: Reduce intake of sour fruits such as olives, sour oranges and unripe pineapples, persimmons and bananas
- Grains: Reduce intake of brown rice, corn, millet and rye.
- Oils: Reduce the use of almond, corn and sesame oils.
- Spices: Avoid chili and cayenne.
- Sweeteners: Avoid large quantities of honey.

## Kapha-balancing Diet

Kapha season is the rainy and cool season that lasts from March through June, depending on location. During kapha season, eat foods that are light and easy to digest. Take warm food and drinks. Eat foods that are pungent, bitter and astringent in taste. Avoid foods that are sweet, salty or sour flavored.

To balance kapha, favor foods that are dry, warm, light, spicy, bitter, astringent:

- Beverages:
- Herbal teas: alfalfa, bancha, barley, blackberry, burdock, chamomile, chicory, clove, cinnamon, dandelion, fenugreek, ginger, hibiscus, jasmine, juniper berry, kukicha, lavender, lemon balm, lemon grass, nettle, passion flower, peppermint, raspberry, red clover, sassafras, spearmint, strawberry, wintergreen, yarrow, yerba mate
  - Juices: aloe vera juice, apple cider, apricot, berry, carrot, cherry, cranberry, grape, mango, peach, pear, pomegranate, prune
  - Other: black tea (spiced), grain beverages
- Condiments: black pepper, chili peppers, chutney, cilantro, dulse, hijiki, horseradish, lemon, mustard (without vinegar), scallions, seaweed, sprouts
- Dairy: cottage cheese (from skimmed goat milk), lassi, non-fat goat milk. Avoid homogenized dairy.
- Food supplements: aloe vera juice, amino acids, barley green, bee pollen, blue-green algae, brewer's yeast, calcium, copper, iron,

magnesium, zinc, royal jelly, spirulina, vitamins A, B, $B_{12}$, C, D, E, EFAs (essential fatty acids found in cold-pressed oils from hemp seed, evening primrose, black currant seed, flax seed and borage oils), whey protein powder (isolate only, not concentrated or hydrolyzed)

• Fruits: apples, applesauce, apricots, berries, cherries, cranberries, dried fruit, guava, peaches, pears, persimmon, pomegranate, prunes, raisins

• Grains (whole): barley, buckwheat, cereals (dry or puffed), corn (organic, non-GMO), couscous, granola, millet, muesli, oat bran, oats, polenta, quinoa, rye, basmati rice, spelt, sprouted wheat bread (Essene style), tapioca, wheat bran

• Legumes (well-cooked and with spices): adzuki beans, black beans, black-eyed peas, chick peas, lentils (red and brown), lima beans, mung beans, mung dal, navy beans, peas (dried), pinto beans, split peas, tur dal, white beans

• Oils: ghee, mustard oil

• Seeds: chia, flax, hemp, popcorn, pumpkin seeds, sunflower seeds

• Spices: all spices except salt, especially fresh ginger

• Sweeteners: fruit juice, honey, stevia

• Vegetables: artichoke, asparagus, beet greens, beets, bitter melon, broccoli, cabbage, carrots, cauliflower, celery, cilantro, corn, daikon radish, dandelion greens, eggplant, fennel (anise), garlic, green beans, green chilies, horseradish, kale, kohlrabi, leafy greens (lettuces), leeks, mushrooms, mustard greens, okra, onions, parsley, peas, hot peppers, prickly pear, rutabaga, spinach, sprouts, summer squash, tomatoes (cooked), turnip greens, turnips, watercress, wheat grass

To balance kapha, reduce foods that are: oily, cold, heavy, sweet, sour:

• Dairy: Butter, cheese, cream, ice cream, sour cream, yogurt and any excess of whole milk are not recommended.

• Fruits: Avoid bananas, coconuts, dates, figs, grapes, limes, mangoes, melons, oranges and pineapples.

- Grains: Reduce intake of rice and wheat.
- Nuts: Avoid nuts.
- Oils: Avoid large amounts of any oil.
- Spices: Avoid salt and salty foods (pickles, chips).
- Sweeteners: Avoid most sugar products.
- Vegetables: Reduce use of cucumbers, okra, sweet potatoes and tomatoes.

**Please see the back of the book for a chart of food guidelines for basic constitutional types.**

# Chapter 11

# Lifestyle and Routine

*Pray with a sincere heart:*
*God, let me remember you constantly throughout the day.*
*Let my every thought, word and deed bring me closer to You.*
*Let me not hurt anyone in thought, word or deed.*
*Be with me in every moment.*

*~ Amma*

Everything in creation has a routine or cycle. Ayurvedic wisdom exalts the use of individualized routines throughout one's life. The *Charaka Samhita* explains, "A wise man interested in long and healthful life, and who seeks happiness, must exercise the highest care in selecting what is wholesome in the matter of food, conduct and behavior." It goes on to state that the average lifespan for a healthy individual is about one hundred years, but will decrease if proper conduct is not followed. Perfect health is a state of balance between the mind, body, spirit and environment. This harmony can be achieved through diet, exercise, lifestyle, meditation, and mental and moral discipline. Nowadays, extra effort is required to maintain health because we are impacted by excessive environmental pollution, food adulteration, untimely working hours and generally unhealthful lifestyles. Ayurvedic regimens are simple, non-invasive, non-traumatic and generally do not interfere with other forms of treatment.

Clear instructions for day-to-day living are offered in Ayurveda's *dinacharya* (daily routine). Likewise, the *ritucharya* (seasonal routine) suggests ways in which we should adapt to the various seasons. When exploring the following routines, it is important to remember that many people are dual dosha. This should be taken into account when choosing and following ayurvedic lifestyle guidelines.

## Dinacharya – Daily Routines for Health

Both vibrant health and Self-realization come through discipline and awareness. Yogis undergo many austerities to attain liberation. To raise our level of health and consciousness, it is essential to control unrestrained desires and drives. Integrating the daily routines of dinacharya is an important step in cultivating discipline and awareness.

*Din* means "day" and *acharya* means "to follow, to find, close to." To follow or be close to the day implies unifying your daily routine with the natural cycle of the sun, moon, earth and the other planets. Following the dinacharya is one of the best means to align with nature. This creates balance and prevents disease. Ultimately, one will find that health and happiness are truly one's most natural state.

The rishis considered daily routine to be a stronger healing force than any other curative medicine. Today society is out of touch with nature. For example, on any given day, very few people know where the moon is in its cycle. In order for us to really heal, we must re-attune ourselves to nature's cycles.

In Ayurveda, time has many meanings and plays an important causative role. The Sanskrit word for "time" also means "transformation." Thus, it is synonymous with change and may be considered the primary cause of change. Time is an important consideration in understanding the prevention, development and elimination of disease. Certain imbalances occur at certain times of the day or in a particular season, which is why dinacharya plays such a vital role.

All cycles are the dynamic interaction of the three principles of life – vata, pitta and kapha (motion, transformation and structure, respectively).

We have already discussed that vata and kapha are cold while pitta is hot. Vata and pitta are light and kapha is heavy. Vata and pitta are mobile while kapha is static. Vata is dry while pitta and kapha are oily and liquid. Just as the heat of pitta reverses the cold of kapha, other qualities increase and decrease as time progresses. Likewise, a certain quality in the environment will build up, and then release or reduce. Nature creates this cycle as a way to constantly restore balance and purify herself. This ebb and flow continuously takes place in the human body as well.

## Dosha Cycles

*If one way is better than another,*
*you may be sure it is nature's way.*

*~ Aristotle*

### First Cycle
6 a.m. to 10 a.m. – Kapha
10 a.m. to 2 p.m. – Pitta
2 p.m. to 6 p.m. – Vata

### Second Cycle
6 p.m. to 10 p.m. – Kapha
10 p.m. to 2 a.m. – Pitta
2 a.m. to 6 a.m. – Vata

It is important to understand that the times listed above as 6 p.m. and 6 a.m. are not fixed; they specifically refer to the exact times of sunset and sunrise. They also vary slightly according to the seasons, longitude and latitude. Based on the above cycles, the recommended daily schedule is divided as follows: morning, noon, evening, dinner and bedtime.

# Arising

Ideally, one should awaken for meditation with or before the sunrise. Sadhaks intent on the goal of Self-realization should arise several hours before the sunrise. In the Vedic tradition, the pre-dawn hours are known as *Brahma Muhurta,* "the time of God." This period, approximately one and a half hours before sunrise, is believed to be the most beneficial time for sadhana, as it is the stillest and quietest time of the day. A healthy person should get up two hours before sunrise. When we wake up during these hours, activity during the day will be more effortless and productive, as the body and mind are alert, clear, light and energetic. Creativity and mental clarity are especially present during these early morning hours. Ayurveda supports the age old adage, "Early to bed and early to rise makes the old man healthy, wealthy and wise." During these early morning hours, the vata element is dominant. By waking up two hours before dawn, one can experience the higher positive vata qualities in nature. The lightness and clarity of vata help to tune the body to the subtle vibrations within nature. This time has the highest level of sattva in the air. Hence, is it the most fresh and pure time of the day.

Some who may take exception to this rule of early-rising are the very young, the old, parents with small children, and people with fevers or diarrhea. These times may also vary slightly for each of the doshas. Vata tends to require more sleep. According to Ayurveda, the ideal sleeping schedule for vata is a 10 p.m. bedtime and a 6 a.m. rising time. While it is also best for a pitta to retire around 10 p.m., a 4 – 5 a.m. rising time is more suitable. Kapha requires the least amount of sleep. A kapha can go to bed at 11 p.m. and wake up at 4 a.m., feeling rested and alert. For a sadhak, a maximum of five to six hours of sleep are recommended regardless of the dosha: six hours for a vata sadhak, five and a half hours for a pitta sadhak, and five hours for a kapha sadhak.

The early morning hours are very conducive for meditation practice; they are times of relative quiet and calm. However, if meditation cannot be practiced before dawn, do not avoid it. Regular meditation is essential for maintaining good health. It helps to rejuvenate and purify the entire nervous system and calms the mind so that deeper awareness, peace and joy may be experienced.

# Elimination

Wastes should be eliminated from the body first thing in the morning. This action helps to revitalize the organism and prepare the body to receive more nutrients. Squatting is the best position for evacuation of the bowels, as it aligns the colon for release of feces. The squatting position also increases the flow of downward moving prana (apana vata).

According to Ayurveda, one should have at least one bowel movement per day. Otherwise, toxins can be reabsorbed into the tissues. To avoid this reabsorption, it is important to drink at least 2-3 liters of water each day. Dehydration is the primary cause of constipation. It is also helpful to eat enough fiber-rich food and good quality oils (such as hemp, flax, olive or sesame oil) and to avoid excessive amounts of raw foods and chilled drinks.

Traditional herbal compounds, such as triphala, can help to restore and maintain the tone of the colon while gently cleansing it on a daily basis. Triphala builds good flora and does not create dependence. However, one must be careful not to abuse other types of laxatives. Even some herbal laxatives (such as cascara sagrada and senna) can weaken the tone of the colon and create dependency.

# Satisfying Natural Urges

As part of a daily regimen, it is essential not to suppress certain natural physical urges like urination, defecation, hunger, thirst, sleep, sneezing, belching, yawning, vomiting, flatulence and panting. For good health, one should satisfy these natural urges instantly;

otherwise various diseases (related to the natural urge) may occur. For example, suppression of the urge to urinate causes pain in the bladder and phallus, and dysuria and distension of the lower abdomen. Suppression of the urge to defecate causes headache, constipation, flatulence, cramps in the abdomen and gripping pain.

## Cleanliness

Habits of cleanliness are very important for good health. These include brushing the teeth, scraping the tongue, gargling, cleansing the mouth and nose, regular massage of the body, application of oil on the head, bathing, trimming of hair and nails, ablution of the feet and the excretory orifices, wearing clean clothes, and the use of aromatherapy.

Early morning bathing is a basic dinacharya practice. In yogic traditions, bathing symbolizes the purification of the soul. From an ayurvedic perspective, it also washes the sweat residue from the pores of the skin, leaving a healthful, radiant glow. Gentle herbal soaps or powders can be used. It is important to avoid unnatural soaps and body care products containing chemicals and unnatural preservatives. These absorb through the skin and cause toxicity in the body.

The daily practice of rubbing the body with oil (abhyanga) can further nourish the skin and deeper tissues. Specific oils also balance each dosha. Vata constitutions should use sesame oil, pitta should use coconut oil, and kapha does best with corn or mustard oil.

Early morning ayurvedic practices include oral hygiene. A thick coating on the tongue indicates ama from improperly digested food in the gastrointestinal tract. One should scrape off this coating with a metallic tongue scraper several times after gently brushing the teeth.

*Neti* and *nasya* are also part of the ayurvedic regime. Neti involves the passing of saltwater through the nose with a neti pot. Nasya is the application of drops of specially medicated oil into each nostril. Neti and nasya remove impure kapha from the sinuses, clear the mind, promote alertness in sadhana, stimulate the flow of prana, and strengthen the neck and shoulders. They are also good for the complexion and stop graying of hair. The physical, mental, emotional and spiritual benefits of both neti and nasya are numerous.

*Gandusha*, or holding fluid in one's mouth, is another recommended practice in which salt water, medicated oil or an herbal decoction is held in the mouth for a while. This action strengthens the teeth, benefits speech and the throat, and helps to cure diseases of the mouth. Sesame oil is particularly beneficial as it contains high levels of calcium, which nourishes the teeth and gums.

## Exercise

Properly performed exercise produces both physical health and mental happiness. To avoid harm, exercise should be tailored to age and prakriti. For most people, yoga asanas and breathing exercises (pranayama) are ideal. (Please see Chapter 15, "Yoga in Ayurveda"). Additionally, walking, swimming, tai chi, chi kung and bicycling are good for most people. Early morning exercise is especially beneficial, as it removes stagnation in the body-mind, strengthens the digestive fire, reduces excess fat and gives an overall feeling of lightness and joy. It also fills the body and mind with prana.

The type of exercise one chooses should be suitable for one's specific constitution. Vata people should exercise regularly in moderation. They excel in sports that require quick bursts of speed and agility. Vata types need less exercise than pittas and kaphas. Pitta individuals should perform moderate exercise, avoiding it during midday and in hot seasons. Pittas excel in competitive sports which require strength, speed and stamina. They should keep in mind the importance of not becoming overly-competitive or overheated. Kapha people should perform heavy exercise. Kaphas do well under pressure in athletic activities, because of their stable and easy-going nature. They require stimulating and vigorous exercise balanced with motivating activities.

Vigorous exercise is not recommended for very weak and emaciated people, after heavy meals, or for anyone with a febrile condition. It is also contraindicated for people who have a tendency to bleed, tuberculosis, heart diseases, asthma or vertigo.

## Abhyanga (Oil Massage)

Typically a self-massage, abhyanga is one of the most important ayurvedic practices to build strength and prevent aging. A central part of dinacharya, it helps to cleanse the body and regulate the doshas. A main cause of aging is the drying of tissue, which results in slower transportation and assimilation of nutrients into the cells of the body. Dryness also slows the elimination of toxic wastes out of the body. Oil massage eliminates this dryness, removes stagnation and nurtures the mind and body. Abhyanga can be performed first thing in the morning 30-60 minutes before bathing, or directly after bathing. Likewise, this can be done in the evening before bed.

When the proper oil is applied, the result is healthful, vibrant skin. Herbal oil massage is beneficial for almost all dosha disorders. Sesame oil suits all dosha types; however vata needs more oil than pitta or kapha.

Vata individuals should massage the whole body with warm sesame oil and give extra attention to the feet, lower back, abdominal area, neck and shoulders. While sesame is best, vata can also use almond, avocado, castor, coconut, mustard, kukui nut and macadamia nut oils.

Pitta individuals should give extra attention to the chest, liver, stomach and head. Sesame oil will slightly increase pitta; thus, the best oils for pitta are coconut or *brahmi thailam* (brahmi in sesame oil).

Kapha types should massage the entire abdomen area, chest and throat, and may also massage the sinuses. Sesame and mustard oils are both suitable for kaphas. Kapha also benefits from dry skinbrushing and the application of dry herbal powders.

All types can finish their daily abhyanga by applying some high-quality essential oils such as rose, sandalwood, frankincense or jasmine to the third eye, throat and heart areas.

## Mental and Moral Discipline

Another important aspect of the daily regimen concerns mental health. According to the *Charak Samhita*, we should exert mental and moral disciplines, including:
- Respect God, teachers, saints and elderly people.
- Be of help to others in times of difficulty.
- Make firm decisions; be fearless, intelligent, brave and forgiving.
- Avoid negative, wicked and greedy people.
- Avoid undesirable places, alcohol and drugs.

Strict mental discipline and adherence to moral values are vital to maintaining mental health. One of the key concepts of Ayurveda demonstrates that abnormal codes of conduct produce stress, and that errors or lack of judgment are at the root of all stress. An improved code of conduct prevents stress and can free the body and mind from physical and mental disorders.

## Spiritual Discipline

*Nowadays it seems that no one has time to go to temples or ashrams or to do any spiritual practice. But if our own child is sick, we are prepared to wait for any length of time in the waiting area of a hospital without getting any sleep. To gain just one foot of land, we will wait outside the courthouse for any number of days in the rain or sun, without even thinking of our husband, wife or children. We can spend hours waiting in a crowded shop to buy a needle for a few cents, but we have*

*no time to pray to God. My children, for those who love God,*
*time for spiritual practice will automatically be available.*

*~ Amma*

*Children, when you sit for meditation, do not think that*
*you can still your mind immediately. At first, you should*
*relax all parts of your body. Loosen your clothes if they*
*are too tight. Make sure that the spine is erect. Then close*
*your eyes and concentrate your mind on your breath.*
*You should be aware of your inhalation and exhalation.*
*Normally we breathe in and out without being aware*
*of it, but it should not be like that; we should become*
*aware of the process. Then the mind will be wakeful.*

*~ Amma*

For anyone concerned with achieving optimal health and spiritual growth, it is essential to have a daily sadhana (spiritual practice). There are infinite numbers of practices. One can meditate, sing bhajans, do mantra japa, read spiritual books, perform selfless service, etc. In a dog-eat-dog world, spiritual practice is the cord of love that binds us to our true Self. Without a direct connection to the Divine, life has no deeper meaning.

There are numerous types of meditation. It is important to practice on a consistent basis. Here is a simple technique. Sit down and go within, turning your attention toward conscious awareness. This practice may last from a few minutes to two hours. It is the most important aspect of dinacharya. Simply be quiet, sit in peace and just be. Meditation is necessary for disciplining the mind and removing the stress of the world. It is best to meditate after morning cleansing and in the evening before bed.

When we experience deep meditation, our body, mind and soul are completely nourished. This spiritual food is so rich that the body needs less food to sustain health. Control of desire, or mental hunger, is the key to longevity and immortality.

The IAM–Integrated Amrita Meditation Technique® is a powerful meditation technique created by Amma to help people find fulfillment in life. The technique refines one's mind, bringing relaxation, concentration, a more expansive sense of self and greater awareness. IAM is taught free of charge all around the world, not only to individuals but also to corporations and correctional institutions. (For more information, go to www.iam-meditation.org.)

## Employment

Work consumes around one-third of the average person's life. Success or failure in one's profession often affects one's self-confidence and feelings of self-worth. It is important that the nature of work align with one's constitution and dharma.

Vata types tend to like work that requires sudden bursts of energy. However, this often leads to exhaustion. In order to create balance they should create routine in their jobs; work that is somewhat repetitive is beneficial. Vata needs a soothing and comforting home and work environment. A perfect vata-type job must have enough excitement to hold their interest and sufficient routine to avoid creating imbalances.

Pitta people, being quite practical, make for good administrators, managers and CEOs. Pittas, by nature, tend to be more aggressive and self-promoting. Self-employment and physical work are often more fulfilling to pittas than the typical nine-to-five desk job. Jobs that require teamwork are balancing for a pitta. They are often workaholics. Usually pitta types often insist on being in the forefront of activity; and they do as much work as they possibly can in a day. They should avoid work that involves excessive heat, i.e. in the hot sun. Pittas benefit from having sufficient challenges in their work without the stress of extreme competition.

Kapha likes stability and balance, however, they should make a consistent, conscious effort to bring change or variety to their jobs and their lives. Otherwise, they can tend toward stagnation or depression. It is good for kaphas to have some physical aspect in their work. Competition and goal-setting also help kapha to break up monotony and stagnation. It is especially important that they have a creative, mentally inspiring and uplifting career. Kaphas usually have long endurance and patience in the workplace, making them good counselors or therapists. Their love and compassion make them excellent healers.

## Bedtime

Meditating before going to sleep promotes sound, peaceful rest. It is best to go to bed around 10 p.m. Massage the soles of the feet with a calming massage or essential oil before going to bed. This simple action will bring calmness and promote wellbeing. Giving thanks and gratitude for the day and all of the experiences and lessons it brought is also calming and rejuvenating before sleep.

One should try to keep the daily routine as close to the recommended dinacharya as possible. The body and mind might resist the change in the beginning, but persistence will bring a much healthier and satisfying life.

Because we have become out of touch with nature, Ayurveda's recommended lifestyles are often far from the average person's way of life. We have forgotten how to live in rhythm with ourselves and with the cycles of nature. While it may seem far from our capabilities, we must strive to move forward with faith and courage. George Bernard Shaw once said, "New opinions often appear first as jokes and fancies, then as blasphemies and treason, then as questions open to discussion, and finally established as truths." If we can be open to change, we open ourselves up to a whole new universe of limitless possibilities.

# Daily Health Awareness

The following is a brief checklist of important and easily observable points to help you monitor and balance your health.

Examine your tongue daily for any signs of ama. If there is a white coating, then the digestive system is working sluggishly and needs to be boosted. This can be done through a short fast or with digestive spices and foods. If the coating is yellow, be careful of pitta-increasing foods such as peppers, wine, alcohol and cayenne. If it is dark brown or black then there may be a fungal infestation. Spots or shaved areas indicate parasites, candida or giardia. A moist, pink tongue is ideal. Examine the tongue for signs of dental impressions along the margins of the tongue. If there are teeth marks then the colon may not be getting enough calcium from the diet or there is malabsorption and poor assimilation. Eating more calcium-rich foods or taking triphala at night before bed may help to resolve this deficiency. However, be careful not to take calcium and vitamin E supplements together, as vitamin E blocks the absorption of the calcium.

If the tongue has cracks, fissures or creases then one may be eating too much dry food. Consider adding ghee to your food. Also, there may be involvement in a repetitive activity (such as typing on a computer) that creates stress along the neck and spine. When performing this type of repetitive work, take frequent breaks and evaluate your work environment, ergonomics, lighting, water intake and air flow.

Pay attention if tartar deposits build up on the teeth. An excess of sweets or lack of sour foods may contribute to the increase of tartar. Teeth that are sensitive to cold, brushing and sweets may indicate that there is too much sour in your diet. If you are drinking citrus juices try to substitute with other juice such as grape, apple or peach.

Stools should be examined for hardness, looseness, floating, frequency, transit time and color. Hardness is associated with dry colon, not enough fluid or too much dry food. Constipation and straining to eliminate may result. Looseness may indicate an imbalance in digestion or intestinal motility, which is often caused by irregular lifestyle. The stool should be well-formed in the shape of a banana. One should have at least one or two regular daily bowel movements, depending on body type. The stool should float. If it does not, it is a sign that the body is producing ama that affects the colon and its ability to absorb nutrients. A stool that has distinct yellow, red or even black color indicates that your digestion is out of balance. Ideal transit time from eating to excretion ranges from 18 to 24 hours. A brown stool without undigested food is best.

Examine the urine daily. If it is frothy, dark yellow or completely clear, then there may be some imbalance in the system. If the urine is dark yellow, there may be too little fluid intake; if it is clear, there might be too much fluid intake. Frothy urine may result from drinking carbonated or other vata-producing substances. Elimination should feel complete.

Examine the skin for color, moisture, lesions, flexibility, softness and tone. Dryness or flaking indicates too many vata influences in the diet, lifestyle and emotions. Abhyanga will be very beneficial. Extreme redness or rashes indicate an excess of pitta. Overly damp or oily skin indicates an excess of kapha. Color aberrations, lesions, loss of tone or flexibility suggest local or systemic imbalances from diet or lifestyle that are sometimes only temporary. If they last for weeks, one should seek professional guidance.

Facial examination also gives indications about health imbalances. Facial examination is a comprehensive system of diagnosis. Below are a few of the most general indicators. It is advised to consult a qualified ayurvedic practitioner for a more complete diagnosis.

Darkness under the eyes indicates weakness in the kidneys and/or adrenals. When the skin on the chin is broken out, it indicates reproductive toxicity. Deep vertical creases above the nose, (between the eyes) represent organ weakness. If the line is on the right side, this shows liver or gall bladder toxicity. If the line is on the left, is represents spleen or pancreatic weakness. If the line is in the center, it shows that the heart or blood pressure in imbalanced.

Women should perform a regular bi-weekly or monthly breast self-exam and men should examine the prostate glands. Seek professional assistance if you feel any abnormalities.

These physical features are readily observed but they are not the only indications of imbalance. The emotions are also valid indicators of imbalance. Anger, worry and excessive feelings of attachment also serve as an alarm system. Excessive thinking causes insomnia and is another valid indication of imbalance in your lifestyle, routine or diet. One should feel an appetite at the appropriate time. If you pay attention to these smaller details (without worrying) you can prevent future problems.

## Ritucharya – Seasonal Routines

*Nature does not hurry,*
*yet everything is accomplished.*

*~ Lao Tzu*

The elements change with each season and thereby affect the doshas. Likewise, both the bodily constitution and its nature change with the seasons. Cold, dry weather increases vata; hot, humid climates increase pitta; cold, wet weather aggravates kapha.

To avoid seasonal imbalances of the doshas, Ayurveda recommends ritucharya (a seasonal routine) to preserve the dosha equilibrium. There is a unique diet, mode of living and routine for each season. These prescribed practices maintain a state of equilibrium in the doshas and assist one in managing the stresses and strains of the changing seasons.

Ayurveda divides the year into six *ritus* (seasons): late summer monsoon (*varsha*), autumn (*sharada*), winter (*hemanta*), late winter (*shishira*), spring (*vasanta*) and summer (*grishma*). These are the traditional seasons in India. Seasons vary depending on where you live. For instance, in northern European countries like Finland, Norway and Sweden, the winter months may last for as many as six to nine months a year.

| DOSHA | Accumulation | Aggravation | Balance |
|-------|-------------|-------------|---------|
| VATA | Summer | Monsoon | Autumn |
| PITTA | Monsoon | Autumn | Winter |
| KAPHA | Winter | Spring | Summer |

## Summer

Summer (grishma) and late summer monsoon (varsha) are the times of heat and fire. They are dominated by the pitta dosha and therefore aggravate pitta while pacifying kapha. In a hot and dry climate, vata can also increase during summer; a humid environment is more suitable for vata types. The pitta of summer reduces near the end of autumn when kapha increases.

In the body, pitta governs the digestive fire, liver, eyes, heart and skin. It also plays a vital role in our creative process and how we perceive the world visually, mentally and emotionally. Thus pitta determines how we digest both the physical nutrients of food as well as the nuances of our life experiences.

During the summer, the inner fire manifests externally as people celebrate life and play joyously outside. However, it is also when inflammatory conditions arise and one must take care not to over-exert, overheat or dehydrate. Summer illnesses include heat stroke, hay fever, prickly heat, dehydration headaches and nausea, and dry, itchy, sunburned skin. Digestive troubles such as acidity, heartburn and ulcers may occur more frequently.

Summer is also a time when many people excessively "party" by drinking alcohol and overeating. This indiscriminate behavior and misuse of the senses can lead to disease. Because the potential for excessive revelry is stronger in summer, it is the best season to practice the principles of viveka and *vairagya*. Viveka means "mindful discrimination" or "awareness." Vairagya means "dispassion" or "nonattachment." Exercising viveka and vairagya does not mean losing love for life; it simply means avoiding the things that do not serve a higher purpose in life. Cultivating these qualities gives us the freedom to live with awareness in the present moment, where the true celebration of life takes place.

As the monsoon season begins in late summer, vata predominates in nature. When bodily vata is aggravated, the digestive fire weakens. One should therefore take care to eat a vata-balancing diet. During the rainy season, one should eat astringent, bitter and pungent foods. Vata constitution should avoid astringent taste even during the rainy season. Easily digestible food should be taken, such as soups and hearty steamed vegetables. Rice, whole wheat and other nutritious whole grains are excellent for balancing vata as well. It is also important to avoid sleeping during daylight hours, spending long hours in the sun and exercising excessively. Regularly taking warm baths and getting warm-oil massages are highly advisable. Do not overindulge in sex. This season presents the perfect time for detoxification programs or panchakarma.

## Summer Seasonal Routine

- Follow a pitta-pacifying diet. Avoid food with pungent, sour and salty tastes. Eat sweet, bitter, astringent, cooling and easily digestible foods. Eat light foods such as dark leafy green vegetables, basmati rice and mung beans. Raw foods such as salads, fruits and berries are ideal. Raw seaweed salads make an excellent summer meal. Raw vegetable juices can be taken abundantly. Fruit smoothies or vegetable juices make great summer breakfasts.
- Make sure to drink sufficient amounts to avoid dehydration. Fresh coconut water and fruit juices are very beneficial, especially aloe

vera, grape, papaya, watermelon, sweet pineapple juice and other
sweet cooling beverages. Cooling herbal teas like peppermint or
fennel are suitable.

- Brush the teeth with cooling, herbal tooth powders or pastes such
  as neem, peppermint and wintergreen.
- Massage with coconut oil during the summer.
- Walk barefoot on the earth.
- Swim in natural bodies of water such as lakes, rivers, oceans and
  waterfalls.
- Yoga asanas should be performed in a cool area out of the direct
  sunlight. Practice should be gentle with lots of standing asanas
  and spinal twists. Surya namaskar can be performed slowly and
  gently. Inversions increase heat and should be minimized.
- Use sweet, cooling and calming essential oils like jasmine, lotus,
  rose, sandalwood, jatamansi and blue chamomile.
- Wash and spray the face frequently with rose water.
- Cooling herbs for the summertime are aloe and amalaki.
- *Shitali* (cooling) pranayama can be performed regularly throughout the summer.

## Autumn

Autumn (Sharad) is the time when vata increases because the qualities of autumn mirror those of vata. The days become dryer and
cooler. The winds start to increase. It is a changing season, and since
change aggravates vata, vata naturally increases. It is important to
protect oneself from excess wind as well as erratic and irrational
behavior during this time. Vata accumulates in the lungs, large
intestine, nails, bones, nerves, skin, joints, hair and brain. Vata
disorders are the largest in number and commonly include constipation, nervousness, anxiety, insomnia, mental instability, speech
disorders, muscular and nerve disorders, indigestion and intestinal
bloating and gas.

## Autumn Seasonal Routine

- Relaxation and stress-free environments are most suitable, especially for those with vata constitutions.
- Alternate nostril breathing without retention before yoga practice helps to calm the mind and relax the nerves.
- Early to bed, early to rise is the best sleeping pattern to follow.
- Warm sesame oil massages are excellent in fall.
- After brushing the teeth, swish warm sesame oil in the mouth for a few minutes. One can also rub the gums with sesame oil using one's finger. Brush teeth with herbal powders or pastes of licorice, fennel or mint.
- Rub sesame oil on the bottom of the feet before bed.
- Turmeric (Curcuma longa) is excellent for reducing vata and balancing the doshas.
- Take warm baths with essential oils, mineral salts and baking soda.
- Yoga asanas can be performed freely. Surya namaskar can be performed slowly with mindfulness. All inversions, especially head and shoulder stands, are extremely helpful in calming vata. Other nurturing and grounding physical disciplines can be practiced (tai chi, chi gong, etc.). Dancing is especially recommended in fall.
- *Chayawanprash* can be taken daily to increase immunity. One teaspoon taken in the morning by itself or with warm spiced milk is an excellent vata tonic.
- A vata-reducing diet is crucial for keeping the dosha under control. It includes eating sweet, sour, salty and mildly spicy foods. Kichari is excellent, especially with root vegetables like beets, carrots, burdock and parsnips. Adding a teaspoon of ghee to kichari increases digestibility and carries the nutrients deep into the tissues. Warm vegetable soups and curries will strengthen the body for the coming cold season. As it is harvest season, an abundance of nurturing foods such as squash, yams, sweet potatoes, pumpkins, zucchini and other vegetables are available. Raw foods, cold drinks, stimulants and most beans should be reduced

or avoided. Organic, non-homogenized and unpasteurized dairy can be taken. Ghee, buttermilk, yogurt and warm spiced milk are excellent tonics for vata. Nuts and seeds can be eaten, as well as the milks of nuts and seeds. Almond, oat, hemp, rice, sunflower and quinoa milks make great milk substitutes. Grains such as oats, basmati rice and quinoa are very beneficial at this time. Herbs such as asafoetida (hing), cardamom, cinnamon, coriander, cumin, fennel and ginger can be taken freely.

- Autumn is a very good time for panchakarma or shatkarma.
- Taking warm turmeric and cardamom milk in the evening is a nourishing and nurturing way to end the day.

# Winter

Early to mid-winter (hemanta) and late winter (shishira) are the seasons when the elements naturally withdraw. It is a time to turn inward and withdraw from external influences; it is a time of rest and rejuvenation. This is also the time when the earth and water elements express their tamasic qualities. This expression of tamas in nature is necessary for the storing of energy that will later manifest as new life in spring. For human beings, this means that the winter period supports introspection, which assists in the development of spiritual, emotional, mental and physical well-being. However, if tamas increases too much, feelings of lethargy or depression may arise. Following kapha-pacifying practices can help counter excessive tamas.

During winter, kapha increases, so kapha individuals should take extra care during this season. Winter's cold and heavy qualities can easily imbalance kapha, resulting in winter health disorders such as common colds, organ weaknesses (especially the kidneys, lungs and pancreas), disturbances of the mucus membranes, bladder problems, blood disorders, increases in the synovial fluids (and other bodily secretions) and weight gain.

Due to the cold, vata also tends to increase in winter, especially in dryer climates. Chilly winds and the drying effects of heating systems also easily aggravate vata. Thus, vata constitutions will also benefit from most of the practices outlined below.

## Winter Seasonal Routine

- Follow a kapha- or vata-pacifying diet depending on your constitution.
- It is okay to sleep a little longer during winter. However, rising before the sun comes up is always beneficial.
- Brush teeth with herbal powders that contain stimulating herbs such as cinnamon, clove and ginger. After brushing the teeth, swish with warm sesame oil for a few minutes. One can also rub the gums with sesame oil using one's finger.
- Daily massages with warm sesame oil are highly beneficial. Let the oil absorb into the body for up to an hour after the massage, then take a hot bath or shower.
- Drink warm water.
- Practicing yoga daily is highly beneficial. Performing twelve vigorous rounds of surya namaskar keeps kapha at bay.
- Make sure to get plenty of exercise, fresh air and sunlight.
- If you are already experienced in pranayama, practice *kapalabhati* or *bhastrika* to dispel cold, dampness and lethargy. If you are not adept in pranayama, you can learn from a qualified teacher.
- Apply nasya (nasal oil) inside the nose each morning.
- Drink warming herbal teas made of ginger, cinnamon, cardamom and black pepper.
- Chayawanprash, an ayurvedic tonic, is an excellent remedy for reducing vata and kapha. It also helps the body to resist colds and promotes general immunity. Taking a heaping teaspoon each morning is an excellent way to start any winter day.

# Spring

Spring (vasanta) is a time of awakening. It is a time for new birth, growth, and planting the seeds of creation. As the spring warmth and light increase, kapha will decrease (except where spring brings rain, which increases kapha). Spring is a time of change, so vata increases during this period despite the increasing warmth. Pitta is balanced. Kapha imbalances are generally prevalent in the spring due to its accumulation during winter.

Traditionally, spring is an excellent time for internal cleansing practices, such as panchakarma or shatkarma. Cleansing the colon is a major part of these techniques. General cleansing enemas can also be easily be administered by oneself at home. Coffee enemas, while not traditional in Ayurveda, are an excellent way to cleanse the colon and liver.

## Spring Seasonal Routine

- Wake up early, several hours before the sun. This helps to dispel kapha, fatigue and lethargy. Additionally, it increases mental awareness, physical strength and digestion.
- Regular massages with warm sesame oil are beneficial. Warm sunflower oil can also be used in the spring.
- Take hot baths and showers. To a bath, add one-quarter cup baking soda, one-half cup Epsom salts (or other mineral salts), and ten drops of an invigorating, therapeutic grade essential oil such as angelica, cardamom, cinnamon, clove, eucalyptus, ginger, lemon, lemongrass, melissa (lemon balm), neroli, orange, sage or thyme.
- Rubbing dry skin with herbal powders or a natural dry skin brush before bathing is quite invigorating.
- Use saunas or sweat lodges regularly to help to burn up accumulated toxins.

- Hot, herbal lemon and ginger tea with honey or tulasi tea with ginger and black pepper can stimulate the digestive fire and burn up accumulated toxins.
- Invigorating yoga asanas such as backbends, spinal twists, hip openers and standing asanas are all beneficial at this time. Doing twelve or more rounds of surya namaskar is a great daily routine.
- Other exercises such as tai chi, chi gong, aikido, bicycling and hiking are encouraged.
- Avoid heavy, oily, salty, sour and sweet food and drinks that can easily aggravate kapha and create ama in the doshas. Light, whole grains (such as basmati or jasmine rice, quinoa, millet and barley) and astringent, pungent and bitter foods are excellent as they are easily digested. Dark leafy greens such as arugula, chard, collards, mustard greens, dandelion, mizuna and kale can be taken at this time. Pulses such as red lentils, aduki beans, mung beans and chickpeas are astringent by nature and an excellent food in the spring. Kichari (mung dhal and basmati rice) is an excellent staple.
- Spring is also a good time to take bitter herbs that cleanse the liver, gall bladder, lymph and blood. Excellent spring herbs are aloe vera, bhumiamalaki, dandelion root, daruharidra (barberry), gentian, guduchi, kutki (katuka), manjistha and turmeric.

# Chapter 12

# Ayurvedic and Yogic Cleansing

*It is good for a seeker to purge the stomach
at least twice a month.
The accumulated feces in the intestines create agitation
and negativity in the mind.
By purging, we clear not only the body, but the mind as well.*

*~ Amma*

*To care for the body is a duty; otherwise the
mind will not be strong and clear.*

*~ Buddha*

One of the most important aspects of Ayurveda is the cleansing and rejuvenation program called panchakarma. Panchakarma is the cornerstone of ayurvedic management of disease. Pancha means "five" and karma means "action." Panchakarma consists of five therapeutic or cleansing treatments. These are specific methods for safely and effectively removing ama from different areas of the body without damaging or weakening the system. Panchakarma gets to the root cause of the problem and re-establishes the essential tridoshic balance in the body. Panchakarma is not only good for alleviating disease, but also helps to maintain excellent health. Additionally, panchakarma works on the subtle body. It helps to burn up old, outdated emotional and mental patterns. Ayurveda often advises undergoing panchakarma during the seasonal changes.

Many factors play a role in the formation of ama: Poor digestion of food, improper food-combinations and choices, poor drinking water, pollution, pesticides in food, and emotional and physical stress. Ama accumulates and spreads throughout the body. These toxins eventually enter into the deeper tissues, organs or channels, thus creating dysfunction, disorder and disease.

The benefits of panchakarma as stated in *Charaka Samhita* are increase of agni, alleviation of disease, restoration and maintenance of health, proper function of all sense organs, proper function of mind and intellect, proper coloration of skin, virility (capacity to produce healthy children), delayed aging and the enjoyment of a healthful life.

Panchakarma is uniquely tailored to meet each individual's needs, according to their constitution and doshic imbalances. The therapies involved in this program effectively loosen ama from the deep tissues so that it can be removed through the body's natural channels of elimination. Before one undertakes the process of panchakarma, a skilled ayurvedic clinician must assess one's weaknesses and determine one's constitution and current state of the doshas. It is important to determine which tissues, channels and organs are imbalanced and need to be addressed. Only then can the clinician successfully design a panchakarma program specifically suited to one's needs.

There are three phases of panchakarma: the preliminary therapies, called *purvakarma*; the five main therapies of panchakarma (*vamana, nasya, virechan, raktamokshana* and *basti*); and post-treatment procedures called *paschatkarma*. Both preparatory and follow-up panchakarma therapies are essential to the success and long-lasting effects of the treatment.

## Purvakarma

Purvakarma prepares the body to rid itself of stored ama. *Snehana* (oleation) is the first step of purvakarma and consists of saturating the body with herbal or medicated oils. Internal oleation with ghee or medicated oil helps to loosen ama and move it from deeper tissues into the gastrointestinal tract. Oils are chosen based on the particular needs and doshic imbalance of the individual. Abhyanga is an individually prepared herbal oil massage designed to deeply penetrate the skin, relax the mind-body, break up impurities and stimulate arterial and lymphatic circulation. It enhances the ability of nutrients to reach starved cells and expedites the removal of ama. The desired result of abhyanga is a heightened state of awareness that will direct the natural internal healing system of the body.

After the massage is completed, *swedana* (sweating) is performed. Swedana is an individually herbalized steam bath intended to dilate the channels so that ama may be more easily removed. Ayurvedic swedana is unique because the head and the heart are kept very cool during the steam bath while the body is heated to remove mental, emotional and physical toxins lodged deeply within the tissues. The cool head and heart provide a sense of calm and openness while the therapeutic steam on the rest of the body can penetrate and cleanse deeply without the body becoming overheated or stressed.

There are several swedana treatments that can be used as adjunct therapies during panchakarma, but the two main types of swedana will be described here. In the first type, a localized application of steam with herbal decoctions or medicated oils is used. This method is extremely effective for certain types of arthritic conditions because it concentrates on specific areas of the body, such as sore joints or muscles, to improve mobility and reduce pain. The second type applies steam evenly to the whole body, except the head, with the use of a sweat box. This method is used to further detoxify the body after abhyanga. It is usually followed by herbal plasters and poultices to help draw toxins out of the pores of the skin.

Purvakarma also uses a therapy called *shirodhara*. *Shiro* means "head" and *dhara* means "the dripping of oil like a thread." In this treatment, warm oil drips in a steady stream across the forehead. It pacifies vata dosha, calms and nourishes the central nervous system, promotes relaxation and tranquility, and improves mental clarity and comprehension. It is especially rejuvenating for prana vata. Shirodhara can actually be performed at the beginning and/ or end of panchakarma depending on the individual, the state of the doshas and dhatus, and the manifested symptoms. Shirodhara is traditionally performed in purvakarma but can be taken on its own or as part of other ayurvedic therapies.

## Panchakarma

Once purvakarma is completed, ama moves down into the gastro-intestinal tract and can be removed with the main panchakarma treatments: vamana, nasya, virechan, raktamokshana and basti. Each of these therapies promotes the removal of ama through the normal channels of elimination.

Vamana (therapeutic emesis) and nasya (nasal administration of medicated oils and herbal preparations) relate to kapha. Virechan (therapeutic purgation) and raktamokshana (therapeutic withdrawal of blood) relate to pitta. Basti (therapeutic herbal enema) relates to vata.

During panchakarma it is essential to follow a personally tailored diet to assist in the removal toxins. Consuming improper foods while undergoing deep cleansing can actually drive the toxins deeper. Traditionally, the staple of the panchakarma diet is kichari with simple vegetables.

## Vamana

Vamana is prescribed when there is congestion in the lungs. It is especially beneficial for people who have repeated cases of bronchitis, colds, cough or asthma. It eliminates the kapha that causes excess mucus. Vamana is typically administered after snehana and swedana. Three to four glasses of licorice or salt water is administered, then vomiting is stimulated by inducing the gag reflex through rubbing the back of the throat and tongue. Once the mucous is released, the patient will feel almost instant relief of symptoms. Usually congestion, wheezing and breathlessness disappear and the sinuses become clear. The traditional preparation of vamana utilizes herbs such as emetic nut, lobelia, licorice and calamus root. It should be performed early in the morning when there is less hydrochloric acid in the stomach.

### Indications for Vamana

Chronic asthma, diabetes, chronic cold, lymphatic congestion, chronic indigestion and edema, also excellent for releasing blocked emotions

### Contraindications for Vamana

People who are very young, very old or very weak; when there is a serious heart disorder

## Nasya

Nasya means "relating to the nose." The nose is the doorway both to the brain and to consciousness. Nasya removes ama from the nasal passages, ears, sinus, throat and eyes. Nasya cleanses by opening the channels of the head and oxygenating the brain. It is extremely useful for vata and kapha disorders, but can be used by pitta as well. It strengthens prana in the body and is excellent for anyone who practices yoga asanas or pranayama.

Prana enters the body through the breath taken in through the nose. Prana is essential for maintaining sensory and motor functions. It governs all mental and intellectual activities, memory and concentration. Deranged prana creates defective functioning of all neurological activities. It manifests as headaches, convulsions, loss of memory and reduced sensory perception. Nasya provides relief for numerous pranic disorders, sinus congestion, migraine headaches, convulsions, and certain eye and ear problems.

There are six main types of nasya:

1. *Pradhamana Nasya* (cleansing nasya) uses dry powders that are blown or inhaled into the nose with a tube. This type of nasya is used for kapha-type diseases involving headaches, heaviness in the head, colds, nasal congestion, sticky eyes, hoarseness of voice due to sticky kapha, sinusitis, cervical lymph adenitis, tumors, worms, some skin diseases, epilepsy, drowsiness, Parkinson's, inflammation of the nasal mucosa, attachment, greed and lust. Traditionally, powders such as brahmi or vaccha are used.

2. *Bruhana Nasya* (nutrition nasya) uses ghee, oils, salt, shatavari ghee, ashwagandha ghee and medicated milks. It is used primarily for vata disorders. It benefits conditions resulting from vata imbalances such as vata-type headaches, migraine headaches, hoarseness, dizziness, heavy eyelids, bursitis, stiff neck, dry sinuses, dry nose, loss of sense of smell, nervousness, fear, emptiness and negativity.

3. *Shaman Nasya* (sedative nasya) uses herbal medicated decoctions, teas and medicated oils. It primarily addresses pitta-type disorders such as thinning of hair, conjunctivitis and ringing in the ears.

4. *Navana Nasya* (decoction nasya) uses a combination of medicated decoctions and oils. It treats vata-pitta or kapha-pitta disorders.

5. *Marshya Nasya* (ghee or oil nasya) is relatively tridoshic and balances the nadis. It is excellent for decreasing stress and increasing mental concentration.

6. *Prati Marshya Nasya* (daily oil nasya) helps to open deep tissues. It can be done everyday and at any time to release stress. Preparations such as *anu thailam* or *brahmi grita* are used.

## Indications for Nasya

Stress, emotional imbalances, stiff neck and shoulders, dry nose, sinus congestion, hoarseness, migraine headaches and convulsions.

## Contraindications for Nasya

Sinus infections, pregnancy, menstruation, after sex, after bathing, after drinking alcohol or eating. Nasya should not be used on children younger than seven years or adults over 80 years of age.

# Virechan

Virechan is a natural, herb-induced purging process. It cleanses the small intestine and pitta-related organs (such as the liver and gall bladder). Virechan removes ama and excess pitta from the body, balancing all metabolic functions. When excess bile (pitta) accumulates in the gall bladder, liver and small intestine, it often results in rashes, skin inflammation, acne, chronic fevers, biliary vomiting, nausea and jaundice. Strong purgative herbs like senna, rhubarb, castor oil, aloe or trivrit are commonly used to induce this cleansing.

## Indications for Virechan:

Skin diseases, chronic fever, enlargement of liver and spleen, thyroid disorders, parasites, anemia, pain in the head, burning of the eyes, thyrglandular swelling, asthma, cough, jaundice, epilepsy, oedema, blood toxicity, stomatitis and hyperacidity.

## Contraindications for Virechan:

Children, very old persons, very weak persons, anal fissures, rectal bleeding, low agni, intestinal ulcers, prolapsed colon, diarrhea and dysentery, haemoptysis (blood in sputum), pregnancy, immediately after childbirth and acute heart disease.

# Basti

Basti is a mild but deeply therapeutic enema. Basti consists of introducing medicated oils or liquids into the colon to be retained and then released. The primary goal of basti is the purification and rejuvenation of the colon, as the colon is connected to all of the other organs and tissues of the body. There are two main types of basti: cleansing and nutritive. The colon is essential for the absorption of nutrients and it is the primary receptacle for waste elimination. It is the seat of vata dosha, which moves the other doshas and all physiological activity. As it balances and nurtures vata, basti has a wide-ranging influence in the body and affects all the doshas, srotas and dhatus.

Vata's predominant site is the colon. Although basti is the most effective treatment of vata disorders, many enemas over a prescribed period of time are sometimes required. Basti relieves constipation, distention, chronic fever, colds, sexual disorders, kidney stones, heart pain, backaches, sciatica and other pains in the joints. Numerous other vata disorders such as arthritis, rheumatism, gout, muscle spasms and headaches may also be treated with basti.

Vata is a significant factor in disease pathogenesis. If vata is controlled through the use of basti, the root cause of most diseases can be eliminated. Vata is the primary force behind the elimination and retention of feces, urine, bile and other excreta.

There are eight general types of basti, each with specific indications and contraindications.

1. *Anuvasana* (oil enema) is used in pure vata disorders and when a person is experiencing extreme hunger or dryness related to vata imbalances.

2. *Niruha-Asthapana* (decoction enema) is used for evacuation of vata, nervous diseases, gastrointestinal conditions, gout, fever, unconsciousness, urinary conditions, appetite, pain, hyperacidity and heart diseases.

3. *Uttara Basti* (urethral for men and vaginal for women) is used for certain semen and ovulation disorders and for problems involving painful urination or bladder infections. This is contraindicated for people with diabetes.

4. *Matra Basti* (daily oil enema) is used in cases of emaciation from stress, overwork, excessive exercise, heavy lifting, walking,

212

excessive or wrong sexual activity and chronic vata disorders. It does not need to be accompanied by any strict dietary restriction or daily routine, and can be administered in all seasons. It gives strength, promotes weight gain and helps elimination of waste products.

5. *Karma Basti* (routine of 30 bastis). May include any type of basti, depending on the person's need.

6. *Kala Basti* (routine of 15 bastis: 10 oil + 5 decoctions)

7. *Yoga Basti* (routine of 8 bastis: 5 oil + 3 decoctions)

8. *Bruhana Basti* (nutritional enema) provides nutrition through the intestines. Traditionally, highly nutritive substances are used, such as warm milk, herbal broth, and herbs like shatavari or ashwagandha.

## Indications for Basti

Constipation, low-back ache, gout, rheumatism, sciatica, arthritis, auto-intoxication, nervous disorders, vata headaches, emaciation and muscular atrophy

## Contraindications for Basti

Diarrhea, rectal bleeding, chronic indigestion, breathlessness, diabetes, fever, emaciation, severe anemia, pulmonary tuberculosis, obesity, low agni, enlarged liver or spleen, unconsciousness, cough, old age or children below the age of seven years

Decoction enemas should be avoided by people with the following conditions: debility, hiccup, hemorrhoids, inflammation of anus, piles, diarrhea, pregnancy, ascites, diabetes and some conditions involving painful or difficult breathing.

Nutritional enemas should be avoided by people with the following conditions: diabetes, obesity, lymphatic obstruction and ascites.

Urethral and vaginal enemas should be avoided by anyone with diabetes.

According to Ayurveda, repeated flushing of water with colonic therapy may weaken the mucous membrane and dry the colon, further disrupting the eliminative function of vata. When medicated oils are used in conjunction with purvakarma therapies, all tissues are nourished and toxins are removed from the whole body as basti removes the ama that has been brought to the colon by the other therapies. The *Charaka Samhita* says that basti provides 50% of the therapeutic benefits of panchakarma. Basti ensures a healthy colon and strong agni.

## Raktamokshana

In the past, panchakarma included raktamokshana, or bloodletting. Traditionally done by applying leeches to the localized area, this treatment was used to remove excess pitta-related ama from the blood and to cure certain blood-related and skin conditions. This method of purification and cleansing of the blood is rarely performed today.

When toxins present in the gastrointestinal tract are absorbed into the blood stream and circulate throughout the body, they create a condition called toxemia. Toxemia is the primary cause of repeated infections, hypertension and many circulatory conditions such as pitta-type skin disorders, utricaria, rashes, herpes, eczema, acne, leukoderma, chronic itching or hives. Raktamokshana is indicated, along with internal medication, to treat these imbalances and in cases of enlarged liver, spleen and gout.

Ayurvedic experts in the west are now establishing new variations of this therapy. One way of performing raktamokshana for oneself is to donate or give blood. Although giving blood does not guarantee that the toxic blood is being removed, it will definitely assist in the production of new blood cells. Extracting a small amount of blood relieves the tension created by pitta-type toxins in the blood. Bloodletting stimulates the spleen to produce antitoxic substances. These stimulate the immune system, thereby neutralizing toxins and allowing for quick cures in many blood disorders. Bloodletting, or giving blood, is contraindicated if there are signs of anemia, edema, extreme weakness, diabetes, and in children and elderly persons.

In modern times, the use of alterative herbs is more commonly practiced. Alterative herbs purify the blood, remove toxins, and possess antibacterial and anti-infective properties. They are excellent in treating tumors, cancers, wounds, sores and many skin and blood-related diseases. Alteratives are also excellent for protecting against infective, contagious diseases and epidemics. The most commonly used alteratives are aloe vera, amalaki, bhumiamalaki, burdock, chaparral, dandelion, echinacea, manjistha, neem, red clover, sandalwood, shallaki, shilajit, turmeric and yellow dock. Women are blessed to have monthly menstruation, though which there is a natural purging of toxins through the blood.

## Indications for Raktamokshana

Pitta disorders, utricaria, rash, acne, eczema, scabies, leucoderma, chronic itching, hives, enlarged liver or spleen, gout

## Contraindications for Raktamokshana

Anemia, edema, weakness, young children, old age, pregnancy, during menstruation

# Paschatkarma

Paschatkarma encompasses the post-panchakarma therapies that include dietary, herbal and lifestyle adjustments and regimes. After panchakarma one should follow a diet and lifestyle that is harmonious to the dosha along with *rasayanas* (rejuvenative herbs) and sufficient rest. Rasayanas consist of herbal and mineral preparations with specific, restorative effects on body and mind. Rasayanas enhance the overall vitality of the body. They nourish and rejuvenate the entire organism and are a crucial part of the paschatkarma procedures.

There are many renewing herbs specifically for one's doshas, dhatus and organs. They must be properly administered along with a rejuvenating diet. It is important to focus on balancing the mind and emotions as well. Following dinacharya is a vital part of this process. Yoga asana, mantra and meditation are also especially beneficial. In addition, breathing fresh, clean air and spending time in nature is extremely rejuvenating to the body, heart, mind and spirit.

Paschatkarma plays an essential role in assisting the body to re-establish a healthy metabolic system and strong immunity. If these post-treatment procedures are neglected, the digestion may not normalize and the production of ama will return. Post-panchakarma diet recommendations include eating light, nourishing foods, such as mung dal soup, basmati rice and cooked vegetables. Other foods are gradually added back into the diet. It is also recommended to return slowly to regular activities to avoid taxing the nervous system, as the body and mind are in a sensitive and sometimes vulnerable state after panchakarma.

## Beyond Panchakarma

There are numerous other methods of cleansing, purifying and rejuvenating that can be used in conjunction with panchakarma and Ayurveda. They may also be used on their own outside of panchakarma. These treatments include *avagaha sweda, elakizhi/kizhi* (name varies in different parts of India), *karnapurna, katti basti, lepana, navakizhi, netra basti/tarpana, pizhichil, shiro basti, shirodhara thala, udwartanam and uro basti.*

Avagaha sweda is a hip bath in a decoction of medicated herbs. Taken after receiving abhyanga, it is used for the treatment of backache, urinary disorders, reproductive disorders and during pregnancy.

Elakizhi or kizhi is the application of medicinal leaves that have been processed in medicated oil. This method is used to combat osteoarthritis, arthritis with swelling, spondylosis, back pain, sports injury, stress and tension.

Karnapurna is the use of medicated herbal fumes to help clean the ears. It is used to alleviate any disorders associated with the ears.

In katti basti, warm, medicated oil is kept over the lower back in an herbal paste reservoir-like dam made of black gram flour. Applications generally last 45-75 minutes depending on the condition and dosha of the individual. It is especially beneficial for lower back pain, muscle spasm, rigidity, lordosis and any type of spinal disorders. It also strengthens the bone tissue.

Lepana is the application of medicated herbal pastes onto affected areas of the body. This therapy is useful in skin diseases, inflammatory conditions, weak muscles, tendon injuries, and bone and spinal disfigurations.

Navakizhi is a deeply cleansing fomentation treatment. Rice is boiled in milk and herbs and then packed in a bolus (cloth bundle). This bolus is then used to massage deeply into the tissues and joints. Navakizhi is often accompanied by oil massage and is excellent for alleviating rheumatism, painful joints and muscles, high blood pressure, high cholesterol and certain skin diseases. The treatment is deeply relaxing, rejuvenating and powerfully detoxifying.

Netra basti/tarpana is the process of keeping medicated ghee over the eyes by using an herbal paste dam made of black gram flour. It is useful in all eye disorders because it nourishes the eyes and removes strain while improving vision. It can be used for prevention of eye problems as well.

Pizhichil is an uninterrupted stream of warmed, medicated oil poured continuously over the body by two ayurvedic therapists as they massage the body simultaneously in unison. The warmth of the oil and synchronicity of the massage combine to create deep tissue cleansing and a heightened state of awareness. Pizhichil is performed according to body type in specific patterns for a period of 60-90 minutes. It is excellent in treating mental tension, physical or emotional stress, weakness of muscles, nervous system disorders, arthritis, rheumatism, paralysis, hemiplagia, sexual debility and infertility.

Shiro basti is a rejuvenative therapy similar in properties to shirodhara. It involves retaining lukewarm medicated oil on the top of the shaved head by fixing a fitted cap firmly around the head. The oil is retained for anywhere from fifteen to sixty minutes depending on the condition and dosha of the individual. This treatment is excellent for memory loss, neurological disorders, schizophrenia, obsessive-compulsive disorder, disorientation, glaucoma, anxiety, stress, paralysis, headache, dry scalp, visual difficulties and insomnia.

Thala involves the application of medicated powder mixed with medicated oil to the top of the head for 20 to 45 minutes. This procedure helps to treat neurological disorders, headache, insomnia, migraine, memory loss, and to improve intelligence.

Udwartanam is a massage that uses a deeply penetrating herbal paste or powder to nourish the lymphatic system. It is applied all over the body (except for the head) in an upwards direction. Great for obesity, low agni, weakness, paralysis and rheumatic symptoms, this powerful, exfoliating treatment conditions the skin while it presses stagnant, lymphatic toxins out of the body.

Uro basti uses the same process as katti basti, but the oil is kept over the chest. This technique is used to treat asthma, respiratory problems, muscular chest pain, heart diseases and to correct pranic disorders.

## Shatkarma

*By the six karmas [shatkarma] one is*
*freed from excesses of the doshas.*

*~ Hatha Yoga Pradipika, verse 36*

Ayurveda and yoga both emphasize cleansing of the body for health and to support spiritual practices. Their methods are similar, and both work by expelling excess dosha and ama, using the body's natural routes of elimination. The yogic method is known in the classical ashtanga tradition as *shatkarma*, or six cleansing measures. These include *basti, dhauti, kapalabhati, nauli, neti and trataka*. These actions have powerful effects on both the physical and energetic bodies (koshas) and on the doshas.

Basti is done just as in Ayurveda but only water is used. Sometimes a medicated herbal oil or tea will be used, but generally it is said that salt water is best as it scrubs out the intestines. Basti generates energy, removes heat, develops strength and control of the abdominal muscles, and massages and tones the organs and nerves.

Dhauti is the cleansing of the gastrointestinal tract by drinking copious amounts of salt water and performing specific asanas. This procedure is performed several times over many hours to clean out the entire gastrointestinal tract. It is very similar to virechan in panchakarma. Another method is called *vamana dhauti*. It is just like vamana in panchakarma but plain salt water is used. Other methods are also employed but require advanced yogic skills.

Kapalabhati means "skull shining." It works primarily upon the third eye, crown and manipura (solar plexus) chakras. It cleanses the nasal sinus area (with its rapid and forced exhalations through the nose), the lungs, blood, tissues and abdomen. Additionally, it lowers high blood pressure and is useful in treatment of colitis, all digestive and reproductive disorders and obesity. In addition to being a purification technique, kapalabhati is a form of pranayama found in both hatha yoga and Ayurveda. Kapalabhati is more purifying and less stimulating than bhastrika, being only slightly warming.

Nauli is intestinal washing or abdominal rolling. This yogic technique requires some practice and skill. The rolling, rotation and agitation of the entire abdomen during nauli gives a deep massage and profound toning to the abdominal muscles and organs. It creates heat in the body, increasing digestive agni and balancing the endocrine functions. This practice also creates changes in emotional disorders, lethargy and diabetes. On a subtle level, it has deep effects on the pranamaya and manomaya koshas, creating mental clarity and power as well as increased prana.

Neti is the process of nasal cleansing. There are two primary methods of performing neti. In *jalaneti,* one uses a small clay or copper pot filled with salt water to flush the sinuses. *Sutraneti* involves using a string coated with ghee that is passed through the nasal canal and brought through the mouth. Neti has a similar effect as nasya. They can be used together to further enhance cleansing actions.

Trataka means "concentration" or "gazing." It is best performed using a ghee lamp or natural candle placed about three feet in front of you. Without blinking or moving, gaze steadily at the candle flame for 15-20 minutes. Follow the breath. Mantras can be repeated silently with the breath. If the eyes feel strained, visualize a light moving from the center of the ajna (third eye) chakra through your eyes to the candle. Relax the eyes and rest the mind. Trataka aids in increasing concentration and in reducing stress and tension. It relaxes and soothes the nervous system.

Ayurveda and yoga complement one another and share many fundamental principles. Practicing both Ayurveda and yoga leads to optimal health, peace and longevity.

**Note: None of the practices or techniques should be attempted on your own. They require professional, experienced guidance. This chapter is for informational purposes only. It is not meant to be an instruction for performing these procedures.**

# Chapter 13

# Subtle Therapies
# (Ancient Alchemy)

*He alone is Fire, He is the Sun,*
*He is Wind, He is the Moon,*
*He is the shining star, He alone is Brahma.*

*~ Yajurveda 32.1*

*We return thanks to our mother, the earth,*
*which sustains us.*
*We return thanks to the rivers and streams,*
*which supply us with water.*
*We return thanks to all herbs,*
*which furnish medicines for the cure of our diseases.*
*We return thanks to the moon and stars,*
*which have given to us their light when the sun was gone.*
*We return thanks to the sun,*
*which has looked upon the earth with a beneficent eye.*
*Lastly, we return thanks to the Great Spirit,*
*in Whom is embodied all goodness,*
*and Who directs all things for the good of Her children.*

*~ Iroquois Prayer*

Since prerecorded history, many civilizations have relied upon gemstones, crystals, colors and fragrances for their healing and spiritual
upliftment. The ancient rishis realized the interconnectedness of all
things in creation. They saw that all that we hear, smell, see, touch

and taste affects our health and consciousness. They understood the unique vibrational frequency of each planet, color, essential oil and gemstone. Using this information, they made in-depth correlations between all of these and used them for physical and spiritual advancement. Gem therapy, color therapy and aromatherapy each constitute an entire healing system requiring numerous volumes of exploration. This section will give a brief overview of each system and how it applies to the framework of Ayurveda.

## Gemstones

The Vedas contain detailed descriptions of the therapeutic benefits of gemstones. They also discuss potencies and prescriptions for safe and effective use. The Vedas declare that both planetary and health imbalances can be harmonized by wearing gems against one's skin or by using them as an ingredient in medicines. In Ayurveda, gems are taken internally in the form of *bhasmas* (purified ash preparations), *pisthis* (powders), gem waters, tinctures, elixirs or essences.

When worn, gems transmit specific vibrational frequencies to the body. They create a protective field and regulate which subtle forces are absorbed. Over time, gemstones in contact with the skin bring about changes in the person's dosha.

In Ayurveda and jyotish (Vedic astrology), the main gemstones that are used for healing purposes are either precious or semiprecious stones of high quality; however, all gemstones have some healing effect. Wearing gemstones to enhance the beneficial effects of planetary influences has been part of Vedic culture for thousands of years.

Ayurveda and jyotish emphasize that it is very important to know the suitability of the gems for the user. In Ayurveda, different gemstones rule over different doshas, organs and dhatus of the body. The stones also have specific healing effects for different disorders. In jyotish, specific stones mirror the planets and their movements. In most instances, the planets, doshas, diseases and gemstones correlate. Jyotish correlates the fingers with the different elements and planets. It is important to know on which finger to place each gemstone and in what setting (gold or silver), in order to achieve maximum benefit. For personal gemstone recommendations, it is advised to consult a qualified jyotishi (Vedic astrologer).

## Gemstones and the Planets

To determine which gemstones to use for emotional, psychological and spiritual purposes, we must look to the stars. Numerous Vedic texts, including the *Brihat Samhita,* the *Agni Purana,* the *Garuda Purana,* the *Ratnapariksha* and the *Devi Bhagavata,* discuss the origins and effects of gemstones. Each of the planets is associated with primary gemstones (listed in bold below), as well as secondary or substitute stones that can be used in addition to or as a replacement for the primary stones. Traditionally, when using a secondary stone it should be of a larger size than the primary gemstone. Precious gemstones worn as rings should be a minimum of two carats and as pendants, five carats. Substitute stones worn as rings need to be a minimum of four carats and pendants should be seven carats or more. For example, if using a peridot ring is used instead of an emerald, the peridot should be around four carats, whereas the emerald may only need to be two or three carats.

### *Planets and Their Gemstones*
**Sun – ruby,** garnet, red spinel, red zircon, red tourmaline, rose quartz or star ruby
**Moon – pearl,** moonstone, clear quartz
**Mars – red coral,** carnelian, red jasper
**Mercury – emerald,** peridot, aquamarine, green zircon, green tourmaline, moldavite, green jade, green agate
**Venus – diamond,** white sapphire, white zircon, white tourmaline, danburite
**Jupiter – yellow sapphire,** topaz, citrine, yellow zircon, yellow tourmaline

**Saturn – blue sapphire,** blue spinel, blue zircon, amethyst, blue tourmaline, lapis lazuli
**Rahu – hessonite (gomeda),** all types of golden garnet, amber
**Ketu – cat's eye,** tiger's eye

## Gemstones and the Doshas

**Gemstones for harmonizing vata:** ruby, pearl, red coral, emerald, yellow sapphire, diamond, gomeda, cat's eye
**Gemstones for harmonizing pitta:** blue sapphire, pearl, red coral, emerald, diamond, ruby
**Gemstones for harmonizing kapha:** ruby, yellow sapphire, cat's eye

## The Healing Properties of Gemstones

• **Ruby:** Ruby gives great warmth and is therefore excellent for vata doshas. It has the ability to increase agni. Ruby increases pitta, which is helpful when pitta is deficient in one's dosha. It alleviates excess vata and kapha. One of the most precious of gems, ruby can easily be the equal to a diamond in value. In India and China, ruby is worn to promote health and happiness. A power ascribed to the ruby is the ability to foretell danger by a loss of color and brilliance. Wearing ruby is said to give good health and longevity. Ruby also increases circulation, vitality and immunity. It is great for increasing the energy of pitta organs like the liver, gallbladder, heart and small intestine. This precious stone helps to build blood, and counteracts weakness, debility and fatigue. It is a powerful rejuvenative and brain tonic. Ruby is used in jyotish for strengthening the heart, improving digestion, promoting circulation, reviving fire and increasing energy. Ruby also strengthens the individual will, promotes independence, gives insight and enhances power. Ruby bhasma treats blood diseases like anemia and skin infections. It promotes the production of new blood cells. Ruby increases circulation and is a powerful heart tonic.

- **Pearl:** Pearl increases kapha, harmonizes vata and reduces pitta. Pearl is one of the best stones for strengthening immunity and building ojas. It works on nourishing all of the dhatus. This precious stone is a great blood purifier and helps with all bleeding disorders. It harmonizes the female reproductive system and increases fertility, vigor and vitality. Pearl's alkalinizing properties help to treat hyper-acidity, ulcers and indigestion. As pearl comes from the deep calm of the ocean floor, it similarly provides a calming effect on the mind, emotions and nervous system. It is soothing to the heart and helps to regulate the flow of prana. Wearing pearl makes us more receptive, open, peaceful and compassionate. Pearl bhasma strengthens bone (asthi) and nerve and bone marrow (majja) dhatus.

- **Red Coral:** As red coral originates from the ocean, it contains the water element. It is an excellent blood purifier and therefore helps pitta. However, it increases agni, and if used in excess, will increase pitta. It is also an excellent stone for vata and kapha doshas. Red coral is said to give the benefic influence of Mars. It gives vitality, vigor, courage and stamina. This stone increases agni and strengthens blood (rakta), nerves and bone marrow (majja), muscle (mamsa) dhatu, bone (asthi) and reproductive (shukra-arthava) dhatus. It is excellent for debilitating diseases, and alleviates appendicitis, arthritis and impotency if used with labradorite. It also strengthens the lungs and is an effective treatment for cough and asthma. Red coral improves energy, calms emotion, gives courage and improves work capacity. It enhances appetite, sexual vitality, personal will power, discipline and intelligence. Red coral bhasma is excellent as an aphrodisiac (vajikarana).

- **Emerald:** Overall, emerald is a tridoshic stone. Emerald has great ability to neutralize vata and alleviate pitta; if worn in excess, it may aggravate kapha. It calms mental agitation, regulates the nervous system, helps to stop nerve pain and improves speech and intelligence. Emerald promotes healing, energizes the breath and strengthens the lungs. It is a powerful immune-boosting stone, and is good for cancer and other degenerative diseases. This gem enhances memory, concentration, creativity (writing, speech and singing), growth and development. It improves lung disorders such as asthma and bronchitis, relieves stagnation, and removes lethargy. Emerald also enhances spiritual practices (sadhana) like mantra, japa, bhajans, hatha yoga and scriptural studies. Emerald is also used for treatment of depression, psychosis, hyperacidity, dyspepsia, stomatitis and obesity. It can be used in conjunction with other stones to enhance the healing of tumors, cysts, cancers and other vata-related disorders. The bhasma of emerald is used to treat all sorts of liver and bone diseases. It is also a powerful nervine and is used in convalescence.

• **Diamond:** Diamond slightly increases kapha, harmonizes vata, and calms and nurtures pitta. It is an excellent tonic for the heart and prana. The diamond is considered the greatest of stones, revered throughout the ages for its great beauty and strength, and also for its powerful, positive, spiritual and physical influences. This gem is said to enhance the wearer with charm and beauty. Physically, it strengthens the reproductive organs and kidneys, and gives protection against severe disease. Diamond is excellent for regulating menstruation. It is beneficial for the nervous system and adrenal glands, while also strengthening ojas. Diamond bestows vitality, longevity and an increase of the divine feminine energy. As diamond rules Venus, it increases passion, desire and creativity, and gives a sense of comfort or nurturing. On a higher level, it bestows divine Love, grace and devotion. The bhasma of diamond is used to treat all types of chronic, debilitating and wasting diseases by increasing immunity, vitality and ojas. It is very costly and was traditionally used only by kings and queens to promote longevity.

• **Yellow Sapphire:** Yellow sapphire is a relatively tridoshic stone. Due to its warming properties, it is an excellent stone for reducing vata. This stone brings blessings, prosperity, benevolence, righteousness, piety and truthfulness. It is excellent for building immunity, strength and longevity. This stone is considered by many to be the most effective for promoting all-around health and well-being. Yellow sapphire also regulates the hormonal system. It is one of the best stones for diabetes and edema. This particular sapphire harmonizes pitta due to its ability to increase ojas and sattvic qualities. It is a great stone for those who have a Guru and are engaged in seva, because it helps the spiritual seeker on the path. Yellow sapphire is not used as a bhasma.

• **Blue Sapphire:** Traditional texts say that blue sapphire must be worn with caution. When used properly, it can have tremendous healing affects, but used wrongly, it can bring calamities. Used correctly, it has the ability to aide in detoxification and immunity. It is also useful for many vata disorders such as weak bones, nervous system disorders, lack of vitality, as well as constipation, epilepsy, paralysis, cancer, immune diseases like HIV and AIDS, psychosis, alcoholism, rage, hypertension, bodily pain, arthritis, rheumatism, vertigo and heart diseases. Blue sapphire clears infections and wards off negative energies. It combats tumors and excess fat, and is good for increasing the entire metabolic process. Blue sapphire strengthens the bones, increases longevity, and helps to calm the nerves and emotions. It promotes peace and detachment. Unless the affects of blue sapphire are known specifically for the individual, it is safer and more affordable to use one of the substitute stones like amethyst or blue zircon. Blue sapphire is not used as a bhasma.

• **Gomeda/Hessonite:** Gomeda contains the fire and ether elements. Overall, gomeda is tridoshic. It calms all types of vata imbalance. Gomeda is the golden color of cow's urine and is a type of golden garnet. Gomeda is a good stone for maintaining balance. It calms the nerves, quiets the mind and relieves depression and mental disorders. This stone is recommended for almost everyone, as it counteracts negative influences, emotions, thoughts and pollution. It gives strength and endurance, and is excellent for immunity and undiagnosed diseases. Gomeda is also beneficial for the endocrine system, respiration, nervousness, indigestion and loss of coordination. This gem reduces stress while promoting intelligence and giving an artistic flair. It is used to avoid unforeseen calamities. It is said to offer protection to people who are in the healing arts field. It also raises consciousness and creativity. Gomeda is not used as a bhasma.

• **Cat's Eye:** Cat's eye has similar properties as ruby. While cat's eye is generally tridoshic, it slightly increases pitta and alleviates vata and kapha. In jyotish, cat's eye is governed by Ketu. Ketu is considered to be like a second Mars, as they have many of the same astrological attributes. This stone is good for promoting psychic and spiritual perception. It is an excellent digestive stimulant. Cat's eye is a good nervine and is helpful for mental disorders. It is even reported to help with hair growth. This stone is used in cases of allergies, brain and breast tumors, and diseases related to stress and environmental toxins. It helps to increase circulation and strengthen the power of the brain, senses and nervous system. Cat's eye increases overall immunity to help combat pathogens, and also helps with meditation and spiritual practices. Cat's eye is not used as a bhasma.

## Properties of the Main Secondary Stones

• **Amethyst:** Amethyst is one of the best stones for reducing excess pitta. Amethyst is extremely cooling and helps to balance high pitta emotions like anger, lust and impatience. It promotes faith, compassion and courage. Amethyst balances the energies of the mind, body and emotions, and brings stability, vigor and peace. This stone also acts as a shield against negativity; additionally, it is excellent against alcohol and drug intoxication.

• **Bloodstone:** Bloodstone is excellent for decreasing pitta. It purifies and oxygenates the blood and strengthens immunity by destroying free radicals. This semiprecious stone is excellent for menstrual disorders. It is also a good stone to use during childbirth as it prevents hemorrhaging. Bloodstone works well for liver and spleen weakness or toxicity, as well as anemic conditions.

• **Citrine:** Citrine is known at the "sunshine stone." It is warming and reduces vata and kapha. It stimulates intuition and higher states of intelligence. This stone increases circulation and digestive fire. It can be used to increase metabolism and combat obesity. Citrine also helps to create material abundance.

• **Fluorite:** Fluorite's properties are similar to those of blue sapphire, but without the possibility of side effects. As it can be cooling, it alleviates pitta but may aggravate kapha. Fluorite emits a soothing and calming energy. It brings mental stability and therefore harmonizes vata. This stone increases the ability to concentrate while promoting clarity and understanding. It calms and rejuvenates the nervous system. Fluorite also protects one from negative vibrations like radioactivity of microwaves, computers, cell phones, electric lines and smog. This stone is excellent for those who work on the computer or who talk on the phone a lot. It is beneficial to keep fluorite near computers, especially along with a plant.

• **Labradorite:** Labradorite is good for reducing kapha, as it is a very active stone. It stimulates productive mental activity while reducing anxiety and stress. As its colors appear to be vibrantly dancing, it inspires creativity and change. This crystal helps to remove blocks and overcome limitations. It assists one to traverse change and move in a positive direction. Labradorite is also beneficial for protection against electromagnetic frequencies that come from computers, television, cell phones, microwaves and other such environmental factors.

• **Lapis Lazuli:** Lapis lazuli can alleviate the stress of mental hyperactivity. Lapis is an excellent stone for all of the doshas, but is especially good for vata dosha. It assists with mental clarity and emotional responsiveness. Lapis enhances serenity and self-acceptance, and attracts success in relationships. It was used by the Egyptians to facilitate seeing deeply into the Self and into the astral spheres of consciousness. It is used to increase one's spiritual vibration and intuition.

• **Moonstone:** Moonstone increases kapha by increasing ojas. It radiates the divine feminine energy of the moon. This stone has the ability to relieve excess heat in the body and mind. Moonstone also soothes the nervous system and reduces mental disturbances. It is one of the best stones to counteract stress and tension.

• **Opal:** Opal is tridoshic but is especially excellent for kapha, as it is a source of inspiration and creativity. It is known as the stone of beauty and charm. Opal stimulates inquisitiveness and initiative. It increases physical energy and mental clarity while protecting against fear, rage and sorrow. It also promotes the qualities of clear mental perspective and inner awakening. Wearing opal helps to alleviate allergy problems due to low immune function. It can also be used to increase faith, compassion and devotion.

• **Rose Quartz:** Rose quartz alleviates vata, calms pitta and, in excess, increases kapha. Rose quartz increases prana, regulates blood pressure, and benefits the circulatory system, making it excellent for heart disease. It also improves the quality of the lymph (rasa) and blood (rakta) dhatus. Emotionally, it creates feelings of calmness, warmth, compassion and understanding, love, patience, and clarity of mind. It helps to harmonize relationships.

## Color Therapy

The colors that we see are light waves absorbed or reflected by everything around us. In nature, a rainbow is light which is refracted by the moisture in the air. The colors of the visible light spectrum are red, orange, yellow, green, blue, indigo and violet. White light consists of all of the colors mixed together. The color of an object depends on how it absorbs and/or reflects light. If an object absorbs all of the light wavelengths, it will appear black. If it reflects all of them, it will appear white.

Colors produce significant changes in our emotions. Each color has its own area of influence in the body and produces physical and mental responses in relation to that area.

Light is absorbed through the eyes as well as through the skin by our sensory nerve endings. The effects of color make it suitable for subtle or spiritual healing. Our chakras and koshas are where healing through colors first takes place. Each chakra and kosha governs particular organs of the body, specific emotions and aspects of the mind. By knowing which color operates through which chakra and their complex interplay, one can balance the chakra, thereby correcting the disease rooted in the particular organ or emotion associated with that chakra.

This principle is equally true for the planets. Just as each planet is governed by gemstones and crystals, they are also governed by certain colors. The planetary colors follow that of their governing gemstone. Sun is associated with red; Moon is associated with white; Mercury is associated with green; Mars, with dark red; Venus, with a transparent-like aqua blue; Jupiter, with yellow; Saturn, with dark blue or black; Rahu, with ultraviolet, dark brown or grey; and Ketu is associated with infrared to multicolored.

## Colors and the Doshas

Anything that emits a color has therapeutic value. The conscious use of color in our lives can assist in creating greater peace and harmony. There are numerous ways to use colors as therapy. The use of colored lamps is one of the most effective methods. This can be easily done by placing colored glass over a light bulb or by using colored bulbs. Nowadays there are companies that sell colored lamp sets with different color slides. Wearing clothes of different colors is of benefit as they impart the healing properties of the specific color. The color of one's house or office can also affect one's health. Nature contains a full spectrum of color. It is very beneficial to frequently visit flower gardens, rivers, forests, mountains, deserts and even just stare at the open sky. Color therapy can even apply to the food we eat.

**Vata Colors:** To balance vata, use warm, heating, calming and moist colors like red, orange, yellow and gold. White and clear to very light shades of blue-green (like aquamarine) are also useful. Neon colors are aggravating as they are overly stimulating. Dark colors will suppress vata.

**Pitta Colors:** Colors that have a cooling and calming nature will balance pitta. White, blue, violet and green are extremely nurturing. For this reason it is very good for pitta-types to spend lots of time in nature with trees and running water. Any bright or stimulating colors will aggravate a pitta.

**Kapha Colors:** To balance kapha, use warm and stimulating colors. Bright colors help to energize slow and stagnated kapha. Similar to vata, reds, oranges, yellows and gold are very beneficial. The colors should be bright and clear.

## Properties of Individual Colors

• **Red:** Red is a hot and stimulating color. It increases pitta while minimizing excess vata and kapha. Red has a vitalizing effect and a positive magnetic energy. In excess or when not well-matched to a person's dosha, it can cause lust, anger, rage, hostility or violence. Red drives toxins out of the body, but can also create too much heat, causing headaches, inflammation, fever, high blood pressure and hot flashes. It governs bone marrow, capillaries and blood vessels. It increases circulation. For stagnant kapha or depleted vata, red can be extremely beneficial, as it is revitalizing and motivates action. It connects to the root chakra and assists in awakening dormant spiritual energy.

• **Orange:** Orange is very warming. Orange soothes vata and kapha. If used in excess, it aggravates pitta. It stimulates the reproductive organs and has a cheering, inspiring effect that makes one optimistic. Orange is also magnetic in a positive way. It energizes and increases positive mental activity. It illuminates and gives the feeling of purity. It is considered a color of renunciation. For this reason, Buddhist and Hindu monks wear orange or saffron colored robes. It increases cellular intelligence, appetite, digestion and effulgence. It relates to the sacral plexus and assists in transcending limited desires.

• **Yellow:** Yellow is warming. Like red and orange, yellow calms vata and kapha and slightly increases pitta. It is a color of joy, activity, inspiration and communication. It strengthens agni. It stimulates the brain and the nerves, inspiring one to gain knowledge and optimism. In traditional Buddhism, yellow is the color of ego death or the transcendental realm. Yellow can be comforting and soothing. It protects against infection, poisons and pollutants. It is the color associated with the solar plexus and helps one to attune to divine will.

• **Green:** Green is refreshing and cooling and brings feelings of harmony and vitality. While generally tridoshic, in excess, it increases kapha. Depending upon the shade of green, it can harmonize kapha, or it can be too cooling. Bright greens harmonize, while dark greens dampen kapha. All shades of green produce calmness and have a restful effect on the eyes. Green is a color of optimism, refreshing and cleansing the body and mind. It alleviates headaches, fever and excessive heat disorders. This color is also good for regulating metabolism, and improving the functioning of the liver, gall bladder and spleen (as they regulate bile and blood, which are forms of pitta). Green possesses tremendous healing power, as it is the color of all plants and of the heart chakra. It strengthens the immune system and invigorates the blood.

• **Blue:** Blue is cold and detached. It is the color of pure mind or consciousness. It is also the color of the throat chakra and of prana. Blue calms and nurtures pitta, while it aggravates vata and is neutral for kapha. It creates serenity and peacefulness, pulling one inward toward meditation. Many retreat centers paint the walls blue to give the feelings of healing, solitude and purity. Dark and rich blue colors have been known to assist with spinal troubles, burns and inflammatory problems. They have been additionally used to reduce anxiety, panic attacks and hysteria. Blue can benefit those with chronic allergies and coughs, since it reduces phlegm. It is also good for the reduction of tumors and cysts.

• **Indigo:** Indigo is cooling and has a calming effect on the nervous system. It is the color of higher consciousness and ajna, the third eye chakra. It relieves pitta and kapha excesses. This color can be used for vata in moderation. It reduces heat, and can be a great comfort for headaches, inflammation and fevers. Indigo has been known to heal burns and poisonous bites, and also has the ability to reduce heart palpitations. It has calming effects both within the body and mind and in the external environment. It assists in meditation; and in many mystic traditions, indigo is the color of the Guru.

• **Violet:** Violet is the color of the Hindu trinity: Brahma, Vishnu and Shiva. This represents the process of creation, sustenance and transformation. It is the color of bliss or higher consciousness. Violet is a cooling color, but also provides a gentle heat to the body. This color subdues pitta and kapha. It is suitable for vata in moderation. Violet stimulates the immune system, builds antibodies and has germicidal qualities. Violet includes light shades of lavender as well as dark purple. Violet is a spiritual color in that it inspires generosity, compassion, detachment and devotion to God. Violet is the color of the crown chakra, helping us to operate from higher states of consciousness.

• **White:** White is the color of purity, contentment and spirituality. White has a tridoshic nature, so it harmonizes all of the doshas. White contains the unity of all colors. It is cooling and nurturing; it is excellent for calming the nervous system, emotions and mind. White can alleviate inflammation and increase mental perception and intelligence. It promotes the awakening of sattvic qualities. White emphasizes the energy of love, purity, compassion and divinity.

## Ayurvedic Aromatherapy

Aromatherapy is one of the oldest forms of natural medicine. For more than 6,000 years, essential oils – the highly concentrated life force of plants – have been used around the world to heal physical and psychological diseases. In the spirit of ecological conservation, it is important to understand the potency of essential oils. It takes very large quantities of plants to make even one drop of essential oil. One drop of essential oil equals in concentration 30 cups of herbal tea. Due to this potency, simply smelling or diffusing oils is a highly effective way by which they can enter the body.

Smelling therapeutic-grade oils enables their essence to pass through the blood-brain barrier and move directly to the limbic brain where emotions, memory and regulatory functions are seated. This action creates an immediate shift in the entire physical body and also brings deep transformation to the mind.

Essential oils are the life force of plants. They are one of the highest sources of antioxidants and protect against free radical damage. They also assist in delivering nutrients inside our bodies. Essential oils make oxygen more available to tissues and cells. This trait is very precious since planetary levels of air pollution, pesticides and chemicals are rising.

Therapeutic grade essential oils naturally offer numerous healing properties such as antiviral, antifungal, antibacterial, antiseptic, anti-depressant, anti-inflammatory, anti-parasitic, immunity stimulating, cell rejuvenating, oxygenating, detoxifying and cleansing.

Keep in mind that the oils are very concentrated plant constituents possessing highly potent medicinal properties. They should be used with intention and utmost respect. When using essential oils with children it is recommended that you dilute the oils at least by half in carrier oil. For use with babies and young children, a diluted drop or two on a cotton ball can be placed near the child for gradual absorption. Pregnant women should not use essential oils during the first trimester. Some oils are contraindicated throughout pregnancy and while breastfeeding.

When applied to the skin directly, the oils penetrate through the pores, enter into the blood stream, affect adjacent organs and circulate instantly to where they are most needed in the body. If you choose to use the oils directly on the skin for healing or other purposes, it is recommended that you use the oils very sparingly and/or dilute the oil in organic almond or jojoba oil. Use essential oils on the body, mix into massage oil, use a compress, drop into bath water, burn in a diffuser or simply smell the bottle to receive numerous therapeutic benefits! Always keep essential oils out of sunlight and store in a cool, dark place.

## Essential Oils for the Doshas

**Vata:** Vata needs warming, fragrant, calming, sweet and relaxing oils in order to stay balanced. Oils best for vata are blue chamomile, cardamom, cinnamon, clove, eucalyptus, frankincense, galbanum, ginger, jasmine, jatamansi, lavender, lemon, lotus, melissa, neroli, orange, patchouli, rhus, rose, sandalwood and tulasi.

**Pitta:** Pitta needs cooling and calming essential oils that nourish and support the body and mind. Oils that balance pitta are chamomile, champaca, helichrysum, Himalayan cedar wood, jasmine, jatamansi, lavender, lemon, lily, lotus, mint (all varities), neroli, oud, rose, sandalwood, St. John's wort, wintergreen and yarrow.

**Kapha:** Kapha needs hot and spicy essential oils. Kapha types benefit from warm, drying and stimulating smells. Oils that help equalize kapha are ajwan, amber, angelica, basil, camphor, cardamom, cinnamon, clove, cypress, eucalyptus, frankincense, galbanum, ginger, helichrysum, hina, jasmine, juniper, keawa, lemongrass, lily, mugwort, myrrh, neroli, oregano, patchouli, ravensara, rose, sage, sandalwood, thyme, tulasi, violet and wintergreen.

## The Healing Properties of Essential Oils

• **Basil (Ocimum basilicum):** Decreases vata and kapha and increases pitta. Basil can be relaxing to muscles, including smooth muscles (those not subject to our voluntary control, such as the heart and digestive system). It may also be used to soothe insect bites when applied topically. Beneficial for mental fatigue, basil can help stimulate and sharpen the sense of smell. Basil oil is an antiseptic, antispasmodic, antibacterial, antiviral, anti-inflammatory, antidepressant, adrenal stimulant and calming agent. Basil has the ability to stimulate hair growth.

• **Birch (Betula lenulta):** Decreases pitta and kapha and increases vata. Birch is good for rheumatism, muscular pain, tendonitis, arthritis, cramps, hypertension, counteracting inflammation, ulcers, cellulite and toxin and fluid accumulation. It has the actions of an antispasmodic, liver stimulant, disinfectant, pain reliever, analgesic, anti-inflammatory, anti-rheumatic and antiseptic.

• **Black Pepper (Piper nigrum):** Decreases vata and kapha and increases pitta. Black pepper essential oil is good for indigestion, low appetite, weak digestive fire, and for removing toxins in the colon and lungs. It can also be used to counter obesity. This oil is an anti-catarrhal, anti-inflammatory, expectorant, analgesic, and is good for blood circulation.

• **Blue Chamomile (Matricaria chamomilla):** Blue chamomile reduces vata and pitta while increasing kapha and ojas. Great for inflammation, nervous system disorders, stress, arthritis, headaches, sore muscles, liver and spleen conditions, menstrual disorders, anger, insomnia and confusion. It is an antispasmodic, analgesic, antiseptic, digestive, nerve sedative and immune-stimulant.

• **Cardamom (Elettaria cardamomum):** Cardamom oil is great for reducing vata and kapha especially in the lungs and large intestine. It increases pitta and the digestive fire. This oil can be used to treat coughs, colds, weak immunity, indigestion, asthma, bronchitis and other vata derangements. It is a stimulant, expectorant, carminative, stomachic, diaphoretic and aphrodisiac.

• **Cedar, Himalayan (Ceodora deodara):** Himalayan cedar wood is tridoshic, and is good for headaches, insomnia, kidney and urinary tract infections, arthritis, and liver and spleen disorders. It is an antiseptic, diuretic, expectorant, nervine and rejuvenative.

• **Cinnamon (Cinnamomum zeylancium):** Cinnamon essential oil increases pitta while reducing vata and kapha. It is excellent as a digestive stimulant and good for lung conditions and congestion. This spicy oil treats infertility and impotency. It is a diaphoretic, anti-helmintic, aphrodisiac, antispasmodic, expectorant, analgesic, diuretic, alterative and carminative all in one.

• **Clary Sage (Salvia sclarea):** Clary sage decreases kapha and has a neutral effect on vata and pitta. It is a good digestive stimulant, as well as a tonic for women's reproductive issues, especially balancing hormones, cramps, premenstrual syndrome and regulating menstruation. Clary sage has an anti-convulsive, antidepressive, antiseptic, antispasmodic, aphrodisiacal, astringent, deodorizing, nervine and sedative nature.

• **Clove (Syzygium aromaticum):** Clove alleviates vata and kapha while increasing pitta. It is good for all coughs, colds and lung problems. This essential oil is also good for toothaches, low blood pressure and reproductive weakness. It is antiseptic, anti-inflammatory, anti-rheumatic, analgesic, expectorant, aphrodisiac and stimulates the immune system.

• **Eucalyptus (Eucalyptus globus, citriodora):** Eucalyptus is one of the best oils to alleviate vata and kapha, while mildly stimulating pitta. It is excellent for treating asthma, bronchitis, excess mucous, infections, congestion, kidney and bladder infections, rheumatism, arthritis and numerous other vata-related disorders. Eucalyptus has many properties, such as analgesic, antiseptic, antispasmodic, decongestant, diuretic, expectorant, antiviral, circulation boosting, anti-fungal and antibacterial.

• **Frankincense (Boswelia thurifera, serrata):** Like most resins, frankincense increases pitta while reducing vata and kapha. It is excellent for cleansing the blood and wounds, as well as for calming the nervous system. Frankincense is also good for lung disorders like bronchitis, colds and congestion. Its actions include antiseptic, astringent, expectorant, sedative, anti-inflammatory, antidepressant, immune stimulating, and calming; it elevates the mind and deepens the breath. It increases purity and is associated with spiritual qualities. Frankincense was traded like money among the Egyptians and Indians. It was one of the gifts offered to Christ at his birth.

• **Geranium (Pelargonium graveolens):** Geranium reduces pitta and kapha and mildly increases vata if used in excess. It is excellent for regulating the menstrual cycle and calming the nervous system, and it is uplifting and emotionally balancing. It is effective in combating stress, fatigue and depression. Geranium can heal skin disorders. Its properties include anti-fungal, analgesic, antidepressant, antiseptic, astringent, deodorant and antibacterial.

• **Helichrysum (Helichrysum angustifolia):** Helichrysum is often called "Immortelle." It is balancing to all three doshas, and is one of the best essential oils to use topically for pain, muscle strain, bruises, inflammation, and sore and tired muscles. It is particularly beneficial for injuries to the bones or muscles, as it speeds up cell regeneration. This oil also supports the lymphatic, endocrine and nervous systems. Helichrysum has healing properties that work on all of the organs, most notably the liver, gall bladder, stomach, spleen and pancreas. It is an antispasmodic, expectorant, anti-coagulant, antiviral, anti-inflammatory and a tissue-regenerating agent. It is additionally helpful with addictions.

• **Jasmine (Jasmine grandiflorum):** Jasmine is calming for pitta and kapha. While beneficial for vata due to its sweet nature, if used in excess it mildly increases vata due to its divinely intoxicating aroma. In general, this oil is uplifting to the spirit and brings a sense of calm, contentment, peace, well-being, courage and confidence. Jasmine can reduce emotional disturbances. It is used to treat weak immunity, poor circulation, fever, burns, skin disorders, cancer, bacterial or viral infections and other immunity-related disorders. It is especially good for the female reproductive system.

- **Lavender (Lavendula angustifolia, officinalis):** Lavender is one of the most widely used essential oils. Due to its numerous medicinal properties, it is one of the best oils to keep with you at all times. It decreases pitta and kapha and is balancing for vata. Lavender is excellent for external skin problems like burns, rashes, eczema, psoriasis, blisters, acne, sexually transmitted diseases, external hemorrhoids and cuts. It can be used to prevent scarring. This oil is also used for athlete's foot, fungus, yeast and bacterial infections. It works by stimulating the immune system. Lavender can also be used for vata diseases like rheumatism, arthritis, lumbago, gout, sciatica, Parkinson's and heart disorders. Its vast properties include being analgesic, anti-convulsive, antidepressant, anti-rheumatic, antiseptic, antispasmodic, antiviral, decongestant, deodorant and restorative. It is also a sedative agent that relieves nervous tension, sleeplessness and irritability. It is one of the most valuable gifts given to us by Mother Nature.

- **Lemon Balm, Melissa (Melissa officinalis):** Melissa reduces pitta and kapha and balances vata. Melissa is excellent for the immune system, allergies, general weakness, lethargy, blood disorders, bacterial and viral infections and as a digestive stimulant. Its many qualities include antidepressant, anti-histaminic, antispasmodic, bactericidal, insect repellent, nervine, immune stimulant, sedative and stomachic.

- **Lemon (Citrus limonum):** Lemon is harmonizing for pitta, vata and kapha. It increases circulation and aids in alertness, concentration and mental clarity. Lemon is an excellent oil to bring along when driving long distances because it is refreshing and revitalizing.

It is useful for staying awake and alert. It is also good for digestive weakness, infectious diseases, bacterial and viral infections, Lyme disease, liver disorders like jaundice and hepatitis, typhoid, malaria, anemia, blood disorders and hypertension. Lemon is one of the strongest antibacterial essential oils.

• **Lotus (Nelumbo nucifera):** There are three main types of lotus: blue, pink and white. They are rare and very expensive. Blue is the rarest and most costly variety. In India, lotus is considered to be one of the most sacred plants. It increases sattvic qualities, while instilling faith and devotion. Lotus decreases pitta and vata while increasing kapha. It is an excellent immune stimulant and is great for the heart and blood. This essential oil helps to alleviate headaches and nausea. It can be used for meditation and to increase love, patience, stillness and compassion. Lotus is the best oil to increase ojas.

• **Myrrh (Commiphora myrrh):** Myrrh, like frankincense, is one of the oldest and most treasured essential oils and resins. Myrrh decreases vata and kapha while stimulating pitta. It is one of the best blood purifiers and immune-stimulants, good for all female reproductive disorders as well as hormonal balancing. This essential oil also treats lung disorders like asthma, bronchitis and whooping cough. Furthermore, it is good for vata derangements like arthritis, rheumatic disorders, gout and insomnia. Myrrh has the properties of being anti-inflammatory, antiseptic, astringent, alterative, rejuvenative, expectorant, revitalizing and sedative in action.

• **Neroli (Citrus aurantium):** Neroli comes from orange flower blossoms. Due to its divine, intoxicating fragrance it is believed to help one connect to the Divine within. It is excellent for mental concentration. Neroli harmonizes the doshas. It is good for circulation and the heart, and use of neroli cures depression, anxiety and nervousness. This essential oil is a great antiseptic, antispasmodic, aphrodisiac, carminative, tonic, stimulant, anti-fungal and antibacterial agent.

- **Patchouli (Pogostemom cablim):** Patchouli decreases vata and pitta while mildly stimulating kapha. It is an excellent fungicide that is useful against bacteria, amoebas and parasites. This oil is also good against skin problems like scabies, ringworm, dermatitis, eczema, dandruff, cracked and dry skin, wrinkles and infections. It is a strong aphrodisiac and tonic for the nervous system and immunity. Patchouli is great for removing stress and nervous tension as it uplifts the spirit. It has antidepressant, anti-inflammatory, antimicrobial, aphrodisiac, antibacterial, deodorant and nervine qualities.

- **Peppermint (Mentha piperita):** Peppermint is cooling, reduces pitta and kapha, and has a neutral effect for vata. It is good for treating headaches and general pains. Peppermint is a stimulant and revitalizer that increases prana flow. It calms acidic stomachs and indigestion and alleviates coughs and congestion. This oil is exceptional for the respiratory tract, and it is often combined with wintergreen, eucalyptus and camphor as a comprehensive treatment for the lungs. Peppermint is often added to toothpastes and shampoos for its cleansing, antiseptic and refreshing nature. It has analgesic, antiseptic, antispasmodic, astringent, expectorant, decongestant, anti-inflammatory, anti-infectious, anti-fungal, digestive and invigorating qualities.

- **Rose (Rose damascena):** The rose is a universal symbol of love. Rose essential oil opens the heart and balances all of the doshas and dhatus, increasing immunity through building love and compassion. Rose is used for all sorts of blood and reproductive disorders because it carries the highest vibrational frequency of any essential oil. It helps to balance hormones and neurological functions, brings relief from depression, sadness, anxiety, worry, fear, grief and nervousness. Rose can be used externally to treat skin disorders. Its vast actions include antidepressant, antiseptic, antispasmodic, alterative, refrigerant, nervine, laxative, astringent, aphrodisiac and rejuvenative.

- **Sandalwood (Santalum album):** Sandalwood is the best essential oil for the mind and meditation because it awakens the third eye while simultaneously calming the nervous system. It is said to be the most spiritual oil, excellent for balancing vata and pitta doshas because it treats all neurological disorders. Sandalwood mildly increases kapha dosha. This oil has a unique effect on vital organs, stimulating the pineal and pituitary glands and nourishing the heart. Due to these actions, prana and ojas become harmonized when this oil is used. Sandalwood is exceptional for fevers, blood toxicity, overheating (sunstroke), skin eruptions, boils, acne, psoriasis, sexually transmitted diseases, immune weakness, depression, fear and reproductive weakness in both men and women. It is an antiseptic, antispasmodic, aphrodisiac, astringent, diuretic, expectorant, tonic, decongestant, sedative, nervine, alterative, antibacterial, insecticide and anti-fungal oil.

• **Tea Tree (Melaleuca):** Tea tree oil is tridoshic, and therefore healing on many levels. It is one of the best immunomodulators available. Tea tree oil can be used on almost any skin disease. Consequently, it is used extensively to treat athlete's foot, candida albicans, vaginal yeast infections, ringworm, fungal infections, and bites from poisonous insects. Tea tree oil is excellent for lung conditions like bronchitis, asthma, tuberculosis, emphysema and congestion. The properties of tea tree oil are antibiotic, antibacterial, anti-fungal, antiviral, expectorant, anti-parasitic, anti-infectious, decongestant and anti-pyretic.

• **Tulasi (Ocimum sanctum):** Tulasi essential oil decreases vata and kapha and slightly increases pitta if used in excess. Tulasi is sattvic by nature and purifies and harmonizes the mind. It assists in clearing out old, stagnant thoughts and emotions. It increases faith, devotion and detachment. Tulasi is uplifting and helps us to overcome sadness and depression. It is used in treatment of lung ailments, especially asthma and bronchitis. It alleviates headaches, fever, sinus congestion, arthritis, rheumatism and brain fog. It is diaphoretic, febrifuge, nervine, antispasmodic, antibacterial, antiseptic, antifungal and emmenagogue.

- **Wintergreen (Gaultheria procumbens):** Wintergreen decreases pitta and kapha and neutralizes vata. This excellent stimulant aids in all sorts of lung disorders. Muscle spasms, inflammation and muscle injuries, and joint and nerve pain are also relieved by wintergreen oil. Internally, wintergreen oil is good for stagnant lymph, blood, edema, sore throats and yeast infections. As it contains natural aspirin, it is also good for headaches. Wintergreen has the properties of a carminative, astringent, analgesic, antispasmodic, expectorant and diuretic agent. It is often used in toothpaste and mouthwash for its antiseptic properties.

- **Ylang Ylang (Cananga odorata):** Ylang ylang reduces vata and pitta, and increases kapha and ojas due to its sweet nature. It is one of the best oils for balancing the menstrual cycle and female hormones. It reduces cramps, tension, repressed or negative emotions and headaches. Ylang ylang is an aphrodisiac that rejuvenates the reproductive system; it is good for infertility and impotency. Its sedative action is good for high blood pressure, stress, anxiety and nervous tension. This oil is also great for repairing aged, cracked and wrinkled skin. It is anti-depressive, sedative, anti-infectious, antiseptic, euphoric and hormonal regulative.

# Chapter 14

# The Healing Powers of Mantras

*In the beginning was the Word. And the Word
was with God and the Word was God.*

*~ The Bible, John 1:1 (KJV)*

*In the present dark age of materialism, the constant repetition
of a mantra is the easiest way to obtain inner purification
and concentration. You can chant your mantra at any time,
anywhere, without observing any rules regarding purity of
body or mind. It can be done while engaged in any task.
Mental purity will come through constant chanting of the
divine name. This is the simplest way. You are trying to cross
the ocean of transmigration, the cycle of birth and death. The
mantra is the oar of the boat; it is the instrument you use
to cross the samsara of your restless mind, with its unending
thought waves. The mantra can also be compared to a ladder
that you climb to reach the heights of God-realization.*

*~ Amma*

## What is a Mantra?

*Om Mantra-Sarayai Namah*

I bow to Her who is the essence of all mantras.

*~ Sri Lalita Sahasranama, verse 846*

*Mantras* intone sounds in their purest and most essential forms. *Mantra japa* (repetition of a mantra) is extraordinarily powerful because it connects us with the original divine energy. When we connect to divine energy, we are relieved of suffering. This is why the meaning of the Sanskrit word *mantra* is, "saving the mind from suffering and illness."

According to Ayurveda, mantras invoke divine energy to flow into us. The way this happens is quite simple. All sentient and non-sentient forms in the universe are composed of different energies, and all the energies in the universe have an associated sound vibration. Modern physics confirms this: all forms in the universe are composed of sound vibrations that emit tangible energy. It follows logically that when we chant sounds associated with divine energy, we too begin to vibrate at the same frequency as the Divine.

Historically, Hinduism and Buddhism have used mantras for spiritual growth and healing. For example, the shamanic tradition of Tibetan Ayurveda has a detailed system of healing using mantras for the treatment of numerous diseases. In ancient India, mastering the chanting of mantras was part of ayurvedic training. Only one who mastered the science of mantras could be called an Ayurveda *acharya* (one proficient in Ayurveda). Vedic texts declare, "By reciting mantras, one can conquer decay, aversion, loss of appetite (dyspepsia), leprosy, disorders of the stomach, cough and asthma. The doer of mantra earns great merit, and in his [or her] next birth attains salvation, which is the portion of the noblest beings." Thus, everything from health and wealth to liberation can be attained by mantra japa.

Historically, mantras were verbally transmitted from master to student when the student was ready. Amma, one of the greatest living masters, offers mantras to those who express interest, while emphasizing that one must be ready to put forth effort once receiving the mantra. She describes the process: "Children, when Amma gives you a mantra, she sows a seed of spirituality within you. She transmits a part of herself into your heart. But, you have to work on it. You have to nurture that seed by meditating, praying and chanting your mantra regularly, without fail. You have to be totally committed." If we commit to chanting our mantra, our entire life will change for the better. Amma explains, "By chanting your mantra, your entire being will be transformed and you will realize your divine nature."

If you have not yet come into contact with a Perfect Master (Satguru) who can transmit a mantra to you directly, you can choose from numerous mantras that can be chanted with great results. They are profoundly effective for all human beings, regardless of one's cultural heritage, spiritual or religious background, age or gender. Amma says, "It is always advisable to obtain a mantra from a Self-realized Master. Until then, we may use one of the mantras of our beloved deity like *Om Namah Shivaya, Om Namo Bhagavate Vasudevaya, Om Namo Narayanaya, Hare Rama Hare Rama Rama Rama Hare Hare Hare Krishna Hare Krishna Krishna Krishna Hare Hare, Hari Om, Om Parashaktyai Namah, Om Shivashaktyaikya Rupinyai Namah,* or the names of Christ, Allah or Buddha."

In order to achieve our spiritual goals, it is vitally important that we practice mantra japa regularly. Effort is required for any undertaking to be successful, and the path of Self-realization is no different. As we put loving effort into our mantra japa practice, grace will flow into us. As more grace comes our way, we find the strength to put forth more effort. Amma says, "The period of sadhana is like climbing a high mountain. You need a lot of strength and energy. Mountain climbers use a rope to pull themselves up. For you, the only rope is japa. Therefore, children, try to repeat your mantra constantly. Once you reach the peak, you can relax and rest forever."

We should attempt to chant our mantra constantly. Mantras can be chanted anywhere, anytime. While bathing, cooking, eating, driving, walking, exercising or shopping, mantra japa can be flowing ceaselessly, either aloud or silently in the mind.

It is important to understand that, while chanting, one should attempt to practice mantra japa with the right attitude. This is because the effectiveness of a mantra depends upon the mental and emotional disposition of the person repeating it. Just like the saying, "Sweetness depends upon the amount of sugar put in," the greater the faith and devotion, the greater the power of the mantra. When we chant with the proper inner disposition, our practice will blossom. The physical vibration unified with the right mental intention increases the influence of the mantra. Hence there is the great metaphysical saying, "Energy flows where intention goes."

Amma suggests, "Do japa with alertness, never mechanically. Each repetition should be like savoring a sweet. In the end, you will reach a state where even if you let go of the mantra, the mantra won't let go of you." For this reason, it is very beneficial to set aside some time each day to sit and repeat mantras and then meditate quietly for some time to feel the vibrations reverberating inside your being.

While mantras can and should be chanted anywhere and anytime, it is good to know that there are specific places that are considered the most conducive to gaining concentration. Any place where an enlightened being has been is sanctified and is therefore an ideal place for chanting. The Vedas also mention the following natural environments as being the best for meditation and mantra japa:

- Flower gardens
- Natural places of solitude
- The middle of a forest
- Any place where no war has taken place
- Any holy place or place of pilgrimage
- Mountain caves
- Underneath a banyan, bilva or peepal tree
- Next to a tulasi plant
- On the banks of a river
- Near a fresh water pond or a spring

Other places conducive for concentrated chanting are near cows, streams, a ghee lamp or a temple. It is also best to chant in the early morning or late afternoon sun, under the full moon or in the presence of a Perfect Master. It is said that doing mantra japa while sitting in a river or stream where the water is up to the navel or the chest is also very purifying. Chanting on the seashore is sattvic and peaceful, and we also get the healing benefits of the negative ions coming from the ocean.

There are many mantras that can be chanted to balance the body, the elements and the chakras. Mantra repetition can enhance spiritual growth, peace and happiness. Some mantras are especially linked to particular planets. Consulting a jyotishi is recommended before using planetary mantras. Below are a few of the divine mantras that can be chanted on a regular basis.

## Divine Mantras

*The mantra should be chanted with great attention. Focus either on the sound of the mantra or on the meaning; or you can concentrate on each syllable of the mantra as you chant. You can also visualize the form of your beloved deity while chanting. Decide the total number of times you will chant the mantra each day. This will help you to do japa with determination. But do not chant heedlessly, just to reach a certain target number. The most important thing is that your mind is one-pointed. Using a mala will help you to count and also to maintain your concentration.*

*~ Amma*

Until the point where it is possible to receive a personal mantra from a Perfect Master like Amma, here are some general mantras. Their meanings are included. These can be chanted regularly.

*Om (Aum):* is the primordial sound, the original manifestation of consciousness. It can be chanted by itself, and is also used at the beginning of any mantra to give it more shakti (spiritual power). *Om* is the sound that precedes creation and lasts beyond the final dissolution. It is the sound that connects and contains all living beings.

*Ma:* represents the Divine Mother, and can be repeated by itself. *Ma* embodies the vibration of divine Love, the Mother of Creation.

*Jai Ma:* "Victory to the Divine Mother" or "Praise the Goddess of the Universe"

*Om Namah Shivaya:* This mantra is one of many ways of praising Lord Shiva. It means "I bow to the Divine Consciousness."

*Om Shivashaktyaikya Rupinyai Namah:* "I bow to Her who is the union of Shiva and Shakti in one form." This mantra is for the union of Shiva and Shakti, or purusha and prakriti. Divine Consciousness and Divine Energy work together to create and sustain the world.

*Om Sri Mata Amritanandamayi Devyai Namah:* This is a mantra for Amma that means "I bow to Amma, the Goddess of Immortal Bliss."

*Om Amritesvaryai Namah:* Another mantra for Amma, it means "I bow to the Goddess of Immortality."

*Om Parashaktyai Namah:* "Salutations to the Goddess who is the Supreme Energy." This mantra is for the Goddess of Creation.

*Om Gam Ganapatayai Namah:* "Salutations to Lord Ganapati." Ganapati is another name for Ganesha, the remover of all obstacles and the son of Shiva and Parvati.

*Om Gam Ganeshaya Namah:* "Salutations to Lord Ganesha," another mantra for Ganesha that helps to remove obstacles and bestow grace.

*Om Sri Hanumate Namah:* "Salutations to the Blessed Lord Hanuman, servant of Lord Rama." This mantra invokes the grace of Hanuman, Son of the Wind, who is endowed with prana. He bestows strength, devotion and faith.

*Om Sri Maha Lakshmyai Namah:* "Salutations to the Great Goddess Lakshmi." This mantra is for the Goddess Lakshmi, the goddess of wealth, beauty and all types of prosperity in the world.

*Om Dum Durgaya Namah:* "Salutations to the Goddess Durga." This mantra is for the Goddess Durga, who destroys the inner obstacles created by ego. Chanting this helps physical, mental, emotional and spiritual problems, and brings protection.

*Om Aim Saraswatyai Namah:* "Salutations to the Goddess Saraswati." The Goddess Saraswati bestows good memory, enhanced learning ability, creativity, knowledge, the power of speech, talent in the arts, including dance and music.

*Om Namo Bhagavate Vasudevaya:* "Salutations to the Supreme Lord Vasudeva." Vasudeva is a name of Lord Vishnu, the sustainer of all life in the world. Chanting this protects a devotee from many troubles and bestows the devotee with peace and prosperity.

*Om Kleem Krishnaya Namah:* "Salutations to the divine Lord Krishna." This mantra is for Lord Krishna, the Avatar, or incarnation of Lord Vishnu. Chanting this bestows love and devotion, and can solve all of the problems that devotees may suffer.

*Om Sri Ramaya Namah:* "Salutations to Lord Rama." This mantra is for Lord Rama, another incarnation of Vishnu, the preserver. It bestows blessings in all aspects of life. The name *Ram* can also be chanted alone.

*Om Krim Kalyai Namah:* "Salutations to the Great Goddess Kali, She who is the remover of darkness." This mantra is for the Goddess Kali who removes the darkness of ego from her devotees.

*Om Mani Padme Hum:* A Buddhist mantra meaning "Om, salutations to the Jewel of Consciousness [the mind], which resides at the heart's lotus."

*Om Tare Tu Tare Ture Svaha:* "Salutations to the Supreme Goddess Tara." A mantra to the Buddhist Goddess Tara, an aspect of Kali or the Divine Mother. She bestows grace and compassion.

*Om Ah Hum Vajra Guru Padma Siddhi Hum:* "I invoke Vajra Guru, Padmasambhava. May your blessings grant Supreme Realization." The mantra of Padmasambhava evokes blessings that help to overcome all obstacles. Padmasambhava was a historical Tibetan Buddhist Master who is said to have been born in a lotus flower. He was a renowned scholar, meditator, healer and Guru.

*Hare Rama, Hare Rama, Rama Rama, Hare Hare, Hare Krishna, Hare Krishna, Krishna Krishna, Hare Hare:* This mantra is for Lord Vishnu, the preserver, in the forms of Rama and Krishna.

*Mahamritunjaya Mantra – Om Tryambakam Yajamahe Sugandhim Pushtivardhanam Urvarukam Iva Bandhanan Mrityor Mukshiya Mamritat:* "We worship the Three-Eyed One, Shiva, who is divinely fragrant and who nourishes all beings. May he liberate us from death for the sake of immortality, just as a cucumber is severed from the bondage of a creeper." *Mritu* means "death" and *jaya* is "victory." Thus, the mantra means "to grant victory over both the ego and death." This powerful mantra can be chanted to attain good health, release from bondage and to solve many other problems. It has been called the greatest reliever from all evils and can be recited at any time like any other maha-mantra (great mantra).

*Gayatri Mantra – Om Bhur Bhuva Svaha, Tat Savitur Varenyam, Bhargo Devasya Dhimahi, Dhi Yo Yonah Prachodayat:* "We meditate upon the spiritual effulgence of that adorable, supreme Divine Reality. Please grant us liberation." The Gayatri mantra is the universal prayer extolled in the Vedas. It is one of the most commonly chanted mantras. It translates: *Om,* we meditate (*dhimahi*) upon the spiritual effulgence (*bhargo*) of that adorable, supreme Divine Reality (*varenyam devasya*), the source (*savitur*) of the physical (*bhur*), the astral (*bhuva*), and the heavenly (*svaha*) spheres of existence. May That (*Tat*) supreme divine being enlighten (*prachodayat*) our (*nah*) intellect (*dhiyo*) (so that we may realize the Supreme Truth).

## Mantras of the Chakras

Each chakra has a *beej* (seed) mantra that activates the chakra's power. These beej mantras assist in healing the physical, emotional, mental and spiritual aspects associated with the chakras. They can be chanted alone or all together.

1. *Muladhara*: *Lam* – Corresponds to the root chakra. Relates to the earth element. It is grounding, calming and gives the feelings of joy, contentment, peace and well-being.
2. *Svadishtana*: *Vam* – Corresponds to the reproductive organs. Relates to the water element, nectar and *ojas*. It inspires creativity, fertility and imagination.
3. *Manipura*: *Ram* – Corresponds to solar plexus and individual willpower and motivation. Relates to the fire element. It increases agni (digestive fire).

4. *Anahata*: *Yam* – Corresponds to the heart and gives enthusiasm and energy to manifest inspirations. Relates to the wind element and prana. Prana governs breath and the heart.
5. *Vishuddha*: *Ham* – Corresponds to the throat and breathing. It is related to the ether/space element. It governs prana and speech.
6. *Ajna*: *Ksham* – Corresponds to the third eye. It increases concentration and awareness, thus enhances meditation.
7. *Sahasrara*: *Om* – Corresponds to the enlightened Self. Chanting *om* leads to Divine Consciousness.

*It is a good practice to write a least one page of your mantra daily. Many people get better concentration by writing than by chanting. Also try to teach children the habit of chanting and neatly writing a mantra. This will also help them to improve their handwriting. The book in which the mantra is written should not be handled carelessly; it should be carefully kept in the meditation or shrine room.*

*~ Amma*

# Chapter 15

# Yoga in Ayurveda

*However much Vedanta we study, without doing sadhana, we
cannot experience Reality. That which we seek is within us, but
to reach it, we have to do sadhana.
To turn the seed into a tree, we have to plant it in the soil,
water it and fertilize it.
It's not enough to just hold it in our hands.*

*~ Amma*

*There is nothing to equal the supreme joy felt by
the Yogi of pure mind who has attained the state
of pure consciousness and overcome death.*

*~ Yoga Vasistha Sara, verse 4.25*

Creating a personal hatha yoga sadhana is extremely helpful on the
path of Self-realization. As explained previously, Ayurveda and yoga
are very closely aligned. Yoga is important for dissolving physical
tension and calming the mind before meditation. It is the perfect
ayurvedic exercise because it rejuvenates the body, improves digestion and removes stress. It can be done by anyone of any age. Yoga
asanas can balance all of the three doshas. Yoga tonifies every area
of the body and cleanses the internal organs of toxins, which is one
of the goals of Ayurveda. Similarly, yoga practitioners can benefit
from the ayurvedic dinacharyas (such as abhyanga, ayurvedic massage), which assist in removing toxins from the body and relaxing
the muscles for yoga practice.

Here is a glance at some of the similarities between yoga and Ayurveda:

- Both are ancient Vedic sciences. Yoga originates in the Yajur Veda. Ayurveda originates in the Atharva Veda and Rig Veda.
- Both recognize that maintaining a healthy body and mind is absolutely necessary for fulfilling the four aims of life (artha, kama, dharma and moksha).
- Both share the same spiritual anatomy and physiology, which consists of 72,000 nadis, seven main chakras, five koshas, the doshas and dhatus.
- Both recognize that the balance of doshas, dhatus and malas is essential for maintaining health.
- Both incorporate diet, herbs, asana, pranayama, meditation, mantra, prayer, puja and rituals for healing the body, mind, emotions and soul.
- Both emphasize physical health as a good foundation for mental, emotional and spiritual well-being.
- Both strive to increase sattva and maintain a balance of prana, tejas and ojas.
- Both incorporate the same spiritual psychology. Ayurveda embraces the shad darshan (six main schools of philosophy), including Patanjali's *Yoga Sutras* and Vedanta. They both understand that attachments are the cause of all suffering and that the ultimate state of health is experienced when we abide in our true nature, the Self, which is dwelling in peace regardless of the state of the physical body.
- Both use specific types of cleansing for the body to encourage the removal of waste products and toxins through their natural routes of elimination. Ayurveda uses panchakarma and yoga uses the shatkarmas.

## Personalized Yoga

Today there are numerous types of hatha yoga classes available around the world. Hatha yoga is the umbrella category containing most contemporary schools of yoga such as Anusara Yoga, Astanga yoga (as taught by Pattabhi Jois), Intregal Yoga, Iyengar Yoga, Sivananda Yoga and Vinyasa Yoga. Modern classes are usually held in large groups. While beneficial, this approach does not deeply address the needs of the individual. For thousands of years, yoga has been taught one-to-one, with the awareness that each person has unique needs. Yoga practices are most beneficial when tailored to support the individual's dosha, state of health and lifestyle. Asana should be practiced under the guidance of an experienced teacher.

For a balanced personal yoga practice, it is important to take into consideration the individual's body structure, prakriti (original constitution) and *vikruti* (present constitutional imbalance). Traditionally, hatha yoga was practiced individually with a master, who also prescribed diet, herbs, pranayama and mantra. Ayurvedic yoga is much more than just physical exercise. It aims at teaching the individual how to live in harmony with themselves, nature and the universe.

## The Benefits of Asanas

*Sadhana should become part of our nature, like brushing our teeth and taking a bath.*

~ *Amma*

According to Ayurveda, there are three main reasons for performing yoga asanas: as exercise for a healthful living regime; as therapy to treat specific disorders in the body and mind; and as a means to return the doshas to their natural state. The ultimate purpose of yoga is spiritual growth and advancement.

Scientific research is now proving that hatha yoga can assist in healing various diseases including arthritis, asthma, back pain, constipation, diabetes, diarrhea, digestive disorders, emotional and mental disorders, heart disease, hormonal imbalances, hypertension, immune weakness, insomnia, migraine headaches, neck pain, physical and mental fatigue, scoliosis, stress, thyroid disorders and numerous others conditions.

Hatha yoga enhances physical health through numerous methods. It strengthens muscles, maintains joint and spine flexibility and integrity, and balances the subtle anatomy (chakras, nadis and koshas). Furthermore, yoga relaxes, rejuvenates, strengthens and energizes the whole body and mind by tonifying and nourishing all of the body systems. Yoga assists in cleansing on all levels of being. On the mental and emotional levels, it harmonizes and stills one's thoughts, and brings self-awareness to the emotional processes. Yoga practice becomes a mirror in which one can examine the Self.

Yoga *chikitsa* (therapy) is often used in conjunction with Ayurveda or as a complimentary form of health care. An ayurvedic practitioner or yoga therapist aims at restoring balance by identifying the underlying causes of illness. The practitioner then helps the patient to develop an appropriate ayurvedic and yoga regime. The foundation and underlying premise of yoga chikitsa is to treat the whole person and bring balance to the doshas.

Yoga chikitsa includes the following: individual dosha assessment, dietary guidelines to restore the balance, lifestyle management, yoga asanas to balance the doshas, and ayurvedic and yogic sadhana recommendations that will bring one into a state of integration. Along with herbs, diet and pranayama, asanas can help to treat almost every disease.

The information presented here is for educational purposes only. It is not meant to replace formal learning from a teacher. All asanas should be performed only under the guidance of an experienced yoga teacher. In the west, there are many weekend and month-long yoga courses that certify one to teach yoga. This is not the traditional method for training and often results in underqualified teachers. It is recommended that yoga teachers have a strong personal and ongoing yoga sadhana. They need to be living a dharmic lifestyle and be dedicated to the upliftment of humanity and creation. They should follow all of the yamas and niyamas to the best of their ability, and should be of excellent character, free from pride. It is important to find a yoga teacher with whom you personally resonate. What is right for one person may not be right for another. Remember the old saying, "One person's medicine is another person's poison." Trust your intuition and let your heart be your guide.

## Ayurvedic Asanas According to Dosha

*Sthira sukham asanam.*

A yoga pose is a steady, comfortable position.

*~ Patanjali's Yoga Sutras, II.46*

*By asana one avoids diseases,*
*by pranayama one avoids adharma,*
*and by pratyahara the Yogi controls his [or her] mental activity.*

*~ Yoga Chudamani, verse 109*

*By a continual practice of yoga for three months, the*
*purification of the nadis takes place. When the nadis have*
*become purified, certain external signs appear on the body*
*of the Yogi. They are lightness of the body, brilliancy of*
*complexion, increase of the agni and leanness of the body,*
*and along with these, absence of restlessness in the body.*

*~ Yoga Tattva, Verses 44-46*

The majority of asanas are balancing to the three doshas. However, there are various asanas and sequences in which they may be practiced that specifically bring a deeper balance to the doshas. The sequences offered below are designed to assist in getting started. Please remember that asana should always be performed with knowledge of correct positioning, breathing, sequencing and counter-balancing.

## Vata Asanas

Vata-predominant individuals should remember to focus on stillness, grounding, strengthening and balancing while doing their practice. This emphasis will assist in calming the mind, strengthening the nervous system and regulating prana. Vatas should focus deeply on the breath while performing asana. This will help to increase prana, awareness and overall strength. The practice space should be free from distractions in a tranquil, nurturing atmosphere. When vatas are harmonious in their yoga asana practice, their muscles will be strong and steady and their joints will move freely without pain or stiffness. They will feel calm, grounded and centered.

### Vata-Pacifying Asanas
*Adho Mukha Svanasana* (Downward Facing Dog Pose)
*Anantasana* (Serpent Pose)
*Ardha Chandrasana* (Half Moon Pose)
*Baddha Konasana* (Bound Angle Pose)
*Bharadvajasana* (Side Legs Sitting Spinal Twist)
*Chaturanga Dandasana* (Plank Pose)
*Dandasana* (Staff Pose)
*Halasana* (Plough Pose)
*Janu Sirsasana* (Head to Knee Pose)
*Jathara Parivartanasana* (Reverse Stomach Pose)
*Konasana* (Open Legs Sitting Forward Bend)
*Marichyasana I, II and III* (Sage Twists)

*Padahastasana* (Hand to Foot Pose)
*Padangustasana* (Big Toe Pose)
*Padottanasana* (Spreading Legs Forward Bend)
*Parivritta Trikonasana* (Revolved Triangle Pose)
*Paripurna Navasana* (Boat Pose)
*Parsvakonasana* (Extended Side Angle Pose)
*Parsvottanasana* (Sideways Stretch)
*Sarvangasana I, II and III* (Shoulder Stands)
*Setu Bandha* (Bridge Pose)
*Shavasana* (Corpse Pose)
*Siddhasana* (Perfected Sitting Pose)
*Sirsasana* (Head Stand)
*Supta Padangusthasana* (Supine Big Toe Pose)
*SuptaVirasana* (Reclined Hero Pose)
*Surya Namaskar* (Sun Salutations)
*Tadasana* (Mountain Pose)
*Trikonasana* (Triangle Pose)
*Upavistha Paschimottanasana* (Sitting Forward Bend – include all variations)
*Urdhva Prasarita Ekapadasana* (Upward Leg Forward Bend Pose)
*Utkatasana* (Chair Pose)
*Uttanasana* (Extension Pose)
*Vasisthasana* (Sideways Plank Pose)
*VirabhadrasanaI, II and III* (Warrior Poses)
*Virasana* (Hero Pose)
*Vriksasana* (Tree Pose)
*Yoga Mudrasana* (Yoga Seal Pose).

## Vata Flow

1. *Surya Namaskar* (Sun Salutation), 6-12 repetitions
2. *Adho Mukha Svanasana* (Downward Facing Dog)
3. *Tadasana* (Mountain Pose)
4. *Utkatasana* (Chair Pose)
5. *Trikonasa* (Triangle Pose)

6. *Parivritta Trikonasana* (Reverse Triangle Pose)
7. *Virabhadrasana I* (Warrior Pose)
8. *Parsvakonasana* (Extended Side Angle Pose)
9. *Padangusthasana* (Foot Big Toe Pose)
10. *Padottanasana* (Spread Leg Forward Bend)
11. *Balasana* (Child's Pose)
12. *Sarvangasana II* (Supported Shoulder Stand)
13. *Halasana* (Plough Pose)
14. *Dandasana* (Staff Pose)
15. *Janu Sirsasana* (Head to Knee Pose)
16. *Virasana* (Hero Pose)
17. *Marichyasana I* and *III* (Sage Twist Pose)
18. *Jathara Parivartanasana* (Reverse Stomach Pose)
19. *Uttanasana* (Extension Pose)
20. *Surya Namaskar* (Sun Salutation), 6-12 repetitions
21. *Shavasana* (Corpse Pose)

## Asanas for Vata-Related Disorders

**Asthma** (respitory dryness, constriction and wheezing): *Adho Mukha Svanasana* (Downward Facing Dog), *Bhujangasana* (Cobra Pose), *Dhanurasana* (Bow Pose), *Halasana* (Plough Pose), *Matsyasana* (Fish Pose), *Paschimottanasana* (Half-Bound Lotus), *Salabhasana* (Locust Pose), *Sarvangasana* (Shoulder Stand), *Sirsasana* (Head Stand) and *Vajrasana* (Thunderbolt Pose)

**Backache:** All standing poses, especially *Virabhadrasana* (Warrior Pose), *Bhujangasana* (Cobra Pose), *Dhanurasana* (Bow Pose), *Halasana* (Plough Pose), *JatharaParivartanasana* (Reverse Stomach Pose), *Salabhasana* (Locust Pose), *Vajrasana* (Thunderbolt Pose) and most spinal twists done gently

**Constipation:** All standing postures, *Eka Pada Apanasana* (Wind Releasing Pose), *Navasana* (Boat Pose), *Sarvangasana* (Shoulder Stand), *Sirsasana* (Head Stand), *Uttana Padasana* (Stretched Leg Pose), *Yoga Mudrasana* (Yoga Seal) and forward bends (standing and sitting)

**Depression** (with fear, anxiety and nervousness): *Balasana* (Child's Pose), *Halasana* (Plough Pose), *Padmasana* (Lotus Pose),

*Shavasana* (Corpse Pose), *Vriksasana* (Tree Pose) and *Yoga Mudrasanasana* (Yoga Seal)

**Flatulence:** Standing forward bends, *AdhoMukhaVriksasana* (Hand Stand), *ArdhaBaddha Padma Paschimottanasana* (Half Bound Lotus with Head to Knee Pose), *Dhanurasana* (Bow Pose), *Janu Sirsasana* (Head to Knee Pose), *Jathara Parivartanasana* (Reverse Stomach Pose), *Mayurasana* (Peacock Pose), *Padahastasana* (Hand to Foot Pose), *Padangusthasana* (Big Toe Pose), *Paripurna Navasana* (Boat Pose), *Salabhasana* (Locust Pose), *Sarvangasana* (Shoulder Stand), *Setu Bandha Sarvangasana* (Bridge Pose from Shoulder Stand), *Sirsasana* (Head Stand) and *Uttanasana* (Intensely Extended Pose)

**Insomnia:** *Adho Mukha Svanasana* (Downward Facing Dog Pose), *Balasana* (Child's Pose), *Bhujangasana* (Cobra Pose), *Savasana* (Corpse Pose) and *Vajrasana* (Thunderbolt Pose)

**Menstrual Disorders** (to encourage proper menstrual flow): *Bhujangasana* (Cobra Pose), *Chakrasana* (Wheel Pose), *Halasana* (Plough Pose) and *Yoga Mudrasanasana* (Yoga Seal)

**Sciatica:** All forward bends, *Adho Mukha Svanasana* (Downward Facing Dog), *Bhujangasana* (Cobra Pose), *Eka Pada Apanasana* (Wind Releasing Pose), *Halasana* (Plough Pose), *Jathara Parivartanasana* (Reverse Stomach Pose), *Sarvangasana* (Shoulder Stand), *Sirsasana* (Head Stand), *Swastikasana* (Cross Legged Forward Bend), *Supta Padangusthasana* (Supine Big Toe Pose), *Vajrasana* (Thunderbolt Pose) and *Yoga Mudrasanasana* (Yoga Seal)

**Sexual Debility:** Poses that lift the body up to rest on the hands, *Bakasana* (Crane Pose), *Halasana* (Plough Pose), *Sarvangasana* (Shoulder Stand), *Utthita Padmasana* (Elevated Lotus Pose) and *Vajrasana* (Thunderbolt Pose)

**Varicose Veins:** *Adho Mukha Vriksasana* (Downward Facing Tree/Hand Stand), *Ardha Chandrasana* (Half Moon Pose), *Bhekasana* (Frog Pose), *Eka Pada Sarvangasana* (One Leg Shoulder Stand), *Salamba Sarvangasana* (Supported Shoulder Stand), *Sarvangasana* (Shoulder Stand), *Shavasana* (Corpse Pose), *Sirsasana* (Head Stand), *Supta Virasana* (Supine Hero Pose), *Vajrasana* (Thunderbolt Pose) and *Virasana* (Hero Pose)

# Pitta Asanas

Pitta individuals need to remain calm and cool, and keep a relaxed intention while doing asanas. Pitta types benefit from cultivating an attitude of forgiveness and surrender, and by offering the fruits of their practice to the Divine. Asana practice generates heat in the body, so it is best for pittas to do yoga asanas at cooler times of the day, such as dawn or dusk. It is also beneficial to place emphasis on asanas that help to release excess heat from the body. These include poses that compress the solar plexus and poses that open the chest. When pittas are harmonious in asana practice they will experience steadfastness, tolerance, patience and a deep feeling of love and compassion. Their bodies will feel cool and their minds calm.

## *Pitta-Pacifying Asanas*
*Adho Mukha Vriksasana* (Hand Stand)
*Anantasana* (Serpent Pose)
*Bandha Sarvangasana* (Shoulder Stand to Bridge)
*Bhujangasana* (Cobra Pose)
*Chandra Namaskar* (Moon Salutations)
*Eka Pada Sarvangasana* (One Leg Extension Shoulder Stand)
*Halasana* (Plough Pose)
*Jathara Parivartanasana* (Reverse Stomach Pose)
*Kraunchasana* (Heron Pose)
*Kurmasana* (Tortoise Pose)
*Makarasana* (Crocodile)
*Marichyasana* (Sage Twist and all variations)
*Parivrittaikapada Sirsasana* (Leg Twist in Head Stand)
*Paschimottanasana* (Full Forward Bend and all variations)
*Sarvangasana* (Shoulder Stand)
*Setu Pada Hastasana* (Hand to Foot Pose)
*Shavasana* (Corpse Pose)
*Siddhasana* (Perfected Sitting Pose)
*Sirsasana* (Head Stand)

*Supta Konasana Sarvangasana* (Open Angle Shoulderstand)
*Surya Namaskar* (Sun Salutations, performed slowly with conscious breath awareness)
*Urdhva Dhanurasana* (Upward Bow Pose)
*Virasana* (Hero Pose)
*Yoga Mudrasana* (Yoga Seal Pose)
*Yoga Nidrasana* (Yogic Sleeping Pose)

## Pitta Flow

1. *Shavasana* (Corpse Pose)
2. *Surya Namaskar* (Sun Salutation), 6-12 repetitions
3. *Tadasana* (Mountain Pose)
4. *Vriksasana* (Tree Pose)
5. *Padottanasana* (Spread Leg Forward Bend)
6. *Adho Mukha Svanasana* (Downward Facing Dog Pose)
7. *Bidalasana* (Cat Pose)
8. *Balasana* (Child's Pose)
9. *Janu Sirsasana* (Head to Knee Pose)
10. *Paschimottanasana* (Full Forward Bend)
11. *Parivritta Janu Sirsasana* (Revolving Head to Knee Pose)
12. *Anantasana* (Serpent Pose)
13. *Supta Padangusthasana* (Supine Big Toe Pose)
14. *Jathara Parivartanasana* (Reverse Stomach Pose)
15. *Sarvangasana III* (Full Shoulder Stand)
16. *Halasana* (Plough Pose)
17. *Adho Mukha Vriksasana* (Hand Stand)
18. *Balasana* (Child's Pose)
19. *Baddha Konasana* (Bound Angle Sitting Pose)
20. *Siddhasana* (Perfected Sitting Pose)
21. *Shavasana* (Corpse Pose)

## Asanas for Pitta-Related Disorders

**Acidity:** All standing postures, especially *Bhujangasana* (Cobra Pose), *Dhanurasana* (Bow Pose), *Paripurna Navasana* (Boat

Pose), *Salabhasana* (Locust Pose), seated spinal twists and *Virabhadrasana I, II* and *III* (Warrior Poses)

**Anger/Hatred:** *Balasana* (Child's Pose), *Dhanurasana* (Bow Pose), *Padmasana* (Lotus Pose), *Sarvangasana* (Shoulder Stand) and *Shavasana* (Corpse Pose)

**Colitis:** *Apanasana* (Wind Releasing Pose), *Bhujangasana* (Cobra Pose), *Dhanurasana* (Bow Pose), *Matsyasana* (Fish Pose) and *Paripurna Navasana* (Boat Pose)

**Hypertension:** All forward bends, *Bhujangasana* (Cobra Pose), *Halasana* (Plough Pose), *Padmasana* (Lotus Pose), *Paripurna Navasana* (Boat Pose), *Sarvangasana* (Shoulder Stand), *Shavasana* (Corpse Pose) and *Siddhasana* (Perfected Sitting Pose)

**Hyperthyroidism:** *Eka Pada Apanasana* (One Leg Wind Releasing Pose), *Karna Pidasana* (Ear to Knee Pose) and *Sarvangasana* (Shoulder Stand)

**Liver** Disorders: Forward bends, all spinal twists, *Apanasana* (Wind Releasing Pose), *Ardha Godha Pitham* (Half Alligator Pose), *Janu Sirsasana* (Head to Knee Pose), *Matsyasana* (Fish Pose), *Padmasana* (Lotus Pose), *Salabhasana* (Locust Pose) and *Sarvangasana III* (Shoulder Stand)

**Malabsorbtion:** *Apanasana* (Wind Releasing Pose), *Matsyasana* (Fish Pose), *Parivritta Trikonasana* (Reverse Triangle Pose) and *Salabhasana* (Locust Pose)

**Migraines:** *Balasana* (Child's Pose), *Matsyasana* (Fish Pose), *Salamba Sarvangasana* (Supported Shoulder Stand) and *Sarvangasana* (Shoulder Stand)

## Kapha Asanas

A kapha person's practice needs to be energetic, warming and stimulating. Vinyasa (a flowing style of yoga) is good for kapha, as it is dynamic and moves fluidly from one pose to the next. In this way, sweating is induced and the heart rate increases. Surya Namaskar is a perfect vinyasa for kapha types. Signs of successful asana practice are normalization of body weight, tonification of muscle mass, free-flowing prana (lack of congestion), balanced energy, and an overall feeling of contentment.

## Kapha-Pacifying Asanas

*Adho Mukha Svanasana* (Downward Facing Dog Pose)
*Baddha Konasana* (Bound Angle Pose)
*Bhujangasana* (Cobra Pose and all variations)
*Ekapadasana* (Upward Leg with Forward Bend Pose)
*Eka Pada Rajakapotasana* (Pigeon Pose)
*Paripurna Navasana* (Boat Pose)
*Parivritta Janu Sirsasana* (Reverse Head to Knee Pose)
*Purvottanasana* (Front Stretched Pose)
*Salabhasana* (Locust Pose)
*Sarvangasana* (Shoulder Stand)
*Sirsasana* (Head Stand)
*Supta Padangusthasana* (Supine Big Toe Pose)
*Surya Namaskar* (Sun Salutation)
*Tadasana* (Mountain Pose)
*Trikonasana* (Triangle Pose)
*Urdhva Dhanurasana* (Upward Bow Pose)
*Vasisthasana* (Sideways Plank Pose)
*Virabhadrasana I, II and III* (Warrior Poses)
*Vriksasana* (Tree Pose)

## Kapha Flow

1. *Surya Namaskar* (Sun Salutation), 12-24 repetitions
2. *Tadasana* (Mountain Pose)
3. *Vriksasana* (Tree Pose)
4. *Virabhadrasana I, II, III* (Warrior Poses)
5. *Trikonasana* (Triangle Pose)
6. *Parivritta Trikonasana* (Reverse Triangle Pose)
7. *Sirsasana* (Head Stand)
8. *Balasana* (Child's Pose)
9. *Adho Mukha Vriksasana* (Hand Stand)

10. *Tadasana* (Mountain Pose)
11. *Ardha Chandrasana* (Half Moon Pose)
12. *Virabhadrasana I* (Warrior Pose)
13. *Chaturanga Dandasana* (Plank Pose)
14. *Vasisthasana* (Side Plank Pose)
15. *Sarvangasana III* (Full Shoulder Stand)
16. *Setu Bandha Sarvangasana* (Bridge Pose from Shoulder Stand)
17. *Navasana* (Boat Pose)
18. *Eka Pada Rajakapotasana* (Pigeon Pose)
19. *Dhanurasana* (Bow Pose)
20. *Surya Namaskar* (Sun Salutations) 6, 12 or 18 repetitions
21. *Shavasana* (Corpse Pose)

## Asanas for Kapha-Related Disorders

All kapha imbalances – asthma, sinus congestion, bronchitis, diabetes, sluggish or weak digestion, sore throat, sinus headache, obesity – can be balanced with the same asanas. Kapha imbalances are rectified through all standing poses, all forward bends.

*Adho Mukha Svanasana* (Downward Facing Dog Pose)
*Bhujangasana* (Cobra Pose)
*Dhanurasana* (Bow Pose)
*Dvipada Viparita Karani* (Inverted Pose)
*Gomukhasana* (Cow Pose)
*Halasana* (Plough Pose)
*Jathara Parivartanasana* (Reverse Stomach Pose)
*Matsyasana* (Fish Pose)
*Mayurasana* (Peacock Pose)
*Paripurna Navasana* (Boat Pose)
*Salabhasana* (Locust Pose)
*Sarvangasana* (Shoulder Stand)
*Simhasana* (Lion Pose)
*Sirsasana* (Head Stand)
*Ustrasana* (Camel Pose)
*Vajrasana* (Thunderbolt Pose) and *Vriksasana* (Tree Pose)

# The Therapeutic Properties of 40 Common Asanas

*When the mind maintains awareness,
without mingling with the senses,
nor the senses with sense impressions,
then Self-awareness blossoms.*

~ *Patanjali Yoga Sutras, II.54*

As we surrender deeper into our spiritual practice, we start awakening to new levels of reality. This can be compared to peeling an onion – beneath each layer is another layer until we reach the center and realize it is empty. It is through that emptiness that we are filled. Until we empty ourselves completely (by removing the layers of ignorance), we must continue diligently with our spiritual practice. Having knowledge of what the benefits of asanas are and why we practice them can inspire us to deepen our yoga practice.

Here is a guide to many of the therapeutic properties of yoga asanas.

*Adho Mukha Svanasana* (**Downward-Facing Dog**). Tridoshic. This asana calms the brain, relieves stress and mild depression, and energizes the body. It stretches the shoulders, hamstrings, calves, arches of the feet and hands while strengthening the arms and legs. It greatly helps to relieve the symptoms of menopause and menstrual discomfort. However, when menstrual flow is heavy, this pose should be avoided; instead, use supine and seated poses. Adho Mukha Svanasana can help prevent osteoporosis and other vata-related bone disorders. It improves digestion by increasing agni and relieves headache, insomnia, back pain and fatigue. This pose is highly therapeutic for high blood pressure, asthma, flat feet, sciatica and sinusitis. It is also reported to provide relief from hangovers.

*Adho Mukha Vriksasana* (**Hand Stand**). Tridoshic. This asana strengthens the shoulders, arms and wrists while stretching the abdominal muscles. It improves the sense of balance, calms the brain and relieves stress and mild depression.

*Ardha Chandrasana* (**Half Moon Pose**). Tridoshic. This asana strengthens the abdomen, ankles, thighs, buttocks and spine. It stretches the groin, hamstrings, calves, shoulders and chest. It can improve coordination and balance, while relieving stress and improving digestion.

*Ardha Matsyendrasana* (**Half Lord of the Fishes Pose**). Tridoshic. This asana has numerous health benefits. It very effectively stimulates the liver and kidneys. It stretches the shoulders, hips and neck while energizing the spine. By stimulating agni, it improves digestion and assimilation. It relieves menstrual discomfort, fatigue, sciatica and backache. Its therapeutic qualities relieve asthma and increase prana flow. It is excellent for promoting fertility. Traditional yoga texts say that Ardha Matsyendrasana increases appetite, destroys most deadly diseases and awakens kundalini shakti.

*Baddha Konasana* (**Bound Angle Pose**). Tridoshic. This asana stimulates abdominal organs, ovaries, prostate gland, bladder, kidneys and heart. It improves general circulation. It stretches the inner thighs, groin and knees. This asana relieves mild depression, anxiety and fatigue. It soothes menstrual discomfort and symptoms of menopause. It alleviates sciatica, high blood pressure, infertility and asthma. It can be practiced until late into pregnancy and is known to help ease childbirth. The traditional yoga texts say that Baddha Konasana destroys disease and eliminates fatigue and exhaustion.

*Bakasana* (**Crane Pose**). Tridoshic. Bakasana strengthens arms and wrists while stretching the upper back. It strengthens the abdominal muscles and opens the groin. It also tones the abdominal organs and increases digestive fire.

*Balasana* (**Child's Pose**). Tridoshic. Child's pose gently stretches the hips, thighs and ankles, while calming the brain and relieving stress, and physical and mental fatigue. It also relieves back and neck pain when done with the head and torso supported.

*Bharadvajasana* (**Bharadvaja's Twist**). Tridoshic. This spinal twist stretches the spine, shoulders and hips while massaging the abdominal organs. It helps to relieve lower backache, neck pain and sciatica as well as deep-seated stress. It greatly improves digestion and is especially good in the second trimester of pregnancy for strengthening the lower back. It is also said to alleviate the pain associated with Carpal Tunnel Syndrome.

*Bhujangasana* (**Cobra Pose**). Tridoshic, increases pitta. Cobra pose strengthens the spine and stretches the chest, lungs, shoulders and abdomen. It tones and firms the buttocks while stimulating the abdominal organs and increasing agni. This action counteracts stress and fatigue by opening the heart and lungs to increase prana flow; therefore, it also has a great therapeutic effect on asthma. The traditional yoga texts say that Bhujangasana increases body heat, destroys disease and awakens kundalini.

*Chaturanga Dandasana* (**Four-Limbed Staff Pose**). Increases pitta, decreases vata and kapha. In this action the arms and wrists are strengthened and the abdomen is toned. This pose is also good for increasing digestive fire.

*Dhanurasana* (**Bow Pose**). Increases vata and pitta, decreases kapha. Dhanurasana stretches the entire front of the body, ankles, thighs, groin, abdomen, chest, throat and the psoas. It also strengthens the back muscles and improves posture. The organs of the abdomen and neck are toned and stimulated here as well.

*Eka Pada Rajakapotasana* (**One-Legged King Pigeon Pose**). Increases vata and pitta, decreases kapha. This asana stretches the thighs, groin, psoas, abdomen, chest, shoulders and neck while stimulating the abdominal organs. It opens the shoulders and chest, increasing prana.

*Garudasana* (**Eagle Pose**). Tridoshic. Eagle pose strengthens and stretches the ankles, calves, thighs, hips, shoulders and upper back. It also improves concentration and balance.

*Gomukhasana* (**Cow Face Pose**). Tridoshic, increases pitta. This asana stretches the ankles, hips, thighs, shoulders, armpits, triceps and chest. It increases prana by opening the chest.

*Halasana* (**Plough Pose**). Tridoshic. This simple asana has many benefits. It calms the brain and mind to reduce stress and fatigue, while stimulating the abdominal organs and the thyroid gland (to increase immunity). It stretches the shoulders and spine and has therapeutic benefits for backache, headache, infertility, insomnia and sinusitis. It also reduces symptoms of menopause.

*Janu Sirsasana* (**Head-to-Knee Pose**). Decreases vata and pitta, increases kapha. Janu Sirsasana calms the brain, helps to relieve mild depression, and stretches the spine, shoulders, hamstrings and groin. It stimulates the liver and kidneys, improves digestion, and helps to relieve symptoms of menopause and menstrual discomfort, anxiety, fatigue, and headache. Therapeutic effects are found on high blood pressure, insomnia and sinusitis. It is excellent during pregnancy (up to the second trimester) as it strengthens the back muscles.

*Kraunchasana* (**Heron Pose**). Tridoshic. This pose stretches the hamstrings and stimulates the abdominal organs and heart, thus increasing the flow of prana.

*Marichyasana I, II and III* (**Pose Dedicated to the Sage Marichi**). Tridoshic. This asana calms the brain and reduces tension while stretching the spine and shoulders and stimulating the the liver, stomach, spleen, pancreas and kidneys. By stimulating the abdominal organs, it increases agni to relieve constipation. It also helps with sciatica, lower back and hip pain, and menstrual cramping.

*Matsyasana* (**Fish Pose**). Tridoshic. It is said that Matsyasana is the destroyer of all diseases. It stretches and stimulates the deep hip flexors (psoas), the muscles between the ribs (intercostals), the abdominal organs and muscles, and the front of the neck and throat. It improves posture by strengthening the muscles of the upper back and the back of the neck.

*Natarajasana* (**Lord of the Dance Pose**). Tridoshic. This asana stretches the shoulders, chest, thighs, groin and abdomen. It strengthens the legs and ankles while improving balance.

*Navasana* (**Boat Pose**). Tridoshic. Boat pose strengthens the abdomen, hip flexors and spine. The kidneys, thyroid, prostate glands and intestines are stimulated. It increases digestive fire and helps to alleviate constipation, stress and nervous tension.

*Padmasana* (**Lotus Pose**). Tridoshic. In the *Yoga Chikitsa* it says that Padmasana destroys all kinds of diseases and awakens Divine Consciousness. It calms the brain, reduces stress and alleviates tension in the body and mind. The pelvis, spine, abdomen and bladder are stimulated. This asana also stretches the ankles, hips and knees. Other benefits include the reduction of menstrual discomfort and sciatic pain. Daily practice of this pose until late into pregnancy is said to help ease childbirth.

*Padottanasana* (**Spread-Legged Forward Bend**). Tridoshic. This position strengthens and stretches the inner and back legs and spine, and tones the abdominal organs. The mind is calmed to reduce stress, and mild back pain is alleviated.

*Parivritta Trikonasana* (**Revolved Triangle Pose**). Tridoshic. This pose strengthens and stretches the legs, hips and spine. As the asana is held, the chest opens to improve breathing and prana flow; it can relieve mild back pain if inflammation is not present. It stimulates the abdominal organs and improves strength and balance.

*Parsvakonasana* (**Extended Side Angle Pose**). Decreases vata and kapha, increases pitta. This asana strengthens and stretches the legs, knees, ankles, groin, spine, chest, lungs and shoulders. It stimulates abdominal organs, increasing stamina and improving digestion and elimination. It also improves balance and concentration.

*Paschimottanasana* (**Sitting Forward Bend**). Decreases vata and pitta, increases kapha. The multiple therapeutic actions of this asana include calming the brain, relieving stress and mild depression, and stretching the spine, shoulders and hamstrings. The liver, kidneys, ovaries and uterus are all stimulated and digestion is improved. It is excellent for relieving the symptoms of menopause and menstrual discomfort as well as soothing headaches, anxiety and fatigue. This asana has healing effects on high blood pressure, infertility, insomnia, obesity, low appetite and sinusitis.

*Salamba Sarvangasana* (**Supported Shoulder Stand**). Tridoshic. This is one of the oldest and most curative asanas of all. The yogic scriptures declare that it can relieve allergies and asthma, stimulate the thyroid, and calm and rejuvenate the nervous system. It is used to pacify almost all vata disorders. In addition, it boosts the immune system, strengthens the heart, calms the mind, helps to relieve stress and mild depression, and stimulates the thyroid, prostate glands and abdominal organs. It stretches the shoulders and neck while toning the legs and buttocks. These actions improve digestion, reduce fatigue and alleviate insomnia. Infertility, sinusitis and menopausal disorders can be treated with this asana.

*Shavasana* (**Corpse Pose**). Tridoshic. Shavasana is the most important yoga asana. It looks easy, but may actually be the hardest asana to master. It requires complete relaxation and surrender. This may sound easy, but in today's world most people do not know how to truly relax. Shavasana means "corpse pose" and the purpose of this asana is to surrender everything. When we have surrendered or have reached complete relaxation, God may come and dance in our hearts freely. Tension keeps the Divine at a distance. Shavasana is calming to the brain and helps to relieve stress and mild depression through deep relaxation. Effects include reduced headache, fatigue, insomnia and blood pressure.

Shavasana should always be practiced after doing yoga asanas. It should be practiced with awareness of breath. It has the potential to relieve any and all tension being held in the body. Vata types can stay in Shavasana for 20 - 30 minutes, pitta types for 15 -25 minutes and kapha types 5 - 15 minutes. This practice allows the energy that was generated and released in the yoga practice to freely flow throughout the body, allowing the body to heal and be nourished. Shavasana is an essential part of any yoga sadhana.

*Simhasana* (**Lion Pose**). Tridoshic. This posture is excellent for relief of tension in the chest and face. One great benefit of this asana is that it stimulates the platysma, a flat, thin, rectangular shaped muscle on the front of the throat. The platysma, when contracted, pulls down on the corners of the mouth and wrinkles the skin of the neck. Simhasana helps to keep the platysma toned as we get older. This asana also increases agni, and tonifies stomach, spleen and pancreas.

*Sirsasana* (**Head Stand**). **Decreases vata and kapha, increases pitta.** Sirsasana calms the brain and helps to relieve stress and mild depression. It invigorates the pituitary and pineal glands and has all of the same properties and healing affects as Sarvangasana. Additionally, it strengthens the lungs, prana, arms, legs, abdominals and spine.

*Supta Padangusthasana* (**Reclining Big Toe Pose**). Tridoshic. This position stretches the hips, thighs, hamstrings, groin and calves, and strengthens the knees. It stimulates the prostate gland, improves digestion, eases backache and sciatic pain, soothes menstrual discomfort, and helps with high blood pressure, flat feet and infertility.

*Tadasana* (**Mountain Pose**). Tridoshic. This asana improves posture, strengthens thighs, knees and ankles, and tones the abdomen and buttocks. It relieves sciatica and flat feet. It is good for centering, especially between other asanas.

*Urdhva Dhanurasana* (**Upward-facing Bow Pose**). Decreases kapha, increases vata and pitta. This asana strengthens the heart arteries and protects them against thickening. It also strengthens and tonifies the spine, and abdominal and back muscles. It regulates the pituitary, pineal and thyroid glands and increases agni. In females, it protects against uterine prolapse and helps with menstrual flow and cramping.

*Ustrasana* (**Camel Pose**). Tridoshic. This is excellent for opening the chest and respiratory system. It benefits all bronchial ailments. It is extremely beneficial for sciatica. It removes stiffness of the back and shoulders while strengthening the lower and mid-back muscles and spine. All of the organs receive an increase in blood flow benefiting their proper functions. Ustrasana alleviates abdominal cramping and helps to regulate menstrual flow.

*Utkatasana* (**Chair Pose**). Decreases vata and kapha, increases pitta. This stance strengthens the ankles, calves, thighs and the spine. It also stretches the shoulders and chest while invigorating the abdominal organs, diaphragm and heart. Prana flow and digestive fire are increased by this asana.

*Uttanasana* (**Intense Forward Bend Pose**). Tridoshic. This forward bend has countless healing benefits. It calms the mind to help relieve stress and mild depression. The liver and kidneys are highly energized and digestion improves in this position. It has curative benefits for headaches, insomnia, asthma, high blood pressure, infertility, osteoporosis and sinusitis. Additionally, it relieves fatigue and symptoms of menopause.

*Utthita Trikonasana* (**Extended Triangle Pose**). Tridoshic. This asana stretches and strengthens the ankles, calves, hamstrings, knees, thighs, hips, groin, shoulders, chest and spine. It tonifies the abdominal organs and thereby improves digestion. It greatly helps to relieve stress, anxiety and nervous tension. It has powerful effects against infertility, osteoporosis, menopause and sciatic pain.

*Virabhadrasana* (Warrior Pose). Decreases vata and kapha, increases pitta. Warrior pose, and all of its variations, strengthen and stretch the ankles, legs, groin, chest, lungs, shoulders and abdominal organs. This dynamic action fuels the digestive fire, stamina and immunity. Practice of this asana relieves backaches, especially through the second trimester of pregnancy. Therapeutic benefits for Carpal Tunnel Syndrome, flat feet, infertility, osteoporosis and sciatica also results from this posture.

*Virasana* (**Hero Pose**). Tridoshic. This posture opens and stretches the thighs, knees, ankles and arches, and leads to improved digestion and relief of gas. Hero pose has excellent healing properties for high blood pressure, asthma and prana imbalances. It also helps to relieve symptoms of menopause, as well as leg swelling during pregnancy.

*Vriksasana* (**Tree Pose**). Tridoshic. Tree pose greatly restores the health of the liver, spleen and kidneys. It strengthens the thighs, calves, ankles and spine while stretching the groin, inner thighs, chest and shoulders. Maintaining this position increases mental concentration and balance; furthermore, it helps to relieve sciatica and improves flat feet.

# Chapter 16

# Stress and Dis-ease

*Children, love can accomplish anything and everything.
Love can cure diseases. Love can heal wounded hearts and
transform human minds. Through love one can overcome all
obstacles. Love can help us renounce all physical, mental and
intellectual tensions and thereby bring peace and happiness.*

~Amma

Humanity has always tried to attain peace and happiness through any and every available means. Nowadays, the need to attain mental peace is more urgent due to the tremendous increase in the stress of modern life. The body, mind, heart and spirit are subjected to the ravages of daily stress, which is the root cause of many diseases. Rapid industrialization, urban crowding, too much competition and excessive hurry are some of the major contributing factors leading to both stress and disease. Worries about physical security and economic difficulties also take a drastic toll on health and longevity.

The body reacts to physical or emotional stress by increasing the production of hormones such as cortisol and epinephrine. These hormones increase heart rate, blood pressure and metabolism to help the body react quickly to a stressful situation. In effect, the body in a state of stress creates extra energy to protect itself. This process is the body's natural "fight or flight" mechanism, and is incredibly useful in truly dangerous situations.

Unfortunately, the type of stress experienced by most people today is not a fleeting occurrence in a harmful situation, but an ongoing state many accept as a natural part of daily life. In fact,

276

many people are unaware of how stressed they really are. Because the extra energy produced by the body under stress cannot be destroyed, it creates imbalance within the whole body-mind system when not properly managed. This imbalance is what leads to disease.

At first, chronic stress can manifest as irritability, nervousness, sleeplessness, headaches and constipation. If these symptoms are not checked, the person may manifest new symptoms such as heart or vein palpitations or high blood pressure. If stress is allowed to continue even further, one may develop hypertension, ischemic heart disease, diabetes mellitus, bronchial asthma, migraines, rheumatoid arthritis, numerous skin conditions such as psoriasis, eczema, hives and acne. Other common manifestations of stress include disturbances of the digestive system, such as ulcerative colitis, peptic ulcers, stomachaches and diarrhea. Because chronic stress depletes and weakens the immune system, it renders one more susceptible to colds and other infections.

Chronic stress creates continuously high levels of cortisol, leading to an increase in appetite and thus weight gain. Being overweight puts one at serious risk for many diseases, especially those of the heart. Furthermore, cortisol also raises the heart rate, increases blood pressure, and increases blood lipid (cholesterol and triglyceride) levels, all of which make one more susceptible to heart attacks and strokes.

At the emotional level, when the body remains in a constant fight-or-flight response, one experiences increased feelings of anxiety, helplessness and depression. This is why chronic stress has been linked with severe depression.

## Stress-related Diseases

The American Psychological Association states that 43% of all adults suffer adverse health effects from stress, and 75–90% of all physician office visits are for stress-related ailments. Stress is linked to the seven leading causes of death: heart disease, cancer, lung disorders, cirrhosis of the liver, suicide, Alzheimer's disease and Diabetes mellitus.

Here is a partial list of conditions known to be directly triggered by stress. This is not a complete list of all stress-related illnesses. Remember, these diseases are not caused solely by stress, but stress is one of the major causes of their onset.

- Addictions
- Alcoholism
- Asthma
- Auto-Immune Disorders
- Bronchitis
- Cancer
- Cirrhosis
- Depression: acute and chronic
- Diabetes
- Fatigue
- Headaches: tension and migraine
- Impaired immune function
- Indigestion
- Insomnia
- Irritable Bowel Syndrome
- Ischemic heart disease
- Peptic ulcers
- Psychoneurosis
- Sexual dysfunction: infertility, impotency, sterility, etc.
- Skin diseases: eczema, psoriasis, dermatitis, etc.
- Stomatitis
- Suicidal tendencies
- Violence

## Types of Stress

External stressors include adverse physical conditions such as exposure to extreme temperatures of hot and cold, and a drastic change in temperature. Other common external stressors are psychological environments such as unpleasant working conditions, school pressures, unhealthful relationships, and having to meet difficult work deadlines. Traumatic life events, such as the death of a loved one, job loss, demotion or promotion, and the ending of a relationship are major external stressors.

Internal stressors can be physical, like bodily infections, or ongoing or unbearable pain. Many factors, such as lifestyle choices, negative thoughts, mental rigidity and self-imposed ideals, can create stress. Lifestyle choices include diet, use of drugs, alcohol and stimulants, sleeping patterns, daily schedules and relationships. Negative thoughts include self-doubt, pessimism, self-criticism, over-analyzing and worrying. Mental rigidity includes unrealistic expectations about ourselves, life and the situations we encounter. It also includes taking things personally, exaggeration, inflexible thinking and unnecessary self-limitations. Self-imposed idealism includes being a perfectionist or workaholic, and trying to please everyone all of the time.

Stress is also created when we are not in harmony with the four goals of life. When one strives to achieve one of the four goals in extreme, balance is disturbed and stress is experienced. This outcome is especially true for those excessively seeking kama and artha. Too often, pleasure and wealth are the primary motivations in life because one wrongly thinks they are the source of lasting happiness. These desires can be used for spiritual growth if harnessed correctly. With awareness, the desire to find a source of lasting happiness can lead us to look within, meditate and reflect on the true nature of things.

## Mental Stress

Mental stress, according to Ayurveda, is caused by an overuse or wrong use of the mental faculties. If you perform intense mental work for many hours a day, or if you work long hours on the computer, it can cause an imbalance in prana vata, the mind-body conductor responsible for brain activity, energy and the mind. The first symptom of prana vata imbalance is losing the ability to cope with basic daily stress. As the person becomes more stressed, the mind becomes hyperactive and the person loses the ability to make clear decisions, think positively, feel enthusiastic, and sleep soundly.

To reduce chronic mental stress, one can control mental activity by monitoring what sensory input is allow to enter into one's minds from television, radio, newspaper, and computers. For example, if one is regularly upset after watching the nightly news, perhaps reducing the amount of television watched is a good idea.

Pacifying prana vata is another way to reduce mental stress. The following measures balance prana vata:

- Go on a vacation somewhere quiet and peaceful.
- Follow a vata-pacifying diet with foods of the sweet, sour and salty tastes.
- Take warm milk and other light dairy products as long as they are pure and organic.
- Give yourself daily abhyanga with warm, vata-pacifying oils.
- Get sufficient rest.
- Avoid stimulants (like caffeine, especially if there is difficulty sleeping) and drink calming herbal teas.
- Meditation and aromatherapy appropriate to the dosha help to relax the mind as well.

### Emotional Stress

Emotional stress can be triggered by difficulties in a relationship, work environment or any stress to the emotional heart. Emotional stress manifests as irritability, anger, lust, depression and emotional instability. It affects sleep differently from mental stress in that it can cause one to wake up during the night, usually at pitta time (10 p.m. – 2 a.m.), and leave one unable to go back to sleep.

Emotional stress disturbs sadhaka pitta, the mind-body conductor responsible for the emotions and functioning of the heart. To balance emotional stress, follow a pitta-pacifying lifestyle and diet. The following practices are also useful:

- Take a relaxing vacation (such as a yoga or meditation retreat).
- Spend time in nature.
- Eat sweet and juicy fruits, especially blueberries, mangoes and dark grapes.
- Follow a pitta-pacifying diet with food of the sweet, bitter and astringent tastes.
- Drink a cup of warm milk with ½ - 1 teaspoon ghee before bed.
- Cook with cooling spices such as cardamom, coriander, cilantro and mint.
- Give yourself daily abhyanga with a cooling oil such as coconut or sandalwood oil.
- Go to bed before 10:00 p.m.

## Physical Stress

Physical stress is caused by wrong use or overuse of the body, such as exercising too much or working for extended periods beyond one's capability. This exertion will cause a person to experience physical fatigue and mental stagnation.

Excessive physical strain can cause the subdoshas to go out of balance. Sleshaka kapha is the subdosha concerned with lubrication of the joints and moisture balance in the skin. Vyana vata is responsible for circulation, nerve impulses and the sense of touch. Tarpaka kapha governs the neurological processes. All of these subdoshas are sensitive to physical strain and lack of exercise. Furthermore, a lack of exercise results in a sluggish and weak digestive fire and the formation of ama (toxins) in the colon. In both types of physical fatigue, the regeneration of cells slows down and the cells become physically tired.

The goal in such cases is to harmonize vata and to strengthen kapha, thus making the body more stable. The following practices are useful:

- Take a long relaxing vacation in nature (not the tourist type).
- Get sufficient rest and moderate exercise (yoga, qigong, tai chi, etc.).

- Follow a vata/kapha-pacifying diet.
- Regularly take warm baths with mineral salt and essential oils.
- Give yourself daily abhyanga with warm sesame or mustard oil.

# Coping with Stress

Identifying unrelieved stress and becoming aware of its effects on our lives is the single most important aspect of managing stress. There are many sources of stress, and there are equally as many possibilities of alleviating it. One should work toward the goals of eliminating the sources of stress and changing one's reactions to stress-provoking situations. One may do this by practicing thoughtful responses to such situations rather than reacting automatically. Here are some helpful guidelines for putting this stress-relieving method into action:

- Be aware of your stressors and your emotional and physical reactions to them.
- Recognize what is changeable and change it.
- Reduce the intensity of your emotional reactions to stress.
- Learn to moderate your physical reactions to stress.
- Build up your physical reserves (ojas).
- Maintain your emotional reserves (prana).

The following are suggested practices from Ayurveda and yoga to reduce stress in daily life:

- *Yoga Nidra* (yogic sleep, a simple guided meditation technique)
- Meditation
- Yoga
- Prayer
- Physical exercise
- Spending time in nature
- Listening to relaxing, peaceful music
- Massage
- Pranayama (gentle, relaxed, conscious breathing)
- Seva (selfless service) to the poor and needy
- Diet

Stress release begins with understanding what pushes you, what your major struggles are, how to put them into perspective, and how to make clear decisions on appropriate actions to take. Although modern society contributes to poor health in alarming ways, simple methods can be used to counteract negative influences and significantly improve health and vitality. Often, simple adjustments in diet and lifestyle can drastically improve our ability to cope with stress. Furthermore, practicing seva is one of the most effective ways of diverting the mind from personal burdens, thus relieving stress. Most people who work full-time jobs but still make time to do some volunteer work each week lead more fulfilling and less stressful lives.

## Herbal Remedies for Combating Stress

Drug companies nowadays are making billions of dollars a year on new drugs to treat stress and stress-related diseases. These drugs only mask the symptoms of stress, and often have many side effects. Ayurveda offers a much more holistic approach. Along with diet, numerous herbs and herbal preparations are available to help us cope with stress in a balanced way.

Herbs for calming the mind, reducing stress and strengthening the nervous system are easily available in most parts of the world. The benefit of taking herbs is that they can be taken safely long-term without side effects. Many of these herbs not only aid in the relief of stress, but also help purify the body of toxins.

Here is a list of the best ayurvedic herbs to use for stress-related diseases, disorders and disharmonies. A detailed, therapeutic description of these herbs can be found in the next chapter, Herbal Medicine.

- Ashwagandha
- Brahmi
- Jatamansi
- Kapikachhu
- Mandukaparni

- Shankapushpi
- Shatavari
- Vaccha

*Aum Sarvesham svastir bhavatu.*
*sarvesham shantir bhavatu.*
*Sarvesham purnam bhavatu.sarvesham mangalam bhavatu.*

May perfection prevail on all.
May peace prevail on all.
May contentment prevail on all.
May auspiciousness prevail on all.

# Chapter 17

# Herbal Medicine

"Doctor, I don't feel very well."
Doctor's response:
2000 BC – "Here, eat this root."
1000 BC – "That root is heathen, say this prayer."
1850 AD – "That prayer is superstition, drink this potion."
1940 AD – "That potion is snake oil, swallow this pill."
2000 AD – "That antibiotic is artificial. Here, eat this root!"

## The Use of Herbs

*We cannot know the purpose of everything. Nature is
a mystery to us. Therefore, we act foolishly and destroy
trees, plants and animals. Many ayurvedic herbs and
plants look to us like useless weeds. Out of ignorance
we destroy them, but a knowledgeable ayurvedic
physician knows how useful and significant they are.*

*- Amma*

Since the beginning of time, all traditional cultures and healing traditions have looked to the plant world as the main source of health, wealth and wellness. In all of the cultures of the world, plants have been used as a source of food, nutrition and medicine for the body, mind and spirit. Ayurveda, the most ancient and developed system of healing, relies on plants for many of its branches of healing.

Herbs have a wide range of effects on our body. Some herbs work as general tonics that cleanse, nourish and rebuild. Others may be used to treat related imbalances or symptoms in a specific system or organ. Due to their unique chemical components, herbs are usually effective in small doses and produce few or no side effects.

Ayurveda uses herbs as preventative medicine, before disease manifests. By strengthening agni (digestive fire) and the immune system, ayurvedic herbal remedies prevent the onset of many diseases and infections. Natural medicines can also increase or boost the immune system when under attack by viruses or bacteria. For serious illnesses such as cancer, AIDS and other autoimmune disorders, herbal treatment can serve as a very effective alternative or complimentary therapy to allopathic treatment. Herbs can provide nourishment and support for the body as it undergoes more intense forms of treatment that may reduce life force.

Herbal treatments are available in a variety of forms, for both internal and external use. Internal forms include taking tinctures, teas, encapsulated or tableted herbs, fresh herbs, dried herbs, flower essences, essential oil dilutions, and medicated wines, pastes, honeys and ghee. External treatments include using herbal and essential oil blends, liniments, powders, pastes, salves and lotions. These may be used topically as hot or cold compresses, as massage oils or as body wraps. Many essential oils are great for putting in baths, or can simply be inhaled.

## The Medicinal Benefits of Plants

Traditional Ayurveda derives all of its medicine from Mother Nature. Herbs are understood to be conscious, living beings that are here to assist humanity. According to Ayurveda, the medicinal value of plants depends largely on how and when they are grown and collected. For this reason, ancient Ayurveda practitioners planted and harvested the herbs according to the placement of the stars. They also used specific mantras during the planting, growing and harvesting times. All these practices increase the medicinal value of the herbs.

After intense observation, experimentation and documentation of hundreds of plants over a period of several thousand years, Ayurveda has come to accurate conclusions about their efficacy. Although the effectiveness of Ayurveda is well known throughout India, the benefits of this ancient wisdom remain relatively unknown to most of the world.

## Using Organic Herbs

Unfortunately, at the present time herbal medicines frequently contain pesticides, herbicides and heavy metals. Amma often reminds us that what used to be medicine has now become poison due to environmental pollution caused by humans. Pesticides, herbicides and heavy metals are proven to cause a wide array of diseases including cancer, brain damage, hair loss and nervous system deterioration, to name just a few.

Many people are suffering health disorders largely due to such chemicals in their air, food, water, home and workplace. It is difficult to heal from a disease caused by chemicals and heavy metals while taking medicines that are also filled with these toxins. If you purchase a non-organic herbal product advertised to help blood circulation or mental clarity, there is no guarantee that it is not also a carcinogenic neurotoxin due to the polluted soil and water that helped it grow.

Amma consistently reminds us that Mother Nature is in a state of major imbalance as a result of humans' lack of respect for Her. When we purchase organic medicines, we support sustainable agriculture, and thus contribute to healing the earth. For these reasons it is strongly encouraged to always use herbs that are organic and free of heavy metals and chemicals. Although properly grown herbs may be more expensive, they are worth it in the long run – benefiting both health and the earth.

# The Properties of Herbs

Ayurvedic herbs are categorized according to their herbal properties and functions. It is important that the ayurvedic practitioner has a proper understanding of which herb to use for a particular disease. A single herb may have multiple properties and one specific property may be present in many herbs.

By analyzing the symptoms and constitution of the patient, the practitioner determines the imbalances in the doshas and selects herbs or herbal formulations to balance them, based on the characteristics of the herbs. Likewise, the ayurvedic practitioner must be able to determine the real source of the patient's imbalance in order to apply the proper treatment. Unfortunately, ayurvedic herbalism is often practiced like allopathy. For example, a particular herb may be given for diarrhea without first determining the cause of the diarrhea. There are dozens of causes and numerous formulas for curing diarrhea. If diarrhea is caused by worms, for example, but it is treated without simultaneously removing the worms, then it is bound to surface again later. It is essential to understand and treat the root of the problem if we wish to permanently correct it.

All plants and herbs contained within Ayurveda's vast pharmacopeia are composed of the mahabhutas (five basic elements), and have been categorized according to the derivatives of these elements. They include: taste (rasa), properties (gunas), potency (virya), taste of the digested product (vipaka), specific properties (prabhavas) and actions (karmas).

There are six rasas: sweet, sour, salty, sharp/pungent, bitter and astringent. Each taste is composed of two of the five elements. The effects of each of the taste groups are as follows:

**Sweet** (madhura): This rasa consists of Earth and Water. It improves complexion, strengthens the body, heals wounds and ulcers, purifies the lymph and the blood.

**Sour** (amla): This rasa consists of Earth and Fire. It is carminative and digestive. It accumulates waste material that is secreted in the tissues, aiding in the process of eliminating the waste from the body.

**Salty** (lavana): This rasa consists of Water and Fire. It is digestive and relaxing. It purifies tissues, separates impurities, accumulates excretions in the system, clears the outlets of the system, and softens all the structures of the body.

**Pungent** (tikta): This rasa consists of Fire and Air. It increases digestive power, purifies the body, prevents obesity, relaxes the ligaments and the system in general, and diminishes formation of breast milk, semen and fat.

**Bitter** (katu): This rasa consists of Air and Ether. It is appetizing, digestive, purifying. It separates and cleanses the doshas, improves secretion of breast milk, reduces the quantity of feces, urine, perspiration, fat, marrow and pus.

**Astringent** (kasaya): It consists of Air and Earth. It heals ulcers, clears all discharges, separates impurities from tissues, and reduces obesity and excessive moisture.

The gunas are grouped in ten complementary pairs: heavy and light, cold and hot, wet/oily and dry, slow and sharp, stable and mobile, soft and hard, clear and sticky/cloudy, smooth and rough, subtle and gross, dense and liquid.

Virya is the energy, power or potency of the herb, determined as either heating or cooling, meaning that it either heats the body or cools it down. The virya of herbs follows the principles of food tastes. Pungent, sour and salty increase heat. Bitter, astringent and sweet cool the body down. Heating herbs increase agni and pitta, while decreasing kapha and vata. Cooling herbs decrease pitta by cleansing the blood, and generally increase vata and kapha.

Vipaka is the post-digestive effect herbs have on the body. The post-digestive effect is expressed in terms of taste; however, it can only be sweet, sour or sharp/pungent. This is because after the digestive process is complete, the six tastes become three: sweet and salty become sweet, sour remains as it is – sour, and bitter, astringent and pungent all become pungent.

Prabhava is the unique property of an herb or a substance (how it acts on the body in addition to the rasa, virya and vipaka). Often this refers to the material's affinity for a certain bodily organ or system. Different herbs may have the same rasa, virya and vipaka and still have a different prabhavas. Usually herbs with prabhava have unique actions that affect the subtle body and mind more than other herbs. They have unique powers that can heal on many levels.

Karma is the action of an herb on the body, as expressed in terms of the three doshas. An herb can increase or decrease any of the doshas.

## The Therapeutic Properties of Herbs

Herbal treatment is a gentle, effective and noninvasive method that works best in situations that are not life-threatening. Please be aware that the following information is for educational and informational purposes only. It is not in any way meant to diagnose, treat or cure any disease, disorder or imbalance. It is best to consult a qualified ayurvedic practitioner about which herbs are suitable for you.

All herbs have specific therapeutic properties that determine their usage. The following is a description of the properties that can accompany specific herbs.

- **Alteratives** cleanse and purify the blood. They remove toxins and have antibacterial and anti-infectious actions. They help restore the body to its normal functioning. Examples: aloe, burdock, garlic, guduchi, manjistha, neem, nettles, red clover, turmeric, yellow dock.
- **Analgesics** relieve muscular tension and pain. Examples: arnica, ginger, helichrysum, mustha, peppermint, solomon seal, tagara, valerian, white willow.
- **Antacids** neutralize acidity and correct pH balance in the stomach, blood and bowels. Examples: chandan, guduchi, kamadudha, moti bhasma, prawal bhasma, shankhabhasma, shatavari.

- **Antibacterials** destroy or stop the growth of bacterial infections. Examples: cat's claw, garlic, haritaki, mahasudarshan, neem, pau d'arco, turmeric.
- **Antibiotics** inhibit the growth and destroy viruses and bacteria. Promote the body's own immune system. Examples: asha, astragalus, chlorella, ginkgo biloba, ginseng, goldenseal, echinacea, mahasudarshan, royal jelly, and both turmeric and neem in large doses.
- **Anti-inflammatories** reduce inflammation. Examples: bringaraj, chandan, kamadudha, kumari, neem, prawal, shankha bhasma and shatavari.
- **Anti-parasitics/Anti-helmintics** remove parasites, worms, bacteria, molds, fungus and yeast from the body. They are excellent in treating candida and other yeast-type infections. Examples: apricot kernel, black walnut, clove, cumin, kutaja, neem, nutmeg, papaya seed extract, vidanga, wormwood.
- **Anti-pyretics** reduce heat in the body, fever and infections with fever. Examples: chandan, chaparral, chickweed, daruharudra, kutki (katuka), mahasudarshan, manjistha, neem, tulasi, turmeric.
- **Antispasmodics** relieve involuntary spasms. Examples: black cohosh, brahmi, jatamansi, kava, lemon balm, mustha, passion flower, sage, shankapushpi, skullcap, tagara, tulasi, calamus (vaccha), valerian.
- **Aphrodisiacs** stimulate and rejuvenate the reproductive organs. They increase virility and ojas. Examples: amalaki, ashwaghanda, bala, damiana, epemedium (horny goat's weed), ginseng, goksura, Kapikachhu, muira puama, passion flower, pippali, shatavari, tongkat ali, vidari, wild yam, yohimbe.
- **Astringents** create firm and condensed tissues and organs. They reduce discharge and secretions from the body. Examples: arjuna, ashoka, ashwaghanda, bala, bayberry, cleaver, cloves, dandelion, eucalyptus, hawthorne berry, rosemary, shepherd's purse, triphala, uva ursi, vidari, witch hazel, yarrow.
- **Bitter tonics** increase digestion. They are naturally drying and help to regulate fire in the body. Almost all bitter herbs are the same

as the anti-pyretics. Examples: chandan, chaparral, chickweed, daruharudra, kutki (katuka), mahasudarshan, manjistha, neem, tulasi, turmeric.

- **Cardiac tonics** strengthen the heart and regulate heart function. Examples: arjuna, gokshura, guduchi, hawthorne berry, punarnava.
- **Carminatives** assist in expelling gas from the intestines. They promote peristalsis, relieving vata dosha. They assist in digestion and increase absorption. Examples: angelica, anise, cardamom, catnip, celery seed, dill, fennel, ginger, hingwastak, parsley, peppermint, pippali, spearmint, thyme, trikatu.
- **Cholegogues** are herbs or substances that promote the flow of bile from the liver and gall bladder. They have a downwards purgation effect. Examples: aloe, bhringaraj, bumiamalaki, guduchi, karavella (bitter gourd), kutki, musta, sandalwood, turmeric.
- **Demulcents** are herbs that soothe the bodily tissues. The word demulcent comes from the Latin verb demulcere meaning "to caress." Something that is demulcent is caressing. A demulcent is an agent, such as oil, that forms a soothing film when administered to the surface of a mucous membrane. It relieves the irritation of the inflamed mucous membrane.
- **Diaphoretics** stimulate perspiration and circulation. They assist in eliminating toxins through the skin. Examples: bilva, garlic, guggulu, pippali, punarnava, sarsaparilla.
- **Diuretics** increase urination through stimulation of kidneys and bladder. They assist in reducing and removing toxins from the body. Examples: bala, bhumyamalaki, dandelion leaf, dashamula, fennel, gokshura, haridra, horsetail, kumari, parsley, punarnava, shankapushpi, tulasi, vanga bhasma, vidanga, yasthi madhu.
- **Emetics** induce vomiting. They assist in cleansing the system of toxins. Examples: emetic nut, vaccha, yasthi madhu.
- **Emmenagogues** promote and regulate healthy menstruation. They treat many female reproductive disorders. Examples: chasteberry (vitex), chitraka, haridra, manjistha, pippali, trikatu, triphala.

- **Emollients** soothe, smooth, soften and protect the skin. Examples: amalaki, bala, comfrey, ginseng, honey, Irish moss, jatamansi, licorice, marshmallow, slippery elm, vidari kanda.
- **Expectorants** promote discharge of phlegm, mucous and kapha from the body. They assist in cleansing the nasal passage, lungs and stomach. Examples: mahasudarshan, pippali, pushkarmula, sitopaladi, talisadi, vaccha, wild cherry bark, yerba santa.
- **Haemostatics** stop internal bleeding or hemorrhaging. They are similar to alterative herbs in that they purify the blood. Examples: cayenne, golden seal, hibiscus, manjistha, marshmallow, mullein, nettles, plantain, turmeric, self-heal.
- **Hepatics** strengthen and tone the liver. Examples: aloe vera, bhumyamalaki, bringaraj, bupleurem, burdock root, dandelion, guduchi, haridra, kumari, kutki, manjistha, milk thistle, neem, shankapushpi leaf.
- **Laxatives** promote healthy bowel movements, counteracting constipation, and removing obstructions of the colon. Examples: buckthorn bark, cascara sagrada, elder berries, kumari, kutki, pippali, psyllium seed, rhubarb, sat isabgol, senna, sitopaladi, triphala, yasthi madhu.
- **Nervines** strengthen and rejuvenate the nervous system. Depending on the specific herb, may have stimulating or sedating properties. They are harmonizing and nourishing for the mind and emotions. Examples: brahmi, chamomile, hops, jatamansi, lemon balm, mandukaparni, oats, passion flower, shankapushpi, St. John's wort, tagara, valerian, tulasi, vervain.
- **Purgatives** promote intense cleansing of the colon, usually through causing diarrhea. Examples: aloe, avipattikar curna, castor, rhubarb, senna.
- **Rejuvenatives** strengthen and restore the body, revitalizing the organs to prevent decay. In Ayurveda there is a whole branch of medicine dedicated to rejuvenation called *rasayanas*. Examples: amalaki, ashwagandha, bala, bibhitaki, brahmi, calamus (vaccha), comfrey, ginseng, gokshura, gotu kola, guggulu, haritaki,

Kapikachhu, makaradwaja bhasma, marshmallow, punarnava, pushkarmula, shring bhasma, shatavari, vidari kanda.

- **Sedatives** calm and tranquilize the body by reducing the functionality of the organ or body part involved. Reduce nervousness. Examples: hops, jatamansi, kava kava, lady's slipper, nutmeg, passion flower, tagara, valerian.
- **Stimulants** increase internal heat, circulation and metabolism. They dispel internal chill and increase all natural functions in the body. Examples: bala, calamus (vaccha), chitraka, ginseng, ginger, kutki, peppermint, pippali, yerba mate, yohimbe.
- **Tonics** are nutritive to the body. They promote weight gain and strength, and nourish the organs and dhatus. Examples: chayawanyaprash, brahmi rasayana, ashwagandha, brahmi, rasa sindhur, amalaki, shilajit, shatavari, bala, ghee, yasthi madhu, pushkarmula, Kapikachhu, muira puama, oat straw and tongkat ali.
- **Vulneraries** aid in healing wounds. They protect against infection and stimulate cell regeneration. Commonly used for cuts, scrapes and burns. Examples: aloe vera, arjuna, bringaraj, neem, nettles, rakta chandan, slippery elm bark, witch hazel.

## Nature's Pharmacy

Plants have an anatomy just as humans do. Each part of the plant works on one of the tissues of the human body. The juiced leaf of the plant works on the plasma (rasa dhatu). The resin or sap of the plant treats the blood (rakta dhatu). The softwood from plants works on the muscle (mamsa dhatu) of the human body. The gum or hard sap of plants treats the fat (meda dhatu). The bark from plants and trees works on the bone (asthi dhatu) of the human body. The leaf of the plant treats the marrow and nerve tissue (majja dhatu). The flowers and fruits of plants work on the reproductive system (shukra/arthava dhatu) of the human body.

| ...ant | Dhatu |
|--------|-------|
| Ju.. .eaf | Rasa / Plasma and Lymph |
| Resin, sap, roots | Rakta / Blood |
| Softwood | Mamsa / Muscle |
| Gum, hard sap | Meda / Fat |
| Bark | Asthi / Bone |
| Leaf | Majja / Marrow and nerve tissue |
| Flowers, fruit | Shukra – Arthava / reproductive organs |

Plants contain the five elements in their different parts. The roots and bark contain the earth and water elements. The flowers are of the fire element. The leaves and fruit of the plant are of the air and ether elements. Each plant also contains its own unique ojas, tejas and prana and transmits specific properties when taken internally.

Some people are healed simply by touching plants or breathing in their subtle vibrations. Tulasi is one such plant that is said to be so powerful that it purifies the atmosphere wherever it grows.

Vata dosha is ruled by plants with sparse leaves, rough and cracked bark, crooked and gnarled branches and very little sap. Pitta is ruled by plants that are bright in color, have bright flowers, sap, moderate strength and are full of heat. Kapha plants are full and abundant in growth, have abundant leaves and sap and are heavy with abundant water content.

## Common Healing Herbs

**Aloe** *(Aloe indica):* The Sanskrit word for aloe is *kumari,* which means "young, female virgin." As its name suggests, it gives an abundance of youthful energy. Traditionally, the juice and leaves are used. This herb is bitter, astringent, pungent and sweet (rasa), sweet (vipaka) and cooling (virya). It alleviates all three of the doshas; furthermore, it is excellent for pain, inflammation and skin-heat disorders. It works on all of the dhatus and has special

295

healing effects on the circulatory, digestive, female reproductive and excretory systems. It is an alterative and bitter tonic that acts as a rejuvenative, emmenagogue and purgative. Additionally, it has a vulnerary action and is an especially good tonic for the liver and spleen. Aloe is one of the best blood purifiers and doubles in potency when combined with turmeric (*haridra*). Together they are extremely valuable in treating tumors, cysts and cancers.

**Amalaki/Amla** *(Phyllanthus embilca/Embilca officinalis):* Amalaki, Indian gooseberry, is often referred to as *dhatri,* which means "nurse." Its healing capacity is compared to a nurse or mother, acting as an all-around tonic and rejuvenator. The roots, seeds and leaves have medicinal value, but it is the fruit that is used primarily. Amalaki contains all tastes except salty. It is mostly sour, sweet (vipaka) and cooling (virya). It alleviates all three doshas; however, it is especially good for pitta disorders. Amalaki works on all the dhatus. It is antacid, anti-inflammatory, antipyretic, alterative, adaptogen, digestive stimulant, mild laxative, hepatoprotective, astringent, haemostatic, antioxidant, cardiotonic, nutritive, tonic and aphrodisiac.

In the *Charaka Samhita,* amalaki is said to bestow long life, intelligence, memory, immunity, health, youth, glow, vigor. It enhances voice, complexion and sexual vigor. Amalaki is used to cure innumerable disorders. It enhances appetite, improves digestion, relieves constipation, counteracts hyperacidity, nourishes the hair and treats liver and spleen diseases. Amalaki is one of three fruits that make up the traditional ayurvedic formula *triphala* (meaning "three fruits").

**Arjuna** *(Terminalia arjuna):* Arjuna is most famous for its abilities to treat heart diseases. Traditionally, the bark is used. It is astringent (rasa), pungent (vipaka) and cooling (virya). It alleviates kapha and pitta doshas. It works on the rasa, rakta, mamsa, asthi and majja dhatus, as well as the circulatory, digestive and

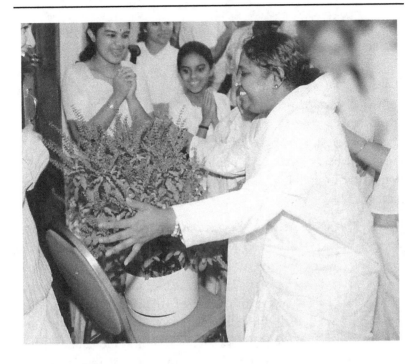

nervous systems. It works directly with the body's prana, and has unique abilities to strengthen the heart muscles. It is used as a heart tonic, circulatory stimulant, alterative, astringent and haemostatic. This herb is one of the best to arrest bleeding both internally and externally. It increases longevity and treats cardiac disease, diabetes mellitus, diarrhea, dysentery and obesity.

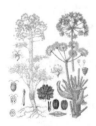

**Asafoetida** *(Ferula asafetida):* Asafoetida is called *hing* or *hingu* in Sanskrit. It is one of the best herbs for the digestive system, removing ama from the gastrointestinal tract. It is pungent and salty (rasa), pungent (vipaka) and warming (virya). It alleviates vata and kapha. This herb penetrates all of the dhatus except the reproductive system (shukra). It benefits the digestive, nervous, respiratory, excretory and circulatory systems. It is stimulating, carminative, antispasmodic, analgesic, anti-helmintic, aphrodisiac and antiseptic.

Asafoetida is excellent in the treatment of worms and parasites. It also alleviates gas and abdominal distention, intestinal colic pain, constipation, arthritis, rheumatism, asthma, cough, convulsions and other nervous system disorders. This herb is very effective at increasing agni. It works especially well with chitraka and trikatu as one of the best digestive stimulants. It is a very common herb used frequently in cooking, and found in most Indian and ayurvedic kitchens.

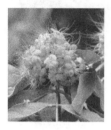

**Ashoka** *(Saraca indica):* Ashoka means "remover of all sorrows." It is one of the most widely used uterine tonics, and is renowned for its ability to stop pain and excess bleeding. The bark, seeds, flowers and fruits of this tree are used medicinally. It is bitter (rasa), pungent (vipaka) and cooling (virya). It reduces pitta and kapha doshas. It works on the rakta, mamsa, meda and asthi dhatus. Ashoka is astringent, alterative, analgesic, diuretic, and cardiac and uterine tonic.

It has a unique effect on the female reproductive channels and the circulatory system. It helps to alleviate all types of bleeding diseases, such as menorrhea and menorrhagia. It is excellent against uterine spasms and associated pain. It also helps to regulate menstruation. Ashoka works on the digestive system to alleviate bleeding piles and hemorrhoids and can also have beneficial effects against colitis and bleeding ulcers. As it works on the circulatory system, it benefits cardiac weakness and arrhythmia. Ashokaristam is a popular formula that is used to treat all types of reproductive weaknesses.

**Ashwagandha** *(Withania somnifera):* Ashwagandha means "smell of a horse" and is said to give the vigor of a horse. It is one of the primary rejuvenatives and aphrodisiacs in ayurvedic medicine. The root of this plant is used alone and in numerous traditional formulas. Its rasa is sweet, astringent and bitter; it has a sweet vipaka and hot virya. It nourishes all of the dhatus. Specifically, it has healing properties for the reproductive, nervous and respiratory systems. This herb increases ojas and prana, and contains nervine, sedative, tonic and astringent properties. It is good as a painkiller and anti-inflammatory agent; thus, it is used in treatment of rheumatic disorders.

Beyond all of these benefits, it also has excellent calming and nourishing effects on the mind, acting as an adaptogen to help the body cope with stress and fatigue. It is also used in large doses as an aphrodisiac. Ashwagandha can be used for any disorders involving general stress, convalescence, weakness or debility.

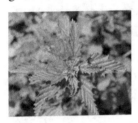

**Bala** *(Sida cordifolia):* Bala means "strength" or "that which strengthens." Along with ashwagandha, it is one of the prime rejuvenatives in the plant world. Traditionally, the leaves, roots and seeds were used, although modern Ayurveda mostly utilizes the root. Bala is sweet (rasa and vipaka) and cooling (virya). It alleviates both pitta and vata doshas. Although it works on all of the dhatus, in the *Charaka Samhita* it is said to have special properties as a rejuvenative for muscle (mamsa dhatu). It is a tonic, rejuvenative, aphrodisiac, demulcent, diuretic, stimulant, nervine, analgesic and is vulnerary in action. It is also extremely beneficial in sexual debility and infertility. Use of bala alleviates all types of vata disorders. It also makes excellent medicinal oil for treatment of arthritis, rheumatism, gout, weak and debilitated muscles, exhaustion, emaciation and convalescence.

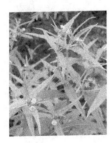

**Bhringaraja** *(Eclipta alba):* In Sanskrit, bhringaraja translates as "that which bestows hair that has the splendid color of a humming bird." It is also called *kesharaja* or "king of the hair," *markava* or "that which prevents premature graying,"

and *kesharanjana* meaning "that which bestows a beautiful tinge to the hair." The whole plant, including the seeds, is incorporated into ayurvedic formulas. Bhringaraja is pungent and bitter tasting (rasa), pungent (vipaka) and hot (virya). It alleviates kapha and vata doshas and is an excellent rejuvenator and tonic. It works on the rasa, rakta, asthi and majja dhatus as well as the circulatory, nervous and digestive systems.

The properties of bhringaraja are alterative, haemostatic, antipyretic, nervine, laxative and vulnerary. In addition to improving the quality of hair it is very beneficial to the eyes and skin. It prevents aging and supports healthy growth and function of the bones, teeth, hair, vision, hearing and mental cognition. It is a potent rejuvenative for the liver and spleen, especially when taken together with brahmi.

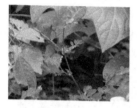

**Bhumyamalaki** *(Phyllanthus niruri):* Bhumyamalaki is said to be one of the best herbs for all liver disorders. It is especially beneficial for viral hepatitis B, jaundice, malaria and cirrhosis (enlargement of liver and spleen). The leaves and juice of the whole plant are used medicinally. It is bitter, astringent and sweet (rasa), sweet (vipaka) and cooling (virya). It works on the rasa, rakta and asthi dhatus, as well as the circulatory, digestive and skeletal systems.

The beneficial actions of this herb are as an alterative, cholagogue, anti-inflammatory, vulnerary and diuretic. In addition to being helpful for the liver, it can be used for eye disease, venereal disease, diabetes, diarrhea, menorrhagia, leucorrhea, urinary tract infections, fever and blood weakness. Bhumyamalaki and amalaki are an excellent combination for treatment of pitta and liver disorders.

**Bibhitaki** *(Terminalia belerica):* Bibhitaki means "the one that keeps you away from disease." The fruit of this tree is used to make an extremely effective laxative and bowel tonic. Its tastes are astringent (rasa), sweet (vipaka) and hot (virya). It has the special potency (prabhava) of a laxative that alleviates all three of the doshas. It works specifically on the rasa, mamsa and asthi dhatus, as well as the respiratory, digestive, excretory and nervous systems. It has rejuvenative properties that are beneficial for the hair, throat and eyes. In addition to being a laxative and rejuvenative, it has astringent, tonic, expectorant, anti-helmintic and antiseptic actions on the body. It is excellent for kapha-type accumulations in the colon, lungs and urinary tract. This herb is an excellent astringent and tonic for the stomach and it increases appetite. It has also been proven worthy in treatment against piles and worms. It is one of the three fruits that make up the ayurvedic formula triphala.

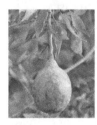

**Bilva** *(Aegle marmelos):* Bilva is sacred to Shiva, and is known as *Shivadruma* or "the tree of Shiva." It is used in *pujas, homas, yagnas* and other traditional ceremonies. This herb is mentioned in all of the ancient ayurvedic texts, as well as in the *Rig Veda* and *Yajur Veda*. Traditionally, the roots, skins, leaves and fruits are used as medicine. The immature fruit has the most beneficial healing properties. It has astringent and bitter tastes (rasa), and is pungent (vipaka) and hot (virya). Although it alleviates all three doshas, due to its hot nature it can increase pitta if taken in excess. It works on rasa, rakta, meda and majja dhatus, as well as the digestive, excretory and nervous systems. It is an astringent and digestive stimulant. This herb is one of the best for treating chronic and acute diarrhea. It corrects weak digestion and malabsorption, thereby increasing agni and small intestine functions. This herb is very effective against worms and parasites, especially when taken with neem and vidanga. The roots and leaves can be added to the fruit and used in treatment of bacterial, typhoid and other types of fevers.

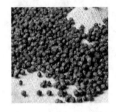

**Black Pepper** *(Piper nigrum):* Due to its hot potency, black pepper is called *marich*, which is another name for the sun in Sanskrit. Black pepper has many healing properties and is used both internally and externally. Black pepper has a pungent taste (rasa), pungent feel (vipaka) and hot effect (virya). It decreases vata and kapha while greatly increasing pitta and the digestive fire. It works on the plasma (rasa), blood (rakta), fat (meda) and marrow-nerve (majja) dhatus, as well as the digestive, circulatory and respiratory systems. It is a stimulant, expectorant, carminative, febrifuge and anti-helmintic. Mixed with sesame oil, it has beneficial healing properties for skin diseases like scabies and leukoderma. A paste application helps to reduce swelling, burning and itching. Black pepper has been proven excellent for treating chronic indigestion, ama in the colon, weak metabolism, congestion, fever and cold extremities.

An ayurvedic formula called trikatu, used to increase digestive fire and metabolism, contains black pepper as one of its main ingredients. Black pepper is a panacea for anorexia, dyspepsia, the enlargement of liver and spleen, and is beneficial for all types of skin diseases. Mixing black pepper with tulasi and honey makes an excellent treatment for fevers.

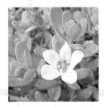

**Brahmi** *(Bacopa monnieri):* The word *brahmi* comes from the Sanskrit word *Brahma*, the "Creator of the Universe." In the *Charaka Samhita*, brahmi is called *samjna sthapana*, meaning "that which restores consciousness." There is much confusion about authentic brahmi. The *Bacopa monnieri* species that is found in south India is said to be true brahmi. In north India, the species *Centella asiatica* (mandukaparni) is often used as brahmi; although it has very similar properties, it is different and inferior to the *Bacopa* variety. Brahmi is bitter and astringent in taste (rasa), sweet after digestion (vipaka) and cold in effect (virya). It has the prabhava to alleviate epilepsy, hysteria, and pitta and vata doshas. It works on the blood (rakta) and marrow and nerve (majja) dhatus. The whole plant is used for this medicine. The leaves are exceptionally good, especially when juiced. Its main properties are rejuvenative, through imparting longevity, memory and intelligence.

This natural brain tonic also acts as a sedative, antispasmodic, alterative and diuretic agent. Brahmi is used to treat a wide range of disorders, including anxiety, panic, fear, nervous system disorders, debility, muscle spasms, paralysis, urinary tract infections, and to boost the immune system. When taken together with bhringaraja it is excellent for the hair. Brahmi should be kept in every household medicine chest. Brahmi thailam can be used in the daily practice of nasya as well as in panchakarma.

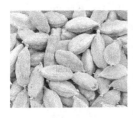

**Cardamom** *(Elettaria cardamomum):* In Sanskrit, cardamom is known as *ela.* The seed and pot are used medicinally. It is pungent and sweet in taste (*rasa*), sweet after digestion (vipaka) and hot in its effect (virya). It is one of the best herbs for alleviating vata and kapha disorders. Cardamom is extremely effective against cough, asthma, tuberculosis and piles. It works on the plasma (rasa), blood (rakta) and marrow and nerve (majja) dhatus as well as the digestive, respiratory, circulatory and nervous systems. This common spice acts as a stimulant, expectorant, carminative, stomachic and diaphoretic. It is one of the best digestive stimulants, as it enkindles agni and destroys kapha in the stomach and lungs. Cardamom oil is used with much benefit on toothaches. Cardamom mixed with ginger, tulasi and honey helps to dissolve blocked phlegm that causes coughs.

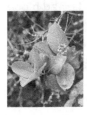

**Chandan** *(Santalum album):* Commonly known as sandalwood, this plant can be used internally and externally. The wood and the volatile oils that come from it can be used medicinally. The powder can be

303

used internally; the essential oil is applied externally. Chandan is widely used for cosmetic purposes, as it rejuvenates the skin and improves complexion. Homes and temples throughout India and Asia use sandalwood for traditional worship (pujas), because it creates sattva and increases the quality of meditation.

This plant is bitter and sweet in taste (rasa), pungent after digestion (vipaka) and cold in its effect (virya). It decreases pitta and vata and it is neutral for kapha except when taken in excess. It works on plasma (rasa), blood (rakta), muscle (mamsa), marrow and nerve (majja) and reproductive (shukra) dhatus, as well as the circulatory, nervous and digestive systems. Sandalwood is alterative, haemostatic, antiseptic, antibacterial, carminative, sedative and refrigerant.

It is very useful for pitta diseases, especially disorders of the blood and skin. It arrests bleeding, relieves body aches, relieves thirst, and counteracts toxins. It is effective against liver disease, jaundice, dysentery, burns, acute gastritis, hyperacidity, eye disorders, cystitis, vaginitis, acne, delirium, vomiting, menorrhagia, hematuria, gonorrhea, sexually transmitted diseases and numerous other disorders. This herb is one of the best to cool and calm the mind, body and nervous system.

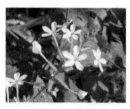

**Chitrak *(Plumbago zeylanica):*** Chitrak is also refereed to as agni (fire), *jvala* (flame) and *aruna* (sun) due to its heating attributes. Traditionally, the root is used for medicinal purposes. Chitrak is pungent and bitter in taste (rasa), pungent after digestion (vipaka) and has a very hot bodily effect (virya). It alleviates vata and kapha by dissolving toxins and greatly increases pitta dosha. In order to be taken internally, it must first be purified in lime juice, otherwise it can be toxic. This herb works especially well on fat (meda) and blood (rakta) dhatus and on the digestive system; consequently, it is one of the best ayurvedic herbs for increasing agni of the liver, spleen and small intestine, which are all pitta organs. Chitrak is excellent for combating weak appetite, constipation, urticaria, indigestion, abdominal distention, bleeding piles, hemorrhoids, parasites, edema, arthritis and numerous other vata and kapha disorders. It should be avoided during pregnancy, as it is a known abortifacient.

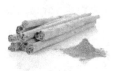

**Cinnamon *(Cinnamomum zeylanica):*** In Sanskrit, cinnamon is called *tvak,* meaning "skin." It is very appropriately named, as the skin of the tree, or bark, is the part used in cooking. This spice is pungent, bitter and sweet in taste (rasa), pungent after digestion (vipaka) and has a hot effect (virya). As it is very warming, it helps to alleviate vata and kapha doshas. Cinnamon works on plasma (rasa), blood (rakta), muscle (mamsa), and marrow and nerve (majja) dhatus, as well as the circulatory, digestive, respiratory and urinary systems. It behaves as a stimulant, digestive, diaphoretic, carminative, alterative, expectorant, diuretic and analgesic agent. This plant is usually chosen to treat diseases caused by ama, heart problems, piles, worms, sinusitis, asthma, cough and disorders of the urinary tract. It is excellent at increasing agni and, combined with ginger, makes an excellent digestive tea.

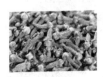

**Clove *(Syzygium aromaticum):*** The Sanskrit name for clove is *lavanga.* The dried flower buds are used for both internal medicine and as essential oil. Clove is pungent and bitter in taste (rasa), pungent after digestion (vipaka) and cold in its final effect (virya). It alleviates kapha and pitta. Clove works on the plasma (rasa), muscle (mamsa), marrow and nerve (majja) and reproductive (shukra) dhatus; its actions include those of a stimulant, expectorant, carminative, analgesic and aphrodisiac. It is primarily used for lung ailments such as colds, cough, asthma, bronchitis and hiccup; additionally, it improves digestive disorders like indigestion or weak digestion. Clove oil rubbed into the gums is very effective against toothaches and gingivitis. As a tea or mixed with other tonic herbs, it helps to counter impotency. Clove is one of the main ingredients in the traditional ayurvedic formula *avipattikar churna,* which is very effective against indigestion and hyperacidity.

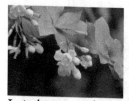

**Daruharidra** *(Berberis aristata):* In western herbology, this herb is called barberry. Its specific prabhava is elimination of ama. All parts of the plant are used for medicinal purposes. It is used both internally and externally. It is bitter and astringent in taste (rasa), pungent after digestion (vipaka) and hot in its overall effect (virya). As a blood purifier it is excellent for alleviating kapha and pitta doshas. It works on plasma (rasa), blood (rakta) and fat (meda) dhatus, as well as the circulatory and digestive systems. Barberry is a strong, bitter tonic and anti-amoebic substance. It is alterative, diaphoretic, rejuvenative, anti-pyretic, laxative, anti-helmintic, antibacterial. This herb is used for healing wounds, debility and general weakness, hemorrhoids, fever, infections, enlargement of liver and spleen, amoebic dysentery, acne, boils, blood-related disorders, jaundice, hepatitis, cervical ulcers, diabetes and obesity.

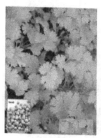

**Dhanyaka** *(Coriandrum sativum):* Known as coriander in the west, dhanyaka is frequently found in Indian kitchens. While it is excellent for cooking, it also possesses great medicinal benefits. The whole plant is used medicinally. It alleviates all three doshas because it helps to digest ama and is beneficial to the heart and mind. It works on the plasma (rasa), blood (rakta) and muscle (mamsa) dhatus, as well as the digestive, respiratory and urinary systems. Coriander is an alterative, diaphoretic, diuretic, carminative and stimulant substance in action. In the *Charaka Samhita,* it is said to improve taste and appetite. It is astringent, bitter and sweet in taste (rasa), sweet after digestion (vipaka) and hot in its effect (virya). Its prabhava is as an appetizer. It is especially effective in alleviating pitta disorders of the digestive tract, urinary system, glandular swelling, cervical adenitis, edema and stomatitis. When made into a paste, coriander alleviates swelling and pain. It can be used to treat allergies, hay fever and immune weaknesses due to accumulation of ama.

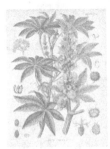

**Eranda** *(Ricinus communis):* Eranda is known in the west as castor. The seeds, roots, leaves and oil are all used for medicinal purposes. Castor is sweet, pungent and astringent in taste (rasa), sweet after digestion (vipaka) and has a hot effect (virya). It alleviates both vata and kapha doshas. This plant is superb for treating vata disorders where ama is involved. It is cathartic, demulcent, analgesic and nervine by nature. Castor oil is applied externally for pain and swelling in cases of arthritis, sciatica, rheumatism, gout, mastitis and many other skin diseases. When applied to the abdomen, it assists in relieving gas and distention. It can be taken internally for a number of vata-related diseases, including arthritis, sciatica, facial palsy, paralysis, body aches, tremors, headaches and constipation. Given with ginger and/or triphala, it makes a very powerful purgative. The juice from the leaves is useful in treating hepatitis and other pitta and blood-related disorders.

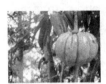

**Garcinia** *(Garcinia cambogia, Mangostana):* This herb is excellent for lipid metabolism, digestive stimulation and weight reduction. The root and fruit of the plant are used medicinally. It is pungent and bitter in taste (rasa), pungent after digestion (vipaka) and has a cold effect (virya). This herb works directly on the digestive system and secondarily on the muscular and nervous systems. It is also useful as a sedative and antispasmodic agent. Well established as a fat-burning herb, garcinia is a very effective herbal medicine for controlling obesity and cholesterol. It works directly on fat (meda) and muscle (mamsa) dhatus. It is known to subdue the appetite, slowing down the conversion of excess carbohydrates into fat.

This plant contains a biologically active compound that is known to inhibit the synthesis of lipids and fatty acids and lower the formation of LDL and triglycerides. Garcinia also contains significant amounts of vitamin C and is used as an immune and heart tonic. It creates thermogenesis, a process wherein internal body heat burns up unwanted fat and toxins. It also helps with catarrhal conditions of the throat. It has a cleansing effect on the urinary system and the uterus. Garcinia also treats insomnia, anxiety, restlessness and other nervous system disorders. It reduces acidity and increases mucosal defense in the gastric areas, justifying its use as an anti-ulcer agent.

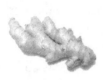

**Ginger *(Zingiber officinale)*:** In India, ginger is known as *sunthi,* which means "dry" and *ardraka,* which means "fresh." Ginger is also called *mahausadhi,* meaning "great medicine" and *visvabhesaja,* meaning "universal medicine." This root is pungent in both the initial and post-digestive tastes (rasa and vipaka) and hot in effect (virya). It alleviates vata and kapha and controls pitta vitiation. Sunthi has the prabhava of being an aphrodisiac, as it increases circulation. It works on all of the dhatus and on the digestive and respiratory systems. Ginger is a stimulant, aphrodisiac, expectorant, carminative, anti-emetic and diaphoretic medicine. It works well against dyspepsia, anorexia, nausea, colds and flu, asthma, cough, heart disease, hemorrhoids and piles. Sunthi, jaggery and sesame combined are an excellent panacea for rheumatic disorders.

It is practical that ginger is used so widely in cooking, as it is extremely supportive for digestion. Ginger is also one of the three ingredients in the famous ayurvedic digestive formulation of trikatu. Mixed with vidanga, it eliminates intestinal worms. The wide variety of its uses makes it another "must have" in any medicine chest.

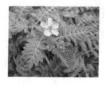

**Gokshura *(Tribulis terrestris)*:** *Go* means "cow" and *kshura* is defined as "scratcher." Gokshura clears and scrapes obstructions from the tissues.

The fruit of this plant is found in numerous ayurvedic formulations. Gokshura is one of the best healing herbs for the urinary and reproductive systems as well as the nervous and respiratory systems. It is sweet in the initial and post-digestive tastes (rasa and vipaka) and cold in effect (virya). It alleviates all three of the doshas. It works on the plasma (rasa), blood (rakta), marrow and nerve (majja) and reproductive (shukra/arthava) dhatus. It behaves as a diuretic, rejuvenative, aphrodisiac, tonic, nervine and analgesic medicine.

Gokshura is used to treat impotency, infertility, seminal debility, venereal diseases, kidney and bladder stones, cystitis, difficult or painful urination, edema, hemorrhoids and numerous other disorders. It has excellent rejuvenative properties for the female reproductive system. When mixed with guggulu (a medicinal tree resin), it is known as gokshuradi guggulu and is one of the best formulas for treating diabetes, gout and sexual debility in both men and women.

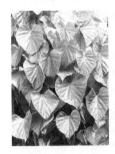 **Guduchi** *(Tinospora cordifolia):* Guduchi means "the one who protects the body." Another name for guduchi is *amrit*, or "nectar." Guduchi is one of the most widely used rejuvenative herbs, as it works on all of the dhatus in the body. It is one of the strongest immune stimulants and harmonizes the functions of all of the organs. Guduchi is also called *vyastha,* or "that which promotes longevity" and *rasyani*, meaning "that which rejuvenates." Guduchi balances all of the doshas. The roots, stems and leaves are used medicinally. It is bitter, pungent and astringent in taste (rasa), sweet after digestion (vipaka) and hot in effect (virya). Guduchi has the special prabhava of being an antitoxin. It also works as a sedative and an antispasmodic agent. This multipurpose herb increases immunity and longevity, enhances memory and overall health, bestows luster to the skin, improves the voice, eyesight and hearing, and boosts energy. It also helps to correct digestive disorders like hyperacidity, colitis, worms, parasites, loss of appetite and vomiting.

Additionally, it helps all liver disorders. Guduchi is excellent for pitta imbalances like fevers and blood disorders.

**Guggulu** *(Commiphora mukul):* Guggulu means "that which protects against disease." Guggulu is bitter, pungent, sweet and astringent in taste (rasa), pungent after digestion (vipaka) and hot in its effect (virya). Guggulu is a resin that alleviates all three of the doshas. It is especially beneficial for vata and kapha disorders, such as arthritis, rheumatism, gout, lumbago, all nervous system disorders, epilepsy, debility, bronchitis, obesity, diabetes, whooping cough, dyspepsia, hemorrhoids, pyorrhea, skin diseases, ulcers, endometriosis, tumors and cancers. When taken in excess, guggulu can slightly increase pitta.

This herb works on all of the dhatus as well as the nervous, circulatory, respiratory and digestive systems. Its actions are rejuvenative, alterative, antiseptic, analgesic, antispasmodic, nervine, expectorant and stimulating. Guggulu is effective in cleansing and healing regimes. There are numerous ayurvedic formulas that contain guggulu as their base, such as triphala guggulu, yogaraj guggulu, rasnadi guggulu, gokshuradi guggulu, kaishore guggulu, amrutadi guggulu, kanchanar guggulu, mahayogaraja guggulu and chandraprabha vatika. Mixed with guduchi, gokshura and sunthi, guggulu alleviates vata-related pain.

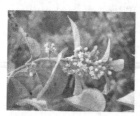

**Gurmar (Gymnema sylvestre):** Gurmar is also known as *Madhuvinashini,* the destroyer of sweet. It is one of the most commonly used plants for treating blood sugar imbalances. It treats a wide variety of diabetes related symptoms. It is used to treat pancreatic secretions including the production of insulin. Its is bitter and astringent (rasa), cooling (virya) and pungent (vipaka). Gurmar is used to alleviate the pitta and kapha dosha. It works on rasa, rakta, medha and shukra and artava dhatus. Its actions are hypoglycaemic, antidiabetic, diuretic and hypocholesterolaemic. Gurmar also helps to alleviate the cravings for sweet foods and reduce appetite. It is therfore very benefical for loosing weight.

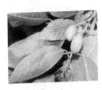

**Haritaki *(Terminalia chebula):*** Haritaki means "that which carries away disease." It is sacred to Shiva (also named Hara), who destroys death. Haritaki has several other names: *abhaya* – fearlessness, *divya* – divine, *jivaniya* – vitalizing, *pranada* – life saving, and *vayahstha* – one that promotes longevity and maintains youth. Haritaki is one of the three ingredients in triphala. The rishi *Vagbhata* praises haritaki as the herb of choice for treating all vata and kapha-related diseases. Haritaki has all tastes (rasa) except salty. It is sweet after digestion (vipaka) and hot in effect (virya). Its prabhava is to balance and harmonize all three doshas. This fruit also works on all of the dhatus. It has laxative, rejuvenative, purgative, expectorant, astringent, tonic and antihelmintic properties.

As medicine, it is used in numerous formulas and for a vast array of diseases. For vata diseases, it is recommended to take with ghee. For pitta diseases, it is recommended to take with jaggery, honey or organic cane sugar. For kapha diseases, it is recommended to take with rock salt. It treats almost all gastrointestinal disorders such as constipation, worms, parasites, hyperacidity, colitis, piles/hemorrhoids, ama, enlargement of liver and spleen, asthma, heart disease, vomiting, jaundice, hepatitis, skin disease, edema, tumors and cancer.

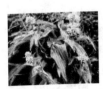

**Jatamansi *(Nardostachys jatamansi):*** The word *jata* means "root" or "tangled knot," like the hair of a *sadhu* or wandering mendicant. As its name implies, the root of this plant is used medicinally. Jatamansi is related to valerian. In *Charaka Samhita* it is classified as an herb that restores consciousness and calms the mind. It is said to have a benevolent effect on any diseases that are psychological in origin.

Jatamansi is bitter, astringent and sweet in taste (rasa), sweet after digestion (vipaka) and cold in effect (virya). This herb alleviates all three doshas, having especially good benefits for kapha and pitta disorders. It has an antipsychotic prabhava. Jatamansi works on the blood (rakta) and marrow and nerve (majja) dhatus, as well as the nervous, muscular and circulatory systems. It has the characteristics of being a cholagogue, sedative, anti-spasmodic, analgesic, anti-inflammatory and emmenagogue agent, and acts as a brain tonic. Additionally, it increases appetite and improves digestion. Not only is this herb very useful in pitta disorders like fevers, hepatitis and cirrhosis, but it also relieves kapha disorders such as cough and asthma. Other disorders jatamansi treats include vertigo, seizures, epilepsy, sexual debility, infertility and impotency. A sattvic herb by nature, it is excellent for enhancing meditation and sadhana. If taken in excessive quantities, jatamansi can cause vomiting and diarrhea with abdominal cramping.

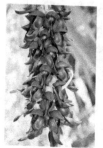

**Kapikachhu** *(Mucuna pruriens):* Kapikachhu is one of the most effective and important ayurvedic aphrodisiacs *(vajikaranas).* It is sweet and bitter in taste (rasa), sweet after digestion (vipaka) and hot in effect (virya). Kapikachhu nourishes all of the dhatus, especially the shukra. The seed of the plant is used medicinally and has a delicious nutty flavor. This herb acts on the nervous, reproductive and respiratory systems. It is a powerful tonifying, rejuvenative and astringent herb. Kapikachhu has many potent medicinal benefits, such as treating general debility and weakness, sexual debility, impotence, infertility, leucorrhea, spermatorrhea, asthma, nervous system debility, paralysis, cervical spondylosis, and multiple sclerosis. Additionally, it is used in the treatment of Parkinson's disease, as it contains substantial amounts of L-dopa, which, as a precursor for L-dopamine, is crucial in its treatment.

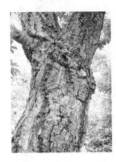

**Katphala** *(Myrica nagi):* In western herbalism, katphala is called bayberry. It is one of the best herbs to eliminate kapha. Katphala is sacred to Shiva and Shakti because of its sattvic nature. It purifies the nadis and allows prana to flow freely through them.It is pungent, bitter and astringent in taste (rasa), pungent after digestion (vipaka) and hot in effect (virya). It alleviates kapha and vata and increases pitta. This herb works on rasa, rakta and majja dhatus, as well as the respiratory, nervous, circulatory and lymphatic systems. It is one of the best herbs for cleansing the lymphatic system. Katphala is a diaphoretic, expectorant, astringent, emetic, antispasmodic and alterative agent. It is used mainly for cough, bronchial asthma, fevers, diabetes, lack of taste, tumors, laryngitis, typhoid, nasal congestion and cardiac debility. This plant should be avoided if there are liver or spleen diseases present.

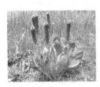

**Katuka/Kutki** *(Picrorhiza kurroa):* This herb is the king of bitter tonics. It is said to be equal to or better than the western herb goldenseal. Katuka has been used for centuries in India to treat fever, indigestion, jaundice and other bacterial or infectious diseases. It is also called *mahausadhi* or "the great medicine" and *dhanvantarigrasta*, the herb "administered by Dhanvantari," the God of Ayurveda. It is bitter in taste (rasa), pungent after digestion (vipaka) and cold in effect (virya). It reduces excess kapha and pitta doshas, and in excess aggravates vata. Katuka works on plasma (rasa), blood (rakta) and fat (meda) dhatus, as well as the digestive, circulatory and urinary systems.

The root of this plant is used medicinally, having strong and bitter tonic with anti-pyretic, alterative, laxative and antibiotic properties. It is one of the best herbs known for detoxifying the blood. It is also an excellent tonic for the liver, spleen, small intestine and all imbalances related to pitta. Katuka also has incredible effects in the treatment of diabetes, viral hepatitis, obesity, parasites, worms, digestive disorders and infectious diseases.

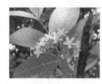

**Kutaja** *(Holarrhena antidysenterica):* As its Latin name implies, kutaja is one of the best herbs for treating dysentery, as well as diarrhea, amoebas, parasites and worms. The bark, root and seed of the plant are commonly used. Kutaja has a pungent, bitter and astringent taste (rasa), becomes pungent after digestion (vipaka) and has a cold effect (virya). It alleviates pitta and kapha. and increases vata. It works on the blood (rakta) and muscle (mamsa) dhatus as well as the digestive, excretory and circulatory systems. This herb has astringent, anti-helmintic and amoebacidal characteristics. It is also good in treatment of bleeding hemorrhoids, malabsorption, colitis and menorrhagia.

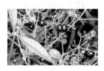

**Manjistha** *(Rubia cordifolia):* Manjistha is considered to be one of the most valuable ayurvedic herbs. The root of this plant is used for cleansing the blood and stopping diarrhea. This herb is bitter, astringent and sweet in taste (rasa), becomes pungent after digestion (vipaka) and hot in its final effect (virya). It alleviates all three doshas. Manjistha works on the rasa, rakta and mamsa dhatus, as well as the circulatory and female reproductive systems. It is alterative, haemostatic, emmenagogue, astringent, diuretic and lithotropic in action. Additionally, it helps prevent and dissolve tumors.

This herb is most beneficial for gastrointestinal disorders like loss of appetite, dyspepsia and worm infestations, as well as being a digestive stimulant. It is one of the best herbs to alleviate ama from kapha and pitta doshas and plasma (rasa) and blood (rakta) dhatus. Manjistha also treats hemorrhoids, eczema, psoriasis, liver and spleen disorders, inflammations, sexually transmitted diseases, menstrual irregularities, amenorrhea, dysmenorrhea, hepatitis and blood disorders. It is used externally in pastes, salves, poultices and creams for wide variety of skin conditions.

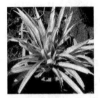

**Musali** *(Asparagus adscendens):* There are two varieties of musali, white *(safed* in Sanskrit) and black *(kali* in Sanskrit). The part of the plant used medicinally is the root. White musali is sweet in initial and post-digestive tastes (rasa and vipaka) and cold in its effect (virya). It alleviates pitta and vata while aggravating kapha. This herb is a rejuvenative, demulcent, aphrodisiac, lithotropic and nutritive tonic. It penetrates all of the dhatus. Safed mainly treats sexual debility, infertility, impotence and spermatorrhea. Black musali is sweet and bitter in taste (rasa), sweet after digestion (vipaka) and hot in its final effect (virya). It has primarily the same medicinal properties as the white musali, and is also used to treat general debility.

**Musta** *(Cyperus rotundus):* Musta was held in high praise by the rishis for its ability to treat numerous illnesses. It is one of the best herbs for almost all female reproductive disorders. Musta works wonders for the regulation of menstruation. It is pungent, bitter and astringent in taste (rasa), pungent after digestion (vipaka) and cold in its overall effect *(virya).* This healing herb alleviates kapha and pitta. The root of this plant is used medicinally. It is an excellent digestive stimulant for pitta dosha. Musta also works on the liver and small intestine by increasing absorption.

In conditions of candida, parasites, worms, bacteria, chronic fever and gastritis, this herb is a fantastic healer. It works on the plasma (rasa), blood (rakta), muscle (mamsa) and marrow and nerve (majja) dhatus, as well as the digestive and circulatory systems. Musta digests and dispels ama. It can be made into a paste and used externally to alleviate skin inflammation, itching, scabies, psoriasis and eczema.

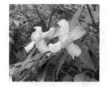 **Nagakeshar** *(Mesua ferrea):* The ancient ayurvedic texts claim there is hardly any digestive disorder that nagakeshar cannot alleviate. It is used for bleeding hemorrhoids, dysentery, loss of appetite, indigestion, excessive thirst, worm infestation, parasites, diarrhea and vomiting. Nagakeshar may also be used to treat menorrhagia, snakebites, sexual debility, cough, asthma and hiccups. It is astringent and bitter in taste (rasa), pungent after digestion (vipaka) and hot in its final effect (virya). Nagakeshar acts to alleviate kapha and pitta doshas; for pitta, it is excellent in treatment of skin diseases and fevers. The whole plant is used for medicinal purposes. Due to its haemostatic and haemopoietic qualities, it helps with cardiac debility and disorders involving the blood vessels.

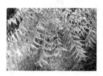 **Neem** *(Azadirachta indica):* In Sanskrit, neem is often referred to as *nimba*, meaning "that which endows good health." It is one of the most powerful blood purifiers and detoxifiers in the ayurvedic pharmacopeia. Neem is bitter and astringent in taste (rasa), pungent after digestion (vipaka) and cold in its total effect (virya). It alleviates pitta and kapha doshas. This herb works on plasma (rasa), blood (rakta) and fat (meda) dhatus as well as on the digestive, circulatory, respiratory and urinary systems. It is a strongly bitter, anti-pyretic, alterative, anti-helmintic, antiseptic and anti-emetic tonic. It is used frequently to treat parasites, worms and bacterial infections.

All parts of the neem plant are used internally and externally for the treatment of skin diseases. The leaves, powder and oil are especially good for applying externally in cases of itching, burning, abscesses, glandular swelling, wounds, inflammation of the joints, rheumatic disorders, ringworm, eczema, psoriasis and scabies. The leaves are used externally for wounds, including open wounds, because neem leaves are an excellent cleanser and healer. Neem also reduces fever while stimulating immunity.

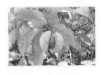

**Nutmeg** *(Myristica fragrans):* Nutmeg is known as *jatiphala* in India. It is one of the best spices for increasing absorption in the small intestine. This spice is also used in aphrodisiac formulas because it has a special ability to prevent premature ejaculation. The seed is the part of the plant used medicinally. It is pungent, astringent and bitter in taste *(rasa)*, pungent after digestion (vipaka) and hot in its final effect (virya). Nutmeg alleviates vata and kapha while stimulating pitta dosha. It works on the lymph (rasa), muscle (mamsa), marrow and nerve (majja) and reproductive (shukra) dhatus, as well as the digestive system. This spice has the properties of an astringent, carminative, sedative, nervine, aphrodisiac and stimulating agent. It is wonderful for digestion and is used often in Indian cooking with a combination of ginger, fenugreek, cinnamon, cardamom and black pepper. As a nervine and sedative, it works wonders on stress and tension. Nutmeg also works well as a painkiller, and together with the western herb white willow bark can greatly alleviate headaches.

**Pippali** *(Piper longum):* Pippali is mentioned in every ayurvedic text. It is a close relative to black pepper, and one of the three herbs that make up the digestive formula trikatu. The dried fruit is used for medicinal purposes. This herb is pungent in taste (rasa) unless fresh, in which case it i s sweet and pungent. It is sweet after digestion (vipaka) and hot in effect (virya). If it is fresh, the virya is cold. Pippali is appetizing, digestive, rejuvenative, aphrodisiac, antipyretic, stimulating, anti-helmintic and a brain tonic. It minimizes vata and kapha doshas while increasing pitta.

This herb affects all of the dhatus except the muscles and bones, as well as the digestive, respiratory and reproductive systems. Pippali treats coughs, colds, constipation, asthma, bronchitis, arthritis, gout, rheumatism, digestive weakness, distention, worms, gas, tumors, impotency, infertility, lumbago, sciatica, epilepsy and paralysis. It is most commonly used to rejuvenate agni and eliminate ama. Taken with other herbs, it increases their effectiveness by enhancing their assimilation.

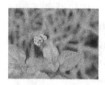 **Punarnava** *(Boerhaavia diffusa):* Punarnava means "what renews the body" or "what restores youth." The leaves and root of this plant were traditionally used by the sages and yogis to promote health, longevity and youthfulness. This herb is pungent, bitter, astringent and sweet at first taste (rasa), becomes pungent (vipaka) and has a hot effect (virya). Punarnava alleviates all three doshas, but can increase pitta if taken in excess. It works primarily on the plasma (rasa) and blood (rakta) dhatus and the circulatory and urinary systems. This herbal medicine is one of the best rejuvenatives for the kidneys and urinary system. It alleviates edema and dysuria. Punarnava is often used in panchakarma during swedana (sweating therapy). It is an excellent blood tonic with alterative, diuretic and rejuvenative properties. This herb can easily dissolve kidney stones and works well in cases of heart disease, hepatitis, hemorrhoids, difficult or burning urination and anemia. Punarnava is often combined with rasna and sunthi as a panacea for rheumatic conditions with swelling and pain. It is quite good for overall debility.

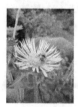 **Pushkarmula** *(Inula racemosa):* In western herbology, pushkarmula is known as elecampane. In some parts of India it is called *svasari* which translates as "the enemy of breathlessness." As its name suggests, it is one of the best herbs to rejuvenate and tone the lungs. Both roots and flowers are used to equalize prana in the body. Pushkarmula is bitter and pungent in taste (rasa), pungent after digestion (vipaka) and is hot in effect (virya). This herb works on all of the dhatus except for the reproductive tissue (shukra). It helps the respiratory, nervous and digestive systems, and is excellent against cough, asthma, bronchitis, cardiac disorders and nervous

system disorders. It is said to be the herb of choice against pleurisy. Pushkarmula is good for anorexia and dyspepsia, as it stimulates agni and destroys ama. In addition, it assists in the healing of skin diseases and wounds and gives strength to combat mental weakness.

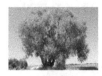 **Sallaki** *(Boswelia serata):* Sallaki is one of the most mentioned herbs in all of the ayurvedic texts. It is a gummy tree resin and is closely related to guggulu and myrrh. This medicine has bitter, sweet and astringent tastes (rasa), pungent feeling after digestion (vipaka) and a cold effect (virya). It brings harmony to vata and kapha doshas. Sallaki works on plasma (rakta), muscle (mamsa), fat (meda) and reproductive (shukra) dhatus, as well as the circulatory, muscular and skeletal systems. It is an alterative, antispasmodic and analgesic agent. This herb is excellent for healing wounds and treating diarrhea, hemorrhoids and blood disorders. Its paste can be used externally for rheumatic complaints, cervical adenitis and to relieve pain and swelling.

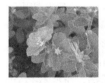 **Shankapushpi** *(Evolvulus alsinodes):* Shankapushpi means "flowers in the shape of a conch." Out of all of the nervines, shankapushpi is said to be the best. It is often used with brahmi, vaccha and jatamansi. The entire plant is used medicinally. This herb is astringent, pungent and bitter in taste (rasa), sweet after digestion (vipaka) and hot in effect (virya). It alleviates all three of the doshas and has a prabhava of alleviating psychosomatic disorders. Shankapushpi works primarily on marrow and nerve (majja) dhatu and on the circulatory system. It is a brain tonic used to promote memory retention and intelligence. As it relaxes the nervous system, it is often included with other aphrodisiac herbs and is said to be an aphrodisiac itself. In women, shankapushpi promotes conception. It is combined with bringaraja and brahmi to promote hair growth. It is used to treat all mental disorders. When the leaves are juiced, it improves appetite and is a mild laxative.

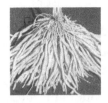

**Shatavari** *(Asparagus racemosus):* Shatavari means "one who possesses one hundred husbands." This general tonic can be given to any person of any constitution. It is often referred to as the "universal rasayana." The root of the plant is used medicinally. Shatavari is sweet and bitter in taste (rasa), sweet after digestion (vipaka) and cold in effect (virya). It works on all of the dhatus as well as the circulatory, reproductive, respiratory and digestive systems. This herb is a rejuvenative, galactogogue, aphrodisiac, anabolic, spermatogenic and *vajikarana* tonic (gives sexual vigor). There are very few disorders for which it cannot be used. It treats weakness in female reproductive organs, general sexual debility, infertility, impotence, menopause, diarrhea, dysentery, ulcers, hyperacidity, dehydration, lung diseases, convalescence, cancer, herpes, leucorrhea, fevers, epilepsy, hysteria, uterine hypoplasia, lumbago, sciatica, inflamed joints and paralysis.

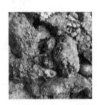

**Shilajit** *(Asphaltum bitumen):* In the classic ayurvedic texts, this herb is called *shilajatu,* but is more commonly known as shilajit. In Sanskrit it means "conqueror of mountains and destroyer of weakness." Shilajit is an organic mineral compound found only in the Himalayas, where the rocks exude a dark brown to black resinous substance. This is decomposition of the plant matter in the rocks from centuries before. The bio-transformed plant matter is squeezed out from the rocks by geothermal pressures. Shilajit is usually found at 1,000-1,500 meters altitude along the Himalayan range.

Shilajit has a bitter and pungent rasa, bitter vipaka and warming virya. It decreases vata and kapha and increases pitta. This herb is mainly used on the marrow and nerve (majja) and reproductive (shukra-arthava) dhatus, and on the urinary system. It is a strong blood purifier, lithotropic, antiseptic, diuretic and rejuvenative tonic.

This herbal medicine has been used for thousands of years to treat all conditions of weakness and debility because it contains immense rejuvenating powers. It is said to have to the power to stop or even reverse the aging process. Many yogis use this herb, as it gives strength, vitality and longevity.

Shilajit helps to lower serum cholesterol, liver cholesterol, serum triglycerides and serum phospholipids. It also increases the healing benefits of other herbs by enhancing their bio-availability. It assists in the delivery of nutrients deep into the tissue and removes deep-seated toxins. Shilajit improves memory and the ability to handle stress. It also reduces recovery time in muscle, bone and nerve injuries. Shilajit stimulates the immune system and reduces chronic fatigue. It is traditionally used as an immunomodulator and for stress-related diseases like high blood pressure and mental and physical fatigue.

In conjunction with turmeric and fenugreek, it has shown great success in the treatment of diabetes. Its antioxidant and anti-inflammatory properties help to decrease and relieve vata-type joint inflammation and pain. Shilajit's effects on the neurotransmitters also seem to help relieve joint pain. Shilajit is also a very powerful antioxidant that is able to cross the blood-brain barrier. It is excellent for anyone who has a regular yoga routine or uses a lot of mental power.

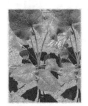

**Tagara** *(Valeriana wallichii):* In western herbology, tagara is called valerian. It is a close relative of jatamansi and they are often used together. Tagara is one of the best herbs for the central nervous system. It is bitter, pungent and sweet in taste (rasa), pungent after digestion (vipaka) and hot in its effect (virya). This herb alleviates all three doshas. It works on plasma (rasa), muscle (mamsa) and marrow and nerve (majja) dhatus, as well as the digestive and respiratory systems. The root of the plant is used medicinally. The properties of tagara are nervine with antispasmodic, anti-epileptic, analgesic, sedative and carminative qualities. It is used in epilepsy, hysteria, headache, delirium, intoxication, neuralgia, multiple sclerosis, convulsions, migraines, vertigo, palpitations, flatulence, abdominal pain, colic, whooping cough, asthma and numerous other disorders.

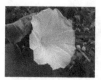

**Trivrit** *(Operculina turpethum):* The *Charaka Samhita* says that trivrit is the best of all laxatives. This root is used extensively by yogis and for pan-chakarma cleansing techniques like virechan (purgation). Trivrit is pungent, bitter, astringent and sweet in taste (rasa), pungent after digestion (vipaka) and hot in its effect (virya). It alleviates pitta and kapha doshas and increases vata. This herb has laxative, anti-pyretic, anti-helmintic, vermicide and lithotropic properties. It works especially well on the plasma (rasa), blood (rakta) and fat (meda) dhatus. Trivrit is used to treat constipation, fever, worm infestation, obesity, liver and spleen disorders, edema, flatulence, jaundice, ascites, gout, rheumatic fever, cough and asthma. For skin disorders, it is often combined with triphala, vidanga and jaggery. Combined with guduchi, sunthi and triphala, it is an excellent medicine for anemia. It can also be used for gynecological and mental disorders.

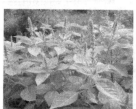

**Tulasi** *(Ocimum sanctum):* Tulasi is considered by many to be the most sacred plant in India. Numerous scriptural injunctions praise the glory of tulasi's healing powers. Tulasi is considered to be the Divine Mother incarnated in plant form, thus She is referred to as Tulasi Devi. Many scriptures sing Her praises:

All of the benefits come because tulasi offers the quality of pure sattva and opens the heart and consciousness. It releases negative ions into the air, purifying air wherever it is grown. Tulasi is pungent and bitter in taste (rasa), pungent after digestion (vipaka) and hot in effect (virya). Tulasi minimizes vata and kapha and only aggravates pitta if taken in excess. It works on the rasa, rakta, majja and shukra dhatus, as well as the nervous, respiratory and digestive systems. It has been said that tulasi harmonizes ojas, tejas and prana. Tulasi has nervine, antispasmodic, febrifugal, antiseptic, diaphoretic and antibacterial properties.

The seeds, leaves and roots all have tremendous medicinal benefits. It is used frequently for stress reduction, immunity and cancer. It is extremely healing for skin diseases, including ringworm infestation. Tulasi increases the potency of any other medicines with which it is taken. It treats excess phlegm, cough, asthma, bronchitis and hiccups. It dissolves ama and thus works on the digestive system. This herb also increases agni and alleviates abdominal distention. Tulasi can also be used to alleviate headaches and increase circulation. It is a must for serious yoga practitioners or meditators, as it promotes clarity of mind, courage, devotion and faith.

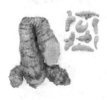 **Turmeric/Haridra** *(Curcuma longa): Haridra* is the Sanskrit name of this root. In many parts of India, it is known as "*haldi,*" which translates, "that which improves the complexion of skin." It is bitter and pungent in taste (rasa), pungent after digestion (vipaka) and hot in effect (virya). Due to its hot virya, it alleviates vata and kapha, and due to its bitter rasa it alleviates pitta.

Turmeric works on all of the dhatus and the digestive, circulatory and respiratory systems. Its main properties are astringent, anti-dermatosic, anti-diabetic, carminative and antibacterial; it also stimulates digestion. It is excellent against all skin diseases including sprains, bruises, wounds, acne, rashes, varicose veins and inflammatory ailments of the joints. It used for treating the lungs, cough, colds, asthma, congestion, constipation, malabsorption, abdominal distention, weak digestive fire, metabolism, blood disorders, diabetes, arthritis, anemia, amenorrhea and kidney weakness. Turmeric should not be used in cases of jaundice or hepatitis. It is one of the best natural antibiotics and it improves intestinal flora. Turmeric and tulasi are wonderful together, as it is said that they both give the energy of the Divine Mother. In addition, turmeric is excellent for yogis to keep their limbs and joints strong and flexible.

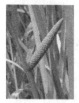

**Vaccha** *(Acorus calamus):* This herb is also called calamus or sweet flag. Vaccha means "to speak." It promotes self-expression and intelligence. The root of the plant is used medicinally to rejuvenate the brain and nervous system, and increase sensitivity and awareness. This herb works by cleansing the subtle nerve channels of toxins. It also augments the metabolic fire of the nervous system. Vaccha is bitter and pungent in taste (rasa), pungent after digestion (vipaka) and hot in effect (virya). It has the prabhava of being a very powerful nervine tonic. This herb alleviates vata and kapha, while slightly increasing pitta. It possesses strong antimicrobial properties, especially against *E.coli, Staphylococcus aureus* and *Aspergillus niger.* Vaccha works on rasa, rakta, meda, majja and shukra dhatus as well as the nervous, respiratory, digestive, circulatory and reproductive systems. It is a stimulant with rejuvenative, expectorant, decongestant, nervine, emetic and antispasmodic properties.

This herb is successfully used in India for the treatment of rheumatism, rheumatic fever, inflamed joints and tendons, pain and swelling, cough, asthma, bronchitis, sinusitis, uterine contractions, ulcers, wounds, headache, earache, tinnitus, arthritis, epilepsy, deafness, hysteria and neuralgia.

It can be used as a powder, juice, paste, fumigation and nasya agent. For epilepsy and other severe vata disorders, vaccha, brahmi and jatamansi mixed with honey work very well. Children can be given vaccha, licorice (yasti madhu) and honey for rejuvenation and as a general nervine tonic.

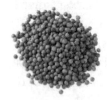

**Vidanga** *(Embelia ribes):* Vidanga is stated in ayurvedic texts to be the most powerful deworming herb. As its main property is anti-helmintic, it is primarily used to treat worms and parasites. It also has carminative, laxative and expectorant qualities, and is used in many of Ayurveda's lung formulas. Most commonly, the fruit of the plant is used, but the leaves, root and bark also have medicinal value. It is pungent in taste (rasa), pungent after digestion (vipaka) and hot in effect (virya). Vidanga works mainly on rakta and meda dhatus and the digestive and excretory systems.

It is used for almost all gastrointestinal disorders, including abdominal pain and ascites. This herb greatly assists in eliminating ama from the colon, and can even be used for loss of appetite, dyspepsia and flatulence. If you take vidanga in large doses (ten grams of the dry powder) in the early morning, and follow with a laxative like triphala in the evening, you can destroy and eliminate all types of worms, including threadworm, tapeworm, roundworm and parasites. As an infusion, vidanga can be used to reduce fever and alleviate excessive thirst and vomiting.

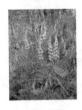 **Yasthi Madhu** *(Glycyrrhiza glabra):* Yasthi madhu, or licorice, is called "honeystick" in Sanskrit. In the *Charaka Samhita,* it is called a vitalizing herb, an herb for oleation, longevity and wounds, beneficial for the throat and an overall rejuvenator. The root of the plant is used medicinally. It is sweet in both initial and post-digestive tastes (rasa and vipaka) and cold in effect (virya). Licorice alleviates pitta and vata disorders. It works on all of the dhatus and the digestive, respiratory, nervous, reproductive and excretory systems.

This herb behaves as a demulcent, expectorant, rejuvenative, laxative, sedative, nervine and emetic tonic. It can be used for cough, colds, bronchitis, sore throats, asthma, laryngitis, ulcers, hyperacidity, abdominal pain, painful or scanty urination and general debility. Although it is heavy, short-term use can alleviate kapha in the stomach and lungs. It is also good for bleeding hemorrhoids. Licorice facilitates the healing of ulcers, gastritis and hyperacidity. It improves skin complexion and restores youthfulness, thus making it excellent for increasing ojas.

## Ayurvedic Formulas

There are numerous herbal medicinal formulations mentioned in the Ayurveda texts. Of all the plants growing in India, six hundred are said to be the most important. From these, all ayurvedic formulations are made, including infusions, decoctions, powders, pills, pastes, poultices, oils and liniments.

Of these, there are five basic methods of preparation: svarasa (juices), kalka (herbal pastes), churna (herbal powders), kvatha (herbal decoctions), phanta (hot herbal infusions) and hima (cold infusions). There are a plethora of other well-known methods of preparations that are commonly used, including milk decoctions, leham or avaleham (medicated jellies), asava and arishta (medicated wines), vati and guti (herbal tablets and pills), thaila (medicated oils) and ghrita (medicated ghee). There are numerous methods of making herbal preparations and each one has unique therapeutic value. For example, arishtams are naturally fermented herbal extracts that address a wide array of conditions such as allergy, anemia, neurological disorders, rheumatic and arthritic symptoms and gastrointestinal problems. Herbs prepared in arishtams have enhanced assimilation and potency.

Here are a few of the most commonly used formulas:

• **Avipattikar:** Avipattikar is one of the best formulas for alleviating vitiated pitta dosha. It reduces hyperacidity. It acts as a mild laxative and removes toxins from the gastrointestinal tract. It has a bitter, pungent and astringent taste (rasa), cooling effect (virya) and sweet post digestion (vipaka). It primarily works on lymph (rasa), blood (rakta) and muscle (mamsa) dhatus. The primary actions of Avipattikar are antacid, antiemetic, carminative, cholagogue, laxative and neuralgic. It alleviates pitta by balancing jathara agni (stomach digestive fire).

- **Chandraprabha:** "That which gives the glow of the moon." It is bitter, sweet, pungent and astringent. It has a heating virya and pungent vipaka. It helps to reduce excess in all doshas. However, used in excess it will increase pitta due to its dry, light and heating properties. It works on rasa, rakta, meda and shukra/artava dhatus. It is composed of guggulu, iron bhasma, cardamom, bay leaf, shilajit, cinnamon, bamboo, guduchi, deodara (cedar), turmeric, pippali, black pepper, chitrak, triphala, vidanga, calamus, ginger, gokshura, sandalwood, salt, as well as numerous other supporting herbs.

It decreases kapha by burning excess ama and reducing high blood sugar levels. It has a potent effect against diabetes. It is a reproductive rejuvenative and increases ojas. Chandraprabha also addresses imbalances related to water-carrying channels. This includes disturbed emotions, menstrual problems (amenorrhea), reproductive problems (such as polycystic ovarian syndrome) and urinary tract issues.

- **Chayawanprash:** Probably the most popular of all formulations is the rejuvenative called chayawanprash. Chayawanprash is excellent for maintaining youthfulness, vigor and vitality. The medicinal benefits of chayawanprash seem endless. The traditional formula of chayawanprash improves skin complexion and fights dermal bacterial infection. It assists in new hair growth and helps absorption of calcium resulting in strong bones and teeth. This herbal blend sharpens the sense organs and increases the digestive fire. It can be used for reproductive weaknesses like impotency and sterility. Furthermore, it is especially good for alleviating cough and asthma, dyspnea, fever, heart diseases, gout, diseases of urine and semen, and disorders of speech. Its strong antioxidant properties heal wounds and strengthen the emaciated. Chayawanprash enhances fertility, regulates menstruation. It improves muscle tone by enhancing protein synthesis, and helps children's development.

Chayawanprash is a powerful free radical scavenger and adaptogen. Taken regularly, it builds immunity, promotes good digestive power and keeps the mind and lungs clear. It is also beneficial for reducing stress, anxiety and depression.

The main ingredient in this formula is amla, the Indian gooseberry. Amla is the small fruit of a citrus tree, and each fruit contains more than 3,000 mg of vitamin C, all of which is completely bioavailable. As mentioned earlier, amla is one of the most powerful rejuvenative herbs used in Ayurveda.

Other ingredients include ghee, sesame oil, honey, raw unrefined sugar, long pepper, cinnamon, cardamom, sandalwood, cloves, giant potato, winter cherry, asparagus, bala, guduchi, gokshura, bhumyamalaki, punarnava, bilva and vadarikand. Additional ingredients may be included as there are numerous home recipes from family lineages, and each recipe is based upon the local availability of herbs. The honey and sugar act as an *anupan,* or vehicle, for the herbs to penetrate deeply into the tissues. Sweet tastes are assimilated quickly into the bloodstream and penetrate cell walls, carrying the active constituents of the chayawanprash.

• **Gokshuradi Guggulu:** Gokshuradi guggulu is a traditional ayurvedic compound used to support the proper function of the genitourinary tract. It strengthens and tones the kidneys, bladder and urethra as well as the reproductive organs. The main ingredient, *gokshura,* is renowned for its rejuvenating action on the kidneys. It also assists in maintaining proper prostate size and function. Combined with *guggulu,* triphala and *trikatu,* it detoxifies the urinary system and maintains healthy urinary composition, thus reducing the risk factors that may lead to stone formation. It is sour, sweet, pungent, bitter and astringent rasa, cooling virya and sweet vipaka. As it is balancing to all doshas, it revitalizes kidneys weakened by vata, calms pitta inflammations, and reduces stones and swelling due to excess kapha.

It is an alterative, anti-bilious, anti-emetic, anti-inflammatory, anti-pyretic, antiviral, appetizer, astringent, carminative, demulcent, depurative, digestant, diuretic, laxative, nutritive, ophthalmic, purgative, refrigerant, rejuvenative, stomachic, tonic and vulnerary formula.

- **Kaishore Guggulu:** Kaishore Guggulu alleviates numerous pitta disorders. It is exceptional for pitta type arthritis where there is pain, inflammation, burning and swelling. It treats muscle, tendon and ligament inflammation. Kaishore Guggulu also treats gout, skin eruptions and infections, lumps and growths. As it purifies toxins it is used in cirrhosis and cancer treatments, especially of liver and breasts. It has a bitter, astringent, sweet and pungent taste (rasa), heating effect (virya) and pungent after digestion (vipaka). It is tri-doshic and works on lymph (rasa), blood (rakta), muscle (mamsa), fat (meda) and bone (ashti) dhatus.

- **Kanchanara Guggulu:** Kanchanara Guggulu is one of the best herbs to reduce glandular swelling. It has an affinity for the lymphatic system and is used to treat swollen lymph nodes, cervical adenitis, scrofula, Hodgkin's disease and swollen glands. Kanchanara Guggulu helps to dissolve growths and fluid based accumulation in the dhatus. It is one of the best herbs for treating thyroid conditions such as hyper or hypothyroidism and goiter. It is also useful in weight issues like obesity and high cholesterol. The taste (rasa) is bitter, pungent, astringent and sweet. It has heating energy (virya) and pungent post digestive effect (vipaka). While it is balancing for all doshas it has an affinity for reducing kapha imbalances. It works on all dhatus.

- **Mahasudarshan:** This is one of the best alterative formulas available. It counteracts fevers and inflammatory conditions by purifying the blood. It greatly decreases kapha and pitta, cleansing excess pitta from lymph, liver and skin. It is bitter, pungent and astringent. It works specifically on rasa and rakta dhatus. Mahasudarshan increases immunity by neutralizing viral and bacterial infections. It has a bitter, pungent and astringent rasa, cooling virya and pungent vipaka. Being bitter, it has a very beneficial effect on the liver.

- **Punarnavadi Guggulu:** Punarnavadi Guggulu is one of the best herbs for reducing vata disorders related to pain and swelling. It is also used to reduce kapha due to its light and dry properties. It has a heating energy (virya) and pungent post digestive (vipaka). Its taste (rasa) is bitter, pungent, sweet and astringent. As a cardiotonic, hypotensive and lithagogue it is a wonderful herbal formulation for heart disorders. It clears excessive fluid from the lymph (rasa) dhatu which alleviates strain on the heart. Its heating property also helps to destroy excess fat and contributes to weight loss. Punarnavadi Guggulu has anti-inflammatory properties that alleviate swelling, stiffness and rigidity thus helping to alleviate arthritic disorders. This formulation also alleviates difficult and painful urination as well as urinary calculi.

• **Sitopaladi Churna:** The "sweet cough" formula, this is an excellent formula for coughs and colds manifesting due to an excess of the three doshas. It clears asthma and allergies and kindles agni. It is an expectorant, anti-allergenic, diaphoretic and bronchodilator. It is sweet and pungent rasa, sweet vipaka, with heating virya. It is primarily for the digestive and respiratory systems.

It contains pippali, cinnamon, vamsa lochana (bamboo manna – the inner part of bamboo), cardamom and rock candy. It can be combined with trikatu to reduce excess mucous and with mahasudarshan to alleviate fever and inflammatory conditions.

• **Trikatu:** Trikatu is one of the most commonly used formulas in ayurvedic medicine. It is used to kindle agni. This herb is made of equal parts long pepper (pippali), ginger (sunthi) and black pepper. As it is very heating, it reduces vata and kapha. Trikatu is known as "the three pungents" and is said to be one hundred times more powerful than any of the three herbs alone. This formula is an expectorant, decongestant and stimulant. It is also used in numerous lung formulas for alleviating asthma, bronchitis, congestion and colds. Trikatu eliminates ama from the body. It is very effective in treating many vata and kapha disorders.

• **Triphala:** Triphala is known as "the three fruits" and is used extensively in Ayurveda. It is said to alleviate literally thousands of diseases from the body. There is a saying in India, "If you have no mother, but you have triphala, everything is going to be all right."

Triphala is harmonizing to all of the doshas and healing to all of the dhatus. It cleanses the colon of ama, gives strength and rejuvenation to the stomach and digestive tract, increases and restores immunity, increases appetite, strengthens the heart, nerves and brain, restores prana, reduces heat and helps with diabetes. Triphala is often used in panchakarma as a purgative. People of all doshic types can use this formula safely.

• **Yogaraj Guggulu:** This is one of the best vata-reducing formulas in the world. It quickly decreases vata in the joints, nerves and muscles. Yogaraj guggulu supports comfortable movement of the joints and muscles and rejuvenates and strengthens the skeletal and neuromuscular systems. It promotes healthy elimination of toxins. It is an alterative, anti-inflammatory, antispasmodic, astringent, carminative, demulcent, depurative, digestant, muscle relaxant, nervine, rejuvenative, stimulant and tonic.

Its rasa is bitter, pungent, astringent and sweet. Its virya is heating with a pungent vipaka. It reduces and balances vata, but in excess may aggravate pitta. It is particularly useful for accumulation of vata in the joints and muscles, which may be indicated by cracking or popping joints, tics, spasms or tremors. (Chronic accumulation may lead to serious conditions such as rheumatism and arthritis.) In vata-type arthritis, the joints may feel cold to the touch and, although not necessarily swollen, they may be dry and painful, especially upon movement. Yogaraj guggulu contains a synergistic blend of detoxifying herbs – including triphala, chitrak and vidanga – that work in conjunction with guggulu to remove excess vata from the joints, nerves and muscles.

## Herbs for the Doshas and Subdoshas

Below is a list of herbs that are typically used to bring harmony to the doshas and subdoshas.

## Vata

ashwagandha, castor (eranda), cinnamon, fenugreek, hing, sesame (tila), tagara, vaccha, white musali, yasthi madhu

## Vata Subdoshas

*Prana* – brahmi, ashwagandha, shatavari, ginseng, jatamansi, shankapushpi

*Udana* – ginger, tulasi, vaccha, jatamansi, yasthi madhu, ashwagandha, sesame oil nasya, castor oil packs

*Samana* – ginger, cardamom, fennel, clove, tulasi, kasturi pills

*Apana* – triphala, psyllium husk (sat isabgol), vidanga, aloe

*Vyana* – ashwagandha, nirgundi, guggulu, jatamansi, tagara

## Pitta

amalaki, chairetta, daruharidra, kutki, lemongrass, manjistha, musta, neem, peppermint, rhubarb (*amlavetasa*)

## Pitta Subdoshas

*Pachaka* – shatavari, amalaki, aloe, daruharidra, yasthi madhu, avipattikar churna, marshmallow, cilantro

*Bhrajaka* – aloe, manjistha, plantain, nettles, red clover, turmeric, dandelion, kutki, bhumiamalaki

*Ranjaka* – bhumiamalaki, guduchi, daruharidra, guggulu, aloe, gotu kola, manjistha, golden seal, amlavetasa, cilantro

*Alochaka* – eyebright, aloe, golden seal, sandalwood, triphala, chamomile

*Sadhaka* – brahmi, gotu kola, jatamansi, yasthi madhu, skullcap, passion flower

## Kapha

bibhitaki, cardamom, chitraka, ginger, guggulu, myrrh, pippali, tulasi, turmeric

## Kapha Subdoshas

*Avalambaka* – bibhitaki, pippali, pushkarmula, guggulu, saffron, thyme, ginger, cayenne, honey, cinnamon, garlic, yasthi madhu, coltsfoot

*Kledaka* – ginger, cinnamon, black pepper, pippali, cayenne, mustard, vaccha, cardamom, fennel, tulasi, trikatu

*Bodhaka* – bayberry, cinnamon, cardamom, ginger, haritaki, peppermint, vaccha, sage

*Sleshaka* – ginger, cayenne, guggulu, myrhh, sallaki, nirgundi, angelica, turmeric, chaparral, garlic

*Tarpaka* – pippali, shilajit, vaccha, shankapushpi, somalata (ma huang/ephedra), haritaki, bibhitaki, brahmi, gotu kola, sage

## Herbs for the Dhatus

This list is very general. Appropriate use of herbs will vary depending on excess and deficiencies of the dhatus, and if the dhatu is sama (with ama) or nirama (without ama). To determine proper usage, please consult with a specialist in Ayurveda.

### Rasa

Vata in Rasa Dhatu – black pepper, ginger, mahasudarshan churna, tulasi

Pitta in Rasa Dhatu – aloe, neem, peppermint

Kapha in Rasa Dhatu – ginger, trikatu

### Rakta

Vata in Rakta Dhatu – amalaki, loha bhasma, shatavari, yasthi madhu

Pitta in Rakta Dhatu – amalaki, ashoka, guduchi, manjistha, neem,

Kapha in Rakta Dhatu – ashoka, daruharidra, kutki, manjistha, myrrh

## Mamsa

Vata in Mamsa Dhatu – ashwagandha, bala
Pitta in Mamsa Dhatu – guduchi, kaishore guggulu, turmeric
Kapha in Mamsa Dhatu – arjuna, kanchanar guggulu, turmeric

## Meda

Vata in Meda Dhatu – ashwagandha, shatavari, vidari kanda, yasthi madhu
Pitta in Meda Dhatu – manjistha, neem, shankapushpi, turmeric
Kapha in Meda Dhatu – kutki, shilajit, triphala

## Asthi

Vata in Asthi Dhatu – ashwagandha, shilajit, yogaraj guggulu
Pitta in Asthi Dhatu – brahmi, kaishore guggulu
Kapha in Asthi Dhatu – gokshuradi guggulu, punarnava guggulu

## Majja

Vata in Majja Dhatu – ashwagandha, jatamansi, vaccha
Pitta in Majja Dhatu – bhringaraja, brahmi, jatamansi
Kapha in Majja Dhatu – brahmi, sallaki, vaccha

## Shukra

Vata in Shukra Dhatu – ashwagandha, bala, Kapikachhu, tongkat ali
Pitta in Shukra Dhatu – ashoka, guduchi, shankapushpi, white musali, shatavari
Kapha in Shukra Dhatu – ashwagandha, gokshura, Kapikachhu, shilajit

## Artava

Vata in Artava Dhatu – ashoka, vadarikand
Pitta in Artava Dhatu – ashoka, shatavari
Kapha in Artava Dhatu – ashoka, chandraprabha

# Chapter 18

# Dharma and the Earth

*Look deep into nature, and then you will
understand everything better.*

*~ Albert Einstein*

*For in the true nature of things, if we rightly consider,
every green tree is far more glorious than
if it were made of gold and silver.*

*~ Rev. Martin Luther King, Jr.*

Thousands of years ago, humans lived in perfect harmony with
nature. Over time, this harmony has been lost. It is impossible
to disrespect Mother Nature and to simultaneously embody true
health and consciousness. The goals of Ayurveda and yoga cannot
be realized without love and respect for Mother Earth.

The modern age has seen such a major decline of dharma that
the environment is in dire need of help. The planet and humanity are at a fragile breaking point where anything could happen.
Resources are quickly diminishing while war and sickness are on the
rise. The human population is increasing at an alarming rate. The
gap between the "haves" and the "have-nots" is increasing. We are
destroying forests, wilderness, rivers, lakes, clean air and nutritious
food. Pollution, desertification and extinction of plants and animals
are rapidly on the rise. The cause of this chaos and destruction is the
human ego. Due to ignorance and pride, the fragile balance of life
on planet Earth is being threatened. All of the other species of life
on the planet are living in balance with nature. It is the humans who

are responsible for the chaos and destruction. If we continue to abuse Mother Earth, She will soon become uninhabitable by humans.

Fortunately, however, it is not too late. There is still hope. If we come together now as a one-world family, united in love, we can restore the lost harmony. We can heal the wounds inflicted on each other and our Mother Earth. We can all eat healthful, nutritious, life-giving foods. It is possible for all beings to live together in peace and happiness with the Earth. Just as the health of a mother greatly affects the health of her nursing baby, the health and happiness of Mother Earth directly affects the health and happiness of Her children – us. It is our dharma to heal our Mother Earth, thus healing ourselves. It is our dharma to heal ourselves, thus healing our Mother Earth.

As Walt Whitman said, "Now I see the secret of the making of the best persons. It is to grow in the open air and to eat and sleep with the Earth." In truth, humans have only one dharma to follow: seeking liberation or union with God, or the Self. All other dharma leads to this one. However, without a habitable planet, this goal is not possible. We can put our priorities in order by asking ourselves what Henry David Thoreau once asked: "What is the use of a house if you haven't got a planet to put it on?" Mother Earth is our home and She is in a state of emergency. She has been screaming and not too many people are listening. It is our current responsibility to preserve the Earth.

As Chief Seattle said, "The Earth does not belong to us, we belong to the Earth." We have an obligation to both our ancestors and our children: to protect what our ancestors have cultivated and to preserve what our children's children will inherit.

Global unification is necessary to restore the lost harmony. By following the principles of eco-dharma, we gain more awareness of how we impact the environment by the products we buy and use. The ancient Cree prophecy says, "Only after the last tree has been cut down, only after the last river has been poisoned, only after the last fish has been caught, only then will one find that money cannot be eaten." We often make money our first priority while neglecting the environment; it is time to seriously re-evaluate our motivations and actions.

On September 27, 2012, the celebration of Amma's 59th birthday, Embracing the World launched the Campaign for Nature Initiative called InDeed. The InDeed Campaign For Nature is a call to help restore the lost balance between humanity and nature through six easy commitments. Embracing the World's InDeed Campaign for Nature has been officially recognized by UNESCO as a project of the United Nations Decade of Education for Sustainable Development. Embracing the World's InDeed Campaign for Nature is all about action. It's about putting Amma's practical suggestions about the way we might use the earth's remaining resources, and the way we interact with the natural world into practice in our own lives and our own communities. It's about what each of us can do, right now, in our own backyard, to help restore the lost harmony between humanity and nature. To learn more about this campaign and what you can do to help preserve nature for the future generations please visit www.embracingtheworld.org/indeed.

*We must not be forced to explore the universe in search of a new home because we have made the Earth inhospitable, even uninhabitable. For if we do not solve the environmental and related social problems that beset us on Earth — pollution, toxic contamination, resource depletion, prejudice, poverty, hunger — those problems will surely accompany us to other worlds.*

*~ Donald G. Kaufman and Cecilia M. Franz,*
*Biosphere 2000: Protecting Our Global Environment, 1996*

*To find the universal elements enough,*
*to find the air and the water exhilarating,*
*to be refreshed by a morning walk or an evening saunter,*
*to be thrilled by the stars at night,*

*to be elated over a bird's nest or a wildflower in spring –*
*these are some of the rewards of the simple life.*

~ *John Burroughs, Naturalist (1837-1921)*

## 108 Tips on How to Help Save the Environment

1. Pray for Peace.
2. Buy energy-efficient appliances and cars.
3. Caulk and weatherstrip doors and windows.
4. Install storm windows.
5. Close off unused areas in your home from heat and air conditioning.
6. Wear warm clothing and turn down heat during winter.
7. Switch to low-wattage or fluorescent light bulbs.
8. Turn off all unnecessary lights.
9. Use cold water instead of hot whenever possible.
10. Opt for small-oven or stove-top cooking when preparing small meals.
11. When using dishwashers and laundry machines, wash full loads rather than partial or overfull loads. Washing machines use 30 to 60 gallons of water for each cycle.
12. Wash clothes only when necessary.
13. Clean the lint screen in clothes dryers.
14. Use moderate amounts of biodegradable, phosphate-free laundry and dish soaps.
15. Install a clothes line in your backyard and let your clothes dry naturally. If you must, dry clothes for 10 minutes in the dryer, pull out the items that can go on hangers and hang them on your shower curtain rod. The remaining clothes dry faster and the others air dry wrinkle-free and last longer.
16. Install an air-assisted or composting toilet.

17. Insulate your water heater. Install water-efficient showerheads and sink-faucet aerators.

18. Take quick showers instead of baths.

19. Make sure water faucets don't drip.

20. Boycott manufacturers that exploit workers, employ child labor, or use toxic chemicals in the manufacturing process. Inquire where clothing and fabrics come from, how they were produced, and by whom.

21. Collect rainwater and gray water for gardening use.

22. Use recycled and rechargeable batteries. Disposable batteries contain toxic chemicals and manufacturing them takes about 50 times as much energy as the batteries produce.

23. Plant deciduous shade trees that block the summer sun but allow the sun's warmth during the winter.

24. Explore getting a solar water heater for your home.

25. Learn how to recycle all of your household goods, from clothing to motor oil to appliances.

26. Set refrigerators to 38°F (3°C) and freezers to 5°F, (-15°C) no colder.

27. Encourage your local recycling center or program to start accepting all types of plastic.

28. Urge local officials to begin roadside pickup of recyclables and hazardous wastes.

29. Encourage friends, neighbors, businesses and local organizations to recycle and to sponsor recycling efforts.

30. Use recycled products, especially paper.

31. Reuse envelopes, jars, paper and plastic bags, scrap paper, etc.

32. Bring your own canvas bags to the grocery store.

33. Encourage local businesses and governments to buy recycled paper.

34. Start a recycling program where you work.

35. Limit or eliminate your use of "disposable" items.

36. Avoid take-out food and drinks. Carry a mug and plastic container in your tote bag, backpack or car. Many places give discounts on drinks if you bring your own mug.

37. Avoid using anything made of plastic foam. It is often made from chlorofluorocarbons (CFC's) which contribute to ozone depletion and never biodegrade.

38. Unplug electronics, such as DVD players, stereos, etc., which have a clock or light on when not in use. They are constantly using electricity when plugged in.

39. Maintain and tune up your vehicle regularly for maximum gas mileage. Keep your car tires inflated to the proper pressure to improve fuel economy and extend the life of the tires.

40. Join a car pool or use public transportation to commute.

41. Write to automobile manufacturers to let them know that you intend to buy the most fuel-efficient car on the road.

42. Reduce your use of air conditioning.

43. Encourage auto centers to install CFC recycling equipment for automobile air conditioners. Freon that is released during servicing becomes both a greenhouse gas and an ozone layer destroyer.

44. Remove unnecessary articles from your car. Each 100 pounds of weight decreases fuel efficiency by 1%.

45. Don't speed; accelerate and slow down gradually.

46. Walk or use a bicycle whenever possible.

47. Urge local governments to enact restrictions on automobile use in congested areas downtown.

48. Enjoy sports and recreational activities that use your muscles rather than gasoline and electricity.

49. Buy products that last.

50. Rent or borrow items that you don't use often.

51. When planning occasions involving gift-giving, why not practice reuse and recycling? Ask guests to bring used items or a recycled gift from home.

52. Use natural fiber clothing, bedding and towels. Use more colored fabrics to avoid the need for bleach. Use old clothing and sheets as cleaning rags.

53. Reuse is a big part of the solution for tackling our waste problem. Maintain and repair the items you own. For example, think of repairing your shoes, bike and knapsack rather than buying new ones.

54. Don't buy aerosols, halon fire extinguishers or other products containing CFCs. Avoid the use of household pesticides.

55. Write to computer chip manufacturers and urge them to stop using CFC-113 (a chlorofluorocarbon that enters the atmosphere and rapidly breaks down ozone) as a solvent.

56. Invest your money in environmentally and socially conscious businesses.

57. Educate yourself about the items you purchase; understand the impact they have on the environment.

58. Use e-mail instead of paper letters.

59. Become vegetarian. Meat production uses a huge quantity of land, soil, water and energy, and one cow emits 200-400 liters of methane per day.

60. Buy locally produced foods; avoid buying foods that must be trucked in from great distances.

61. Read labels. Eat organic and less-processed foods.

62. Start a garden. Plant an organic garden instead of a lawn.

63. Watering your garden with an underground drip system. Water at night to limit evaporation.

64. Plant trees. Strategically located, trees can reduce heating and cooling bills, help prevent soil erosion and reduce air pollution.

65. Compost kitchen and garden waste or give it to a friend who can.

66. Inform schools, hospitals, airlines, restaurants and the media of your environmental and food concerns.

67. Stay informed about the condition of the Earth.

68. Talk to friends, relatives and co-workers about preventing global climate change.

69. Read and support publications that educate about long-term sustainability.

70. Start a global climate change study group.

71. Educate children about sustainable living practices.

72. Photocopy this list (on recycled or tree-free post consumer paper, or email it) and send it to everyone you know.

73. Buy energy-efficient products from companies that help protect the environment.

74. Get involved in local tree-planting programs.

75. Join an environmental organization. If they're not already addressing climate change, get them involved.

76. Support zero population growth.

77. Adapt to the local climate as much as possible rather than trying to isolate yourself from it.

78. Donate money to environmental organizations.

79. Support programs and products that aim to save rainforests.

80. Support solar and renewable energy development.

81. Work to protect local watershed areas.

82. Pave as little as possible.

83. Learn more about biodynamic and sustainable agriculture.

84. Encourage sewage plants to compost their sludge.

85. Encourage your power companies to supply wind power. (It is available in most states.)

86. Shorten your shower by a minute or two and you'll save up to 150 gallons of water per month.

87. Support disarmament and the redirection of military funds to environmental restoration.

88. Write letters to the editors of local newspapers expressing your concern about climate change and environmental issues.

89. Support electoral candidates who run on environmental platforms.

90. Attend city council meetings and speak out for action on climate change issues.

91. Use a water filter instead of drinking bottled water.

92. Never let water run unnecessarily. Wash dishes in a basin of water rather than under a running faucet. Turn off the faucet while you brush your teeth. If you just wet and rinse your toothbrush instead of letting the water run, you will save nine gallons of water each time you brush. When shaving, filling the basin instead of letting the water run will save 14 gallons of water.

93. Compost your leaves and yard waste, which will improve your garden's soil. Minimize the use of garden chemicals by weeding.

94. In place of watching TV or listening to the stereo, spend time reading, writing, telling stories and making music.

95. Use a water-efficient showerhead. They're inexpensive, easy to install, and can save you up to 750 gallons of water a month.

96. Strive to establish good communications with friends, neighbors and family; include learning conflict resolution skills.

97. Spend time seeing, hearing and rejoicing in the beauty of the Earth. Feel your love for the Earth. Make serving the Earth your first priority.

98. Learn about the simpler, less resource-intensive lifestyles of aboriginal and native people.

99. Spend time with children enjoying and appreciating nature.

100. Think often about the kind of Earth you would like to see for your grandchildren's grandchildren.

101. While doing small things, think big. Think about redesigning cities, restructuring the economy, re-conceiving humanity's role on the Earth.

102. Plant tulasi and other medicinal herbs.

103. Visualize a healthful planet.

104. Breathe.

105. Meditate.

106. Awaken.

107. Serve.

108. Love.

*He that plants a tree is a servant of God,*
*he provides a kindness for many generations,*
*and faces that he hath not seen shall bless him.*

*~ Henry Van Dyke*

*Study nature, love nature, stay close to*
*nature. It will never fail you.*

*~ Frank Lloyd Wright*

# Chapter 19

# Mother Nature

*God is in everything, not just in human beings. God is
in mountains, rivers and trees, in birds and animals,
in clouds, the sun, the moon and the stars.*

~Amma

*One thing we know: our God is also your God.
The Earth is precious to Him.*

~ Chief Seattle

The whole world is currently in the midst of a massive ecological and
spiritual crisis. This crisis is manifesting as the growing destruction
of our natural environment, the overwhelming stress of our daily
lives, the unending conflicts and wars between nations, and the
unhappiness and discontent most people feel in their daily lives. The
terrorism and natural disasters plaguing the world are a reflection
of a much deeper problem – humanity is out of balance with itself
and its environment.

Humanity has certainly made many great technological and
scientific advances. However, our planet's natural resources of air,
water and food are running short. On May 25th, 2010, Amma gave
a speech at the State University of New York at Buffalo, where she
explained the absolute necessity of unifying science, technology
and spirituality:

"Knowledge is like a river. Its nature is to constantly flow.
Wherever it can flow, it does so, nourishing culture. On the other
hand, the same knowledge, if devoid of values, becomes a source

of destruction for the world. When values and knowledge become one, there can be no more powerful instrument for the welfare of humankind. Today, physicists have even begun investigating the possibility that the essential substratum of the manifest universe and the individual are one and the same. We are standing on the threshold of a new era wherein material science and spirituality will move forward hand in hand. It is Amma's prayer that we expand our minds to embrace both scientific knowledge and spiritual wisdom. We can no longer afford to see these two streams of knowledge as flowing in opposite directions. In truth, they complement one another. If we merge these streams, we will find that we are able to create a mighty river – a river whose waters can remove suffering and spread life to all of humanity."

The human species has overpopulated the earth so much that all life on the planet suffers from the effects. We have hoarded and consumed so much of the planet's resources that Mother Earth herself is suffering. Numerous species have lost their homes or even become extinct as a result of our actions. We must put an end to this senseless destruction. Amma tells us, "The never-ending stream of love that flows from a true believer toward the entire Creation will have a gentle, soothing effect on nature. Our love is the best protection of nature. My children, one of our priorities should be to preserve nature. We must put an end to the practice of destroying the environment for our selfish, short-term needs."

We continue to fail in understanding the laws of nature and the interdependence of all creatures. We are currently on a fast-moving collision course of destruction, rather than treading lightly on a path of love and compassion. We are devouring our world with unprecedented greed and lust for power. In this greed, we are rapidly diminishing what little usable resources remain on Earth. As of yet, we have failed to comprehend that the ultimate result of this is destruction. Amma also tells us, "It is when our selfishness increases that we begin to lose our innocence. When this happens, we become estranged from nature and begin to exploit her. We don't know what a terrible threat we have become to her. By harming nature, we are paving the way for our own destruction. In truth, the progress and prosperity of humanity depend solely on the good that people do for nature."

If this current environmental and spiritual crisis serves as an awakening, it can help us to realize a higher level of human potential, unifying science and technology with nature and spirituality. Without such an awakening, we face an imminent global environmental catastrophe that will devastate humanity as well as the natural environment upon which all life depends. What will manifest depends on each of us, and the love and compassion that we put into our thoughts, words and actions.

Amma says, "Life is filled with God's light, but only through optimism will you experience that light. Look at the optimism of nature. Nothing can stop it. Every aspect of nature tirelessly contributes its share to life. The participation of a little bird, an animal, a tree or a flower is always complete. No matter what the hardships, they continue to try wholeheartedly."

At the present moment, our collective consciousness is like a light smothered in endless darkness, the infinite caged within the finite. We urgently need to escape our self-imposed limitations. Our hearts and minds have unlimited capacity to open up to the highest levels of consciousness. The real purpose of yoga, Ayurveda and this precious human birth is to unite our consciousness with the Divine. May we move forward with true awareness, in the light of love, filled with compassion for nature, humanity and all sentient beings.

## Nature Sutras

This is a compilation of poetry and teachings about Mother Nature. It is a call for the restoration of the lost harmony between humanity and nature. May it serve as inspiration to awaken inner love for nature.

*I remember a hundred lovely lakes, and recall the fragrant breath of pine and fir and cedar and poplar trees. The trail has strung upon it, as upon a thread of silk, opalescent dawns and saffron sunsets. It has given me blessed release from care and worry and the troubled thinking of our modern day. It has been a return to the primitive and the peaceful. Whenever the pressure of our complex city life thins my blood and benumbs my brain, I seek relief in the trail; and when I hear the coyote wailing to the yellow dawn, my cares fall from me – I am happy. ~ Hamlin Garland*

*I only went out for a walk and finally concluded to stay out till sundown, for going out, I found, was really going in. ~John Muir*

*Just as nature creates the favorable circumstances for a coconut to become a coconut tree, and for a seed to transform itself into a huge fruit tree, nature creates the necessary circumstances through which the individual soul can reach the Supreme Being and merge in eternal union with Him. ~Amma*

*The color of the mountains is Buddha's body; the sound of running water is his great speech. ~ Dogen*

*Nature is the art of God. ~ Dante Alighieri*

*Man's heart away from nature becomes hard. ~Standing Bear*

*How glorious a greeting the sun gives the mountains! ~John Muir*

*Adopt the pace of nature: her secret is
patience.* ~Ralph Waldo Emerson

*Climb the mountains and get their good tidings. Nature's peace
will flow into you as sunshine flows into trees. The winds will
blow their own freshness into you, and the storms their energy,
while cares will drop off like autumn leaves.* ~John Muir

*God writes the gospel not in the Bible alone, but on trees
and flowers and clouds and stars.* ~Martin Luther

*I believe that there is a subtle magnetism in
nature, which, if we unconsciously yield to it, will
direct us aright.* ~Henry David Thoreau

*When we live harmoniously with nature in love and unity,
we will have the strength to overcome any crisis.* ~Amma

*Forget not that the earth delights to feel your bare feet and
the winds long to play with your hair.* ~Kahlil Gibran

*I thank you God for most this amazing day:
for the leaping greenly spirit of trees
and a blue true dream of sky;
and for everything which is natural
which is infinite
which is yes.* ~e.e. cummings

*Nature is our first Mother. She nurtures us throughout our
lives. Our birth mother may allow us to sit on her lap for
a couple of years, but Mother Nature patiently bears our
weight our entire life. Just as a child is obligated to his birth*

*mother, we should feel an obligation and responsibility toward Mother Nature. If we forget this responsibility, it is equal to forgetting our own Self. If we forget nature, we will cease to exist, for to do so is to walk toward death. ~Amma*

*The poetry of earth is never dead. ~John Keats*

*In wilderness I sense the miracle of life, and behind it our scientific accomplishments fade to trivia. ~Charles A. Lindbergh*

*The human spirit needs places where nature has not been rearranged by the hand of man. ~Author Unknown*

*The sun, with all those planets revolving around it and dependent on it, can still ripen a bunch of grapes as if it had nothing else in the universe to do. ~Galileo*

*I believe a leaf of grass is no less than the journey-work of the stars. ~Walt Whitman*

*Everybody needs beauty as well as bread, places to play in and pray in, where nature may heal and give strength to body and soul. ~John Muir*

*Great things are done when men and mountains meet. This is not done by jostling in the street. ~William Blake*

*To me, a lush carpet of pine needles or spongy grass is more welcome than the most luxurious Persian rug. ~Helen Keller*

*Life becomes fulfilled when humankind and nature move together, hand in hand in harmony.* ~Amma

*Shall I not have intelligence with the earth? Am I not partly leaves and vegetable mould myself?* ~Henry David Thoreau

*One touch of nature makes the whole world kin.* ~William Shakespeare

*And this, our life, exempt from public haunt, finds tongues in trees, books in the running brooks, sermons in stones, and good in everything.* ~William Shakespeare

*Those who dwell among the beauties and mysteries of the earth are never alone or weary of life.* ~Rachel Carson

*Nature is man's teacher. She unfolds her treasures to his search, unseals his eye, illumines his mind, and purifies his heart; an influence breathes from all the sights and sounds of her existence.* ~Alfred Billings Street

*Let us permit nature to have her way. She understands her business better than we do.* ~Michel de Montaigne

*Look at nature. Nature is a textbook from which we must learn. Each object is a page of that book. Each and every object in nature teaches us something.* ~Amma

*I go to nature to be soothed and healed, and to have my senses put in order.* ~John Burroughs

*Nature will bear the closest inspection. She invites us
to lay our eye level with her smallest leaf, and take an
insect view of its plain.* ~Henry David Thoreau

*Nature is full of genius, full of divinity, so that not a snowflake
escapes its fashioning hand.* ~Henry David Thoreau

*There is a sufficiency in the world, in nature, for man's
need but not for man's greed.* ~Mohandas K. Gandhi

*If one way be better than another, that you
may be sure is nature's way.* ~Aristotle

*Nature is the art of God.* ~Thomas Browne

*It is now the urgent duty of all human beings to please
nature by performing selfless actions endowed with
mutual love, faith and sincerity. When this is done,
nature will bless you back with abundance.* ~Amma

## Conclusion – A New Beginning

The ultimate goal of life, Self-realization, should become our primary focus. This precious human birth must not be wasted on sense pleasures and material pursuits alone. Instead, let us use this life to get free from the cycles of birth and death. Now is the only time there is. Turn inward and uncover the truth and beauty that remain hidden deep within.

Ayurveda and yoga are invaluable tools that will help us on this journey. When the body and mind have been purified, we will see clearly the nature of the universe and the Self. We must put forth effort for grace to flow. We must strengthen our hearts and minds to be unwavering from the goal. May Amma's Grace and Love ever be with us.

*Let us stand together and show the world that compassion, love and concern for our fellow beings have not completely vanished from the face of this earth. Let us build a new world of peace and harmony by remaining deeply rooted in the universal values that have nourished humanity since time immemorial. Let us say goodbye to war and brutality forever, reducing them to the stuff of fairytales. Let us be remembered in the future as the generation of peace.*

*~ Amma*

*Shakti do jagadambe, bhakti do jagadambe,*
*prema do jagadambe ma.*
*Mujhe visvas dekar raksa karo, Amritesvari jagadambe ma.*

Divine Mother, give me strength,
Divine Mother, give me devotion,
Divine Mother, give me pure love.
O Divine Mother, protect me by giving me perfect faith.
O immortal Goddess, Mother of the Universe.
~ *Shakti Do Jagadambe, verse I, Bhajanamritam Vol. IV*

*Suddhosi buddhosi Naranjanosi,*
*Samasara maya parivarjitosi,*
*Samsara svaranam,*
*Jaja moha nayjan,*
*Najannaprejhur*
*Trisatsvarupi.*

O beloved child, thou art the ever-pure,
the ever-awakened, the ever-spotless.
Thou art completely free from maya,
free from the illusion of this earth-life.
Already thou art awakened.

~ *Sage Madalasa*

# Self-Examination Charts

These charts enable you to determine your individual constitution. Accurately determining your constitution will assist you in following a proper lifestyle regime. Balancing your doshas is essential to living a happy and healthful life.

Please do not make definitive conclusions about yourself based on these charts. They are generalizations meant for educational purposes and as a guide for self-examination. On each line, place a checkmark next to the aspect that applies most to you. To ensure accuracy, please be as honest as possible with yourself. Remember that no one is purely one type. .

For more specific diagnosis, please see an experienced ayurvedic practitioner who can perform an in-depth diagnosis.

## Prakriti – Your Individual Constitution

| Aspects | Vata | Pitta | Kapha |
|---|---|---|---|
| Activity | very active | moderate | slow |
| Appetite | low, variable | strong | steady |
| Body frame | thin | medium | large |
| Body weight | light | moderate | heavy |
| Concentration | short-term only, poor | above average, good | long-term, excellent |
| Disease pattern | nervous, anxiety, pain | heat-related | mucous-related |
| Dreams | fearful, active | angry, fiery | watery, calm |
| Elimination | dry, hard, constipated | oily, loose, soft | oily, thick, slow |
| Emotions | fearful, insecure | angry, irritable | attached, greedy |

| | | | |
|---|---|---|---|
| Endurance | fair | good | high |
| Eyes | small, dry, active | sharp, penetrating | big, attractive |
| Hair color | brown, black | red/grey | dark |
| Hair quantity | average | thin | thick |
| Hair type | dry | medium thickness | oily |
| Memory | good short-term | good | good long-term |
| Mental | quick, restless | sharp, aggressive | calm, steady, stable |
| Pulse pattern | swan, feeble, thready | frog, moderate, jumping | swan, broad, slow |
| Skin | dry, rough | soft, oily | thick, oily |
| Sleep | light, disturbed | sound, medium | deep, long |
| Strength | fair | above average | excellent |
| Talking | rapid, scattered | clear, fast, sharp | slow, clear, sweet |
| Teeth | protruding, crooked | medium-sized, soft | large, strong |
| Thirst | variable | excessive | slight |
| Thoughts | erratic | consistent | steady pace, focused |
| Voice | high-pitched, feeble | medium-pitched | low-pitched |
| Totals: | | | |

# Subdosha Charts

Place a checkmark next to the description that applies to you.

| Vata | |
|---|---|
| **Prana Vata** | |
| anxiety | |
| asthma | |
| dehydration | |
| emaciation | |
| hiccups | |
| hoarseness | |
| insomnia | |
| loss of voice | |
| senility | |
| shortness of breath | |
| tension headaches | |
| tuberculosis | |
| wasting | |
| worry | |
| **Total Prana Vata** | |
| | |
| **Udana Vata** | |
| cancer | |
| dry cough | |
| dry eyes | |
| earaches | |

| | |
|---|---|
| fatigue | |
| lack of enthusiasm | |
| overexcitement | |
| sore throat | |
| speech defects | |
| stuttering | |
| tonsillitis | |
| weakness | |
| **Total Udana Vata** | |
| | |
| **Samana Vata** | |
| dehydration | |
| diarrhea | |
| indigestion | |
| low energy | |
| poor nutrition | |
| rapid digestion | |
| slow digestion | |
| **Total Samana Vata** | |
| | |
| **Apana Vata** | |
| birth trauma, difficult birth | |
| constipation | |
| diabetes | |
| diarrhea | |

| | | | | |
|---|---|---|---|---|
| dysmenorrhea | | anemia | |
| low back pain | | anger | |
| menstrual disorders | | blood disorders | |
| sexual dysfunction | | hostility | |
| stillbirth | | jaundice | |
| **Total Apana Vata** | | liver disease | |
| | | low blood pressure | |
| **Vyana Vata** | | rashes | |
| arthritis | | Total Ranjaka Pitta | |
| frequent blinking | | | |
| heart irregularities | | **Sadhaka Pitta** | |
| joint cracking | | Emotional disturbance | |
| joint pain | | Heart attack | |
| nervousness | | Indecision | |
| poor circulation | | Low intelligence | |
| Total Vyana Vata | | Poor memory | |
| | | **Total Sadhaka Pitta** | |
| *Pitta* | | | |
| **Pachaka Pitta** | | **Alochaka Pitta** | |
| acidity | | Eye diseases | |
| addictions | | Red/irritated eyes | |
| cravings | | Anger | |
| heartburn | | Vision problems | |
| indigestion | | **Total Alochaka Pitta** | |
| ulcers | | | |
| Total Pachaka Pitta | | **Bhrajaka Pitta** | |
| | | Acne | |
| **Ranjaka Pitta** | | All skin disorders | |

| | | | | |
|---|---|---|---|---|
| Boils/Abscesses | | | **Bodhaka Kapha** | |
| Hot skin | | | Diabetes | |
| Inflammation | | | Food sensitivity | |
| Poor memory | | | General congestion | |
| Rashes | | | Loss of taste | |
| Skin cancer | | | Obesity | |
| **Total Bhrajaka Pitta** | | | **Total Bodhaka Kapha** | |
| | | | | |
| *Kapha* | | | **Tarpaka Kapha** | |
| **Kledaka Kapha** | | | Depression | |
| Bloating | | | Headaches | |
| Excess mucous in stomach | | | Impairment of senses | |
| | | | Irritability | |
| Slow digestion | | | Loss of smell | |
| **Total Kledaka Kapha** | | | Sinus problems | |
| | | | **Total Tarpaka Kapha** | |
| **Avalambaka Kapha** | | | | |
| Asthma | | | **Sleshaka Kapha** | |
| Back pain | | | Chest congestion | |
| Chest/lung congestion | | | Lethargy | |
| Heart pain | | | Loose joints | |
| Lethargy | | | Stiffness of joints and body | |
| Stiffness | | | Swelling | |
| **Total Avalambaka Kapha** | | | **Total Sleshaka Kapha** | |

# Three Gunas Constitutional Chart

Place a checkmark next to the one that most accurately applies to you. Again, be honest with yourself. If the result is not how you wish it to be, you can use this as a tool for self-improvement, growth and inner expansion.

| Aspects | Satva | Rajas | Tamas |
|---|---|---|---|
| Alcohol | never | occasionally | often |
| Anger | rarely | occasionally | often |
| Attachment | little | moderate | high |
| Cleanliness | high | moderate | low |
| Concentration | strong | moderate | lacking, poor |
| Contentment | usually | occasionally | never |
| Creativity | high | moderate | poor |
| Daily exercise | always | occasionally | rarely |
| Depression | rarely/never | occasionally | often |
| Desire/lust | little | moderate | excessive |
| Detachment | high | moderate | low/none |
| Diet | pure vegetarian/ vegan | some meat | diet high in meat |
| Discrimination | high | moderate | low/none |
| Drugs | never | occasionally | often |
| Fear | rarely | occasionally | often |
| Forgiveness | easily | forgives with time | holds grudges |
| Greed | little | moderate | high |
| Love | unconditional | personal | selfish, lacking |
| Mantra/prayer | daily | occasionally | never |
| Meditation | daily | occasionally | never |
| Memory | strong | moderate | poor |
| Non-coveting | always | moderate/ occasionally | rarely |

| | | | |
|---|---|---|---|
| **Non-stealing** | always | occasionally | rarely |
| **Non-violence** | always | occasionally | rarely |
| **Peace of mind** | almost always | moderate/ occasionally | rarely |
| **Pride/ego** | modest/humble | fluctuating | vanity |
| **Self-discipline** | high | moderate | low/none |
| **Self-study/ reflection** | high | moderate | low/none |
| **Sense control** | good | moderate | weak |
| **Sensory input** | calm, pure | mixed | disturbed |
| **Seva (selfless service)** | regularly | moderate/ occasionally | poor/rarely |
| **Speech** | peaceful, serene | excited, agi-tated | lifeless, dull |
| **Spiritual study** | daily | occasionally | never |
| **Truthfulness** | always | usually | rarely |
| **Will power** | strong | fluctuates | weak |
| **Work ethic** | selfless | personal gain | lazy |
| **Totals** | | | |

# Food Charts

* means eat in moderation
** means eat rarely

| Vata | | | |
|---|---|---|---|
| **FRUITS –**<br>**Advisable**<br>*Most sweet fruit* | **FRUITS –**<br>**Avoid**<br>*Most dried fruit* | **VEGETABLES**<br>**–**<br>**Advisable**<br>*In general, veg-*<br>*etables should be*<br>*cooked.* | **VEGETABLES**<br>**–**<br>**Avoid**<br>*Frozen, raw or*<br>*dried vegetables* |
| • apples (cooked)<br>• applesauce<br>• apricots<br>• avocado<br>• bananas<br>• berries<br>• cherries<br>• coconut<br>• dates (fresh)<br>• figs (fresh)<br>• grapefruit<br>• grapes<br>• kiwi<br>• lemons<br>• limes<br>• mangoes<br>• melons<br>• oranges<br>• papayas<br>• peaches<br>• pineapple<br>• plums<br>• prunes (soaked) | • apples (raw)<br>• cranberries<br>• dates (dry)<br>• figs (dry)<br>• pears<br>• pomegranates<br>• prunes (dry)<br>• raisins (dry)<br>• watermelon | • asparagus<br>• beets<br>• cabbage (cooked)<br>• carrots<br>• cauliflower*<br>• cilantro<br>• cucumber<br>• daikon radish*<br>• fennel (anise)<br>• garlic<br>• green beans<br>• green chilies<br>• Jerusalem artichoke*<br>• leafy greens *<br>• leeks<br>• lettuce*<br>• mustard greens*<br>• okra<br>• olives, black<br>• onions (cooked)* | • artichoke<br>• beet greens**<br>• bitter melon<br>• broccoli<br>• Brussels sprouts<br>• burdock root<br>• cabbage (raw)<br>• cauliflower (raw)<br>• celery<br>• corn (fresh)**<br>• dandelion greens<br>• eggplant<br>• horseradish**<br>• kale<br>• kohlrabi<br>• olives, green<br>• onions (raw)<br>• peppers, sweet and hot |

| Vata | | | |
|---|---|---|---|
| **FRUITS –** Advisable *Most sweet fruit* | **FRUITS –** Avoid *Most dried fruit* | **VEGETABLES –** Advisable *In general, vegetables should be cooked.* | **VEGETABLES –** Avoid *Frozen, raw or dried vegetables* |
| • raisins (soaked) • rhubarb • strawberries • tamarind | | • parsley* • parsnip • peas (cooked) • potatoes, sweet• pumpkin • radishes (cooked)* • rutabaga • spaghetti squash* • spinach* | • potatoes, white • prickly pear (fruit and leaves) • radish (raw) • sprouts • tomatoes (cooked)** • turnips • wheat grass |

| Vata | | | |
|---|---|---|---|
| **LEGUMES –** Advisable | **LEGUMES –** Avoid | **DAIRY –** Advisable *Most dairy is good.* | **DAIRY –** Avoid |
| • lentils (red)* • mung beans • mung dal • soy cheese* • soy milk* • soy sauce* • soy sausages* • tofu* • tur dal • urad dal | • adzuki beans • black beans • black-eyed peas • chick peas (garbanzo beans) • kidney beans • lentils, (brown) • lima beans | • butter • buttermilk • cheese (hard)* • cheese (soft) • cottage cheese • cow's milk • ghee • goat's cheese • goat's milk | • cow's milk (powdered) • goat's milk (powdered) • yogurt (plain, frozen or with fruit) |

| Vata | | | |
|------|---|---|---|
| **LEGUMES – Advisable** | **LEGUMES – Avoid** | **DAIRY – Advisable** *Most dairy is good.* | **DAIRY – Avoid** |
| | • miso** <br> • navy beans <br> • peas (dried) <br> • pinto beans <br> • soybeans <br> • soy flour <br> • soy powder <br> • split peas <br> • tempeh <br> • white beans | • ice cream* <br> • sour cream*• <br> yogurt <br> (diluted and <br> spiced)* | |

| Vata | | | |
|------|---|---|---|
| **NUTS – Advisable** *In moderation* | **NUTS – Avoid** | **SEEDS – Advisable** | **SEEDS – Avoid** |
| • almonds <br> • black walnuts <br> • brazil nuts <br> • cashews <br> • charole <br> • coconut <br> • filberts <br> • hazelnuts <br> • macadamia <br> nuts <br> • peanuts <br> • pecans <br> • pine nuts <br> • pistachios <br> • walnuts | • none | • chia <br> • flax <br> • halva <br> • hemp <br> • pumpkin <br> • sesame <br> • sunflower <br> • tahini | • popcorn <br> • psyllium** |

| Vata | | | |
|---|---|---|---|
| GRAINS – Advisable | GRAINS – Avoid | BEVERAGES – Advisable | BEVERAGES – Avoid |
| • amaranth* <br> • durham flour <br> • oats (cooked) <br> • pancakes <br> • quinoa <br> • rice (all kinds) <br> • seitan (wheat meat) <br> • sprouted wheat bread (Essene) <br> • wheat | • barley <br> • bread (made with yeast) <br> • buckwheat <br> • cereals (cold, dry or puffed) <br> • corn <br> • couscous <br> • crackers <br> • granola <br> • millet <br> • muesli <br> • oat bran <br> • oats (dry) <br> • pasta** <br> • polenta** <br> • rice cakes** <br> • rye <br> • sago <br> • spelt <br> • tapioca <br> • wheat bran | • alcohol (beer or wine)* <br> • almond milk <br> • aloe vera juice <br> • apple cider <br> • apricot juice <br> • berry juice (except for cranberry) <br> • carob* <br> • carrot juice <br> • cherry juice <br> • grain beverage (coffee substitute) <br> • grape juice <br> • grapefruit juice <br> • hot spiced milk <br> • lemonade <br> • mango juice <br> • miso broth <br> • orange juice <br> • papaya juice <br> • peach nectar <br> • pineapple juice <br> • rice milk <br> • sour juices <br> • soy milk (hot and well-spiced)* | • apple juice <br> • black tea <br> • caffeinated beverages <br> • carbonated drinks <br> • chocolate milk <br> • coffee <br> • cold dairy drinks <br> • cranberry juice <br> • iced tea <br> • icy cold drinks <br> • herbal teas: alfalfa** barley** basil** blackberry borage** burdock cinnamon** corn silk dandelion ginseng hibiscus hops** jasmine** lemon balm** <br> • mixed vegetable juice |

| | Vata | | |
|---|---|---|---|
| **GRAINS –** Advisable | **GRAINS –** Avoid | **BEVERAGES** – Advisable | **BEVERAGES** – Avoid |
| | | • herbal teas: ajwan bancha catnip* chamomile chicory chrysanthe-mum* clove | • pear juice<br>• pomegranate juice<br>• prune juice**<br>• soy milk (cold)<br>• tomato juice**<br>• vegetable bouillon |

| | Vata | | |
|---|---|---|---|
| **OILS –** Advisable<br>*Most suitable at top* | **OILS –** Avoid | **SPICES –** Advisable<br>*Almost all spices are good.* | **SPICES –** Avoid |
| • sesame<br>• ghee<br>• olive<br>• most other oils<br>*External use only:*<br>• coconut<br>• avocado | • flax seed | • ajwan<br>• allspice<br>• almond extract<br>• anise<br>• asafoetida (hing)<br>• basil<br>• bay leaf<br>• black pepper<br>• cardamom<br>• cayenne*<br>• cinnamon<br>• cloves<br>• coriander<br>• cumin<br>• curry leaves<br>• dill | • caraway |

| Vata | | | |
|---|---|---|---|
| OILS –<br>**Advisable**<br>*Most suitable<br>at top* | OILS –<br>**Avoid** | SPICES –<br>**Advisable**<br>*Almost all spices<br>are good.* | SPICES –<br>**Avoid** |
| | | • fennel<br>• fenugreek*<br>• garlic<br>• ginger<br>• mace<br>• marjoram<br>• mint<br>• mustard seeds<br>• nutmeg<br>• orange peel<br>• oregano<br>• paprika<br>• parsley<br>• peppermint<br>• pippali<br>• poppy seeds<br>• rosemary<br>• saffron<br>• savory<br>• spearmint<br>• star anise<br>• tarragon<br>• thyme<br>• turmeric<br>• vanilla<br>• wintergreen | |

| Vata | | | |
|---|---|---|---|
| CONDI-MENTS – Advisable | CONDI-MENTS – Avoid | SWEETEN-ERS – Advisable | SWEETEN-ERS – Avoid |
| • chutney, mango (sweet or spicy)<br>• cilantro*<br>• dulse<br>• gomasio<br>• hijiki<br>• kelp<br>• ketchup<br>• kombu<br>• lemon<br>• lime<br>• mayonnaise<br>• mustard<br>• pickles (lime pickle, mango pickle)<br>• salt<br>• scallions<br>• seaweed<br>• soy sauce<br>• sprouts*<br>• tamari | • chocolate<br>• horseradish | • barley malt<br>• fructose<br>• fruit juice concentrate<br>• honey (raw and unpro-cessed<br>• jaggery<br>• molasses<br>• rice syrup<br>• sucanat<br>• turbinado | • maple syrup**<br>• white sugar |

| Vata | |
|------|------|
| **FOOD SUPPLEMENTS –** Advisable | **FOOD SUPPLEMENTS –** Avoid |
| • aloe vera juice* <br> • amino acids <br> • bee pollen <br> • minerals: calcium, copper, iron, magnesium, zinc <br> • royal jelly <br> • spirulina <br> • blue-green algae <br> • vitamins A, B, B$_{12}$, C, D and E | • barley green <br> • brewer's yeast |

| Pitta | | | |
|-------|-------|-------|-------|
| **FRUITS –** Advisable <br> *Most sweet fruit* | **FRUITS –** Avoid <br> *Most sour fruit* | **VEGETABLES – Advisable** <br> *Most sweet and bitter vegetables* | **VEGETABLES – Avoid** <br> *Most pungent vegetables* |
| • apples (sweet) <br> • applesauce <br> • apricots (sweet) <br> • avocado <br> • berries (sweet) <br> • cherries (sweet) <br> • coconut <br> • dates <br> • figs <br> • grapes (red and purple) <br> • limes* | • apples (sour) <br> • apricots (sour) <br> • bananas <br> • berries (sour) <br> • cherries (sour) <br> • cranberries <br> • grapefruit <br> • grapes (green) <br> • kiwi** <br> • lemons <br> • mangoes (green) <br> • oranges (sour) | • artichoke <br> • asparagus <br> • beets (cooked) <br> • bitter melon <br> • broccoli <br> • Brussels sprouts <br> • cabbage <br> • carrots (cooked) <br> • carrots (raw)* <br> • cauliflower <br> • celery <br> • cilantro <br> • cucumber | • beet greens <br> • beets, raw <br> • burdock root <br> • corn (fresh)** <br> • daikon radish <br> • eggplant** <br> • garlic <br> • green chilies <br> • horseradish <br> • kohlrabi** <br> • leeks (raw) <br> • mustard greens <br> • olives (green) <br> • onions (raw) |

| Pitta | | | |
|---|---|---|---|
| FRUITS – Advisable<br>*Most sweet fruit* | FRUITS – Avoid<br>*Most sour fruit* | VEGETABLES – Advisable<br>*Most sweet and bitter vegetables* | VEGETABLES – Avoid<br>*Most pungent vegetables* |
| • mangoes (ripe)<br>• melons<br>• oranges (sweet)<br>• papayas*<br>• pears<br>• pineapple (sweet)<br>• pomegranates<br>• prunes<br>• raisins<br>• watermelon | • peaches<br>• persimmons<br>• pineapple (sour)<br>• plums (sour)<br>• prickly pear<br>• rhubarb<br>• strawberries<br>• tamarind | • dandelion greens<br>• fennel (anise)<br>• green beans<br>• Jerusalem artichokes<br>• kale<br>• leafy greens<br>• leeks (cooked)<br>• lettuce<br>• okra<br>• olives (black)<br>• onions (cooked)<br>• parsley<br>• parsnips<br>• peas<br>• peppers (sweet)<br>• potatoes (sweet, white) | • peppers (hot)<br>• radishes (raw)<br>• spinach (cooked)**<br>• spinach (raw)<br>• tomatoes<br>• turnip greens<br>• turnips |

| | | *Pitta* | |
|---|---|---|---|
| **LEGUMES –** Advisable | **LEGUMES –** Avoid | **DAIRY –** Advisable | **DAIRY – Avoid** |
| • adzuki beans<br>• black beans<br>• black-eyed peas<br>• chick peas (garbanzo beans)<br>• kidney beans<br>• lentils (brown, red)<br>• lima beans<br>• mung beans<br>• mung dal<br>• navy beans<br>• peas (dried)<br>• pinto beans<br>• soy beans<br>• soy cheese<br>• soy flour*<br>• soy milk<br>• soy powder*<br>• split peas<br>• tempeh<br>• tofu<br>• white beans | • miso<br>• soy sauce<br>• soy sausages<br>• tur dal<br>• urad dal | • butter (unsalted)<br>• cheese (soft, not aged, unsalted)<br>• cottage cheese<br>• cow's milk<br>• ghee<br>• goat's cheese (soft and unsalted)<br>• goat's milk<br>• ice cream<br>• yogurt (freshly made and diluted)* | • butter (salted)<br>• buttermilk<br>• cheese (hard)<br>• sour cream<br>• yogurt (plain, frozen or with fruit) |

| Pitta | | | |
|---|---|---|---|
| **GRAINS – Advisable** | **GRAINS – Avoid** | **BEVERAGES – Advisable** | **BEVERAGES – Avoid** |
| • amaranth<br>• barley<br>• cereal, dry<br>• couscous<br>• crackers<br>• durham flour<br>• granola<br>• oat bran<br>• oats (cooked)<br>• pancakes<br>• pasta<br>• rice (basmati, white, wild)<br>• rice cakes<br>• sago<br>• seitan (wheat meat)<br>• spelt<br>• sprouted wheat bread (Essene)<br>• tapioca<br>• wheat<br>• wheat bran | • bread (with yeast)<br>• buckwheat<br>• corn<br>• millet<br>• muesli**<br>• oats (dry)<br>• polenta**<br>• quinoa<br>• rice (brown)**<br>• rye | • almond milk<br>• aloe vera juice<br>• apple juice<br>• apricot juice<br>• berry juice (sweet)<br>• carob<br>• cherry juice (sweet)<br>• cool dairy drinks<br>• grain beverage (coffee substitute)<br>• grape juice<br>• hot, spiced milk*<br>• mango juice<br>• miso broth*<br>• mixed vegetable juice<br>• orange juice*<br>• peach nectar<br>• pear juice<br>• pomegranate juice<br>• prune juice<br>• rice milk<br>• soy milk<br>• vegetable bouillon<br>• herbal teas: alfalfa bancha | • apple cider<br>• berry juice (sour)<br>• caffeinated beverages<br>• carbonated drinks<br>• carrot juice<br>• cherry juice (sour)<br>• chocolate milk<br>• coffee<br>• cranberry juice<br>• grapefruit juice<br>• iced tea<br>• iced drinks<br>• lemonade<br>• papaya juice<br>• tomato juice<br>• sour juices<br>• herbal teas: ajwan basil** cinnamon* clove eucalyptus fenugreek ginger (dry) ginseng hawthorne hyssop |

| | | *Pitta* | |
|---|---|---|---|
| **GRAINS –** Advisable | **GRAINS –** Avoid | **BEVERAGES –** Advisable | **BEVERAGES –** Avoid |
| | | barley<br>blackberry<br>borage<br>burdock<br>catnip<br>chamomile | juniper berry<br>pennyroyal |

| | | *Pitta* | |
|---|---|---|---|
| **NUTS –** Advisable | **NUTS –** Avoid | **SEEDS –** Advisable | **SEEDS – Avoid** |
| • almonds (soaked and peeled)<br>• charole<br>• coconut | • almonds (with skin)<br>• black walnuts<br>• brazil nuts<br>• cashews<br>• filberts<br>• hazelnuts<br>• macadamia nuts<br>• peanuts<br>• pecans<br>• pine nuts<br>• pistachios<br>• walnuts | • flax<br>• halva<br>• hemp<br>• popcorn (no salt, buttered)<br>• psyllium<br>• pumpkin*<br>• sunflower | • chia<br>• sesame<br>• tahini |

| Pitta | | | |
|---|---|---|---|
| OILS – Advisable *Most suitable at top* | OILS – Avoid | SPICES – Advisable | SPICES – Avoid |
| • sunflower<br>• ghee<br>• canola<br>• olive<br>• soy<br>• flax seed<br>• primrose<br>• walnut<br>*External use only:*<br>• avocado<br>• coconut | • almond<br>• apricot<br>• corn<br>• safflower<br>• sesame | • basil (fresh)<br>• black pepper*<br>• caraway*<br>• cardamom*<br>• cinnamon<br>• coriander<br>• cumin<br>• curry leaves<br>• dill<br>• fennel<br>• ginger (fresh)<br>• mint<br>• neem leaves*<br>• orange peel*<br>• parsley*<br>• peppermint<br>• saffron<br>• spearmint<br>• tarragon*<br>• turmeric<br>• vanilla*<br>• wintergreen | • ajwan<br>• allspice<br>• almond extract<br>• anise<br>• asafoetida (hing)<br>• basil (dry)<br>• bay leaf<br>• cayenne<br>• cloves<br>• fenugreek<br>• garlic<br>• ginger (dry)<br>• mace<br>• marjoram<br>• mustard seeds<br>• nutmeg<br>• oregano<br>• paprika<br>• pippali<br>• poppy seeds<br>• rosemary<br>• sage<br>• savory<br>• star anise<br>• thyme |

| Pitta | | | |
|---|---|---|---|
| CONDI-MENTS – Advisable | CONDI-MENTS – Avoid | SWEETEN-ERS – Advisable | SWEETEN-ERS – Avoid |
| • black pepper*<br>• chutney, mango (sweet)<br>• cilantro*<br>• dulse*<br>• hijiki<br>• kombu*<br>• lime*<br>• sprouts<br>• tamari* | • chili pepper<br>• chocolate<br>• chutney, mango (spicy)<br>• gomasio<br>• horseradish<br>• kelp<br>• ketchup<br>• lemon<br>• lime pickle<br>• mango pickle<br>• mayonnaise<br>• mustard<br>• pickles<br>• salt**<br>• scallions<br>• seaweed<br>• soy sauce<br>• vinegar | • barley malt<br>• fructose<br>• fruit juice concentrate<br>• maple syrup<br>• rice syrup<br>• sucanat<br>• turbinado | • honey** (raw, unprocessed)<br>• jaggery<br>• molasses<br>• white sugar** |

| Pitta | |
|---|---|
| FOOD SUPPLEMENTS – Advisable | FOOD SUPPLEMENTS – Avoid |
| • aloe vera juice<br>• barley green<br>• brewer's yeast<br>• minerals: calcium, magnesium, zinc<br>• spirulina<br>• blue-green algae<br>• vitamins D and E | • amino acids<br>• bee pollen**<br>• royal jelly**<br>• minerals: copper, iron, vitamins A, B, $B_{12}$, and C |

| Kapha | | | |
|---|---|---|---|
| FRUITS – Advisable<br>*Most astringent fruit* | FRUITS – Avoid<br>*Most sweet and sour fruit* | VEGETABLES – Advisable<br>*Most bitter and pungent veg-etables* | VEGETABLES – Avoid<br>*Most sweet and juicy vegetables* |
| • apples<br>• applesauce<br>• apricots<br>• berries<br>• cherries<br>• cranberries<br>• figs (dry)*<br>• grapes*<br>• lemons*<br>• limes*<br>• peaches<br>• pears<br>• persimmons<br>• pomegranates<br>• prunes<br>• raisins<br>• strawberries* | • avocado<br>• bananas<br>• coconut<br>• dates<br>• figs (fresh)<br>• grapefruit<br>• kiwi<br>• mangoes**<br>• melons<br>• oranges<br>• papayas<br>• pineapple<br>• plums<br>• rhubarb<br>• tamarind<br>• watermelon | • artichoke<br>• asparagus<br>• beet greens<br>• beets<br>• bitter melon<br>• broccoli<br>• Brussels sprouts<br>• burdock root<br>• cabbage<br>• carrots<br>• cauliflower<br>• celery<br>• cilantro<br>• corn<br>• daikon radish<br>• dandelion greens<br>• eggplant<br>• fennel (anise)<br>• garlic<br>• green beans<br>• green chilies<br>• horseradish<br>• Jerusalem artichoke<br>• kale<br>• kohlrabi<br>• leafy greens<br>• leeks<br>• lettuce | • cucumber<br>• olives<br>• parsnips**<br>• potatoes (sweet)<br>• squash (winter)<br>• taro root<br>• tomatoes (raw)<br>• zucchini |

| | Kapha | | |
|---|---|---|---|
| **FRUITS –** Advisable *Most astringent fruit* | **FRUITS –** Avoid *Most sweet and sour fruit* | **VEGETABLES –** Advisable *Most bitter and pungent vegetables* | **VEGETABLES –** Avoid *Most sweet and juicy vegetables* |
| | | • mustard greens<br>• okra<br>• onions<br>• pumpkin | |

| | Kapha | | |
|---|---|---|---|
| **LEGUMES –** Advisable | **LEGUMES –** Avoid | **DAIRY –** Advisable | **DAIRY –** Avoid |
| • adzuki beans<br>• black beans<br>• black-eyed peas<br>• chick peas (garbanzo beans)<br>• lentils (red and brown)<br>• lima beans<br>• mung beans*<br>• mung dal*<br>• navy beans<br>• peas (dried)<br>• pinto beans<br>• soy milk<br>• soy sausages<br>• split peas<br>• tempeh<br>• tofu (cooked)*<br>• tur dal<br>• white beans | • kidney beans<br>• miso<br>• soy beans<br>• soy cheese<br>• soy flour<br>• soy powder<br>• soy sauce<br>• tofu (raw)<br>• urad dal | • buttermilk*<br>• cottage cheese (from skimmed goat's milk)<br>• ghee*<br>• goat's cheese (unsalted and not aged)*<br>• goat's milk (skim)<br>• yogurt (diluted) | • butter (salted)<br>• butter (unsalted)**<br>• cheese (soft and hard)<br>• cow's milk<br>• ice cream<br>• sour cream<br>• yogurt (plain, frozen or with fruit) |

| Kapha | | | |
|---|---|---|---|
| **NUTS –**<br>**Advisable**<br>*In moderation* | **NUTS – Avoid** | **SEEDS –**<br>**Advisable** | **SEEDS –**<br>**Avoid** |
| • almonds<br>• black walnuts<br>• brazil nuts<br>• cashews<br>• charole<br>• coconut<br>• filberts<br>• hazelnuts<br>• macadamia<br>  nuts<br>• peanuts<br>• pecans<br>• pine nuts<br>• pistachios<br>• walnuts | • none | • chia<br>• flax<br>• halva<br>• hemp<br>• pumpkin<br>• sesame<br>• sunflower<br>• tahini | • popcorn<br>• psyllium** |

| Kapha | | | |
|---|---|---|---|
| **GRAINS –**<br>**Advisable** | **GRAINS –**<br>**Avoid** | **BEVERAGES**<br>**– Advisable** | **BEVERAGES**<br>**– Avoid** |
| • amaranth*<br>• barley<br>• buckwheat<br>• cereal (cold,<br>  dry or puffed)<br>• corn<br>• couscous<br>• crackers<br>• durham<br>  flour*<br>• granola<br>• millet<br>• muesli | • bread (made<br>  with yeast)<br>• oats (cooked)<br>• pancakes<br>• pasta**<br>• rice (brown,<br>  white)<br>• rice cakes**<br>• wheat | • aloe vera juice<br>• apple cider<br>• apple juice*<br>• apricot juice<br>• berry juice<br>• black tea<br>  (spiced)<br>• carob<br>• carrot juice<br>• cherry juice<br>  (sweet)<br>• cranberry<br>  juice | • almond milk<br>• caffeinated<br>  beverages**<br>• carbonated<br>  drinks<br>• cherry juice<br>  (sour)<br>• coffee<br>• dairy drinks<br>  (cold)<br>• grapefruit<br>  juice |

| Kapha | | | |
|---|---|---|---|
| **GRAINS – Advisable** | **GRAINS – Avoid** | **BEVERAGES – Advisable** | **BEVERAGES – Avoid** |
| • oat bran<br>• oats (dry)<br>• polenta<br>• quinoa*<br>• rice (basmati, wild)*<br>• rye<br>• sango<br>• seitan (wheat meat)<br>• spelt*<br>• sprouted wheat bread (Essene)<br>• tapioca<br>• wheat bran | | • hot spiced milk*<br>• grain beverage (substitute coffee )<br>• grape juice<br>• herbal teas: alfalfa<br>bancha<br>barley<br>blackberry<br>burdock<br>chamomile<br>chicory<br>cinnamon<br>clove<br>• mango juice<br>• peach nectar<br>• pear juice<br>• pineapple juice*<br>• pomegranate juice<br>• prune juice<br>• soy milk (hot and well-spiced) | • herbal teas: marshmallow<br>rosehip**<br>• iced tea<br>• icy cold drinks<br>• lemonade<br>• miso broth<br>• orange juice<br>• papaya juice<br>• rice milk<br>• sour juices<br>• soy milk (cold)<br>• tomato juice |

| Kapha | | | |
|---|---|---|---|
| OILS – Advisable *Most suitable at top* | OILS – Avoid | SPICES – Advisable *All spices are good.* | SPICES – Avoid |
| • corn<br>• canola<br>• sunflower<br>• ghee<br>• almond | • apricot<br>• avocado<br>• coconut<br>• flax seed**<br>• olive<br>• primrose<br>• safflower<br>• sesame<br>• soy<br>• walnut | • ajwan<br>• allspice<br>• almond extract<br>• anise<br>• asafoetida (hing)<br>• basil<br>• bay leaf<br>• black pepper<br>• caraway<br>• cardamom<br>• cayenne<br>• cinnamon<br>• cloves<br>• coriander<br>• cumin<br>• curry leaves<br>• dill<br>• fennel*<br>• fenugreek<br>• garlic<br>• ginger<br>• mace<br>• marjoram<br>• mint<br>• mustard seeds<br>• neem leaves<br>• nutmeg<br>• orange peel<br>• oregano<br>• paprika | |

| Kapha | | | |
|---|---|---|---|
| **OILS – Advisable** *Most suitable at top* | **OILS – Avoid** | **SPICES – Advisable** *All spices are good.* | **SPICES – Avoid** |
| | | • parsley <br> • peppermint <br> • pippali <br> • poppy seeds <br> • rosemary <br> • saffron <br> • sage <br> • savory <br> • spearmint <br> • tarragon <br> • thyme <br> • turmeric <br> • vanilla* | |

| Kapha | | | |
|---|---|---|---|
| **CONDI-MENTS – Advisable** | **CONDI-MENTS – Avoid** | **SWEETEN-ERS – Advisable** | **SWEETEN-ERS – Avoid** |
| • black pepper <br> • chili peppers <br> • chutney, mango (spicy) <br> • cilantro <br> • dulse* <br> • hijiki* <br> • horseradish <br> • lemon* <br> • mustard (without vinegar) <br> • scallions <br> • seaweed* <br> • sprouts* | • chocolate <br> • chutney, mango (sweet) <br> • gomasio <br> • kelp <br> • ketchup** <br> • lime <br> • mayonnaise <br> • pickles <br> • salt <br> • soy sauce <br> • tamari <br> • vinegar | • fruit juice concentrate <br> • honey (raw, unprocessed) | • barley malt <br> • fructose <br> • jaggery <br> • maple syrup <br> • molasses <br> • rice syrup <br> • sucanat <br> • turbinado sugar <br> • white sugar |

| Kapha | |
|---|---|
| **FOOD SUPPLEMENTS –** Advisable | **FOOD SUPPLEMENTS –** Avoid |
| • aloe vera juice<br>• amino acids<br>• barley green<br>• bee pollen<br>• brewer's yeast<br>• minerals: calcium, copper, iron, magnesium, zinc<br>• royal jelly<br>• spirulina<br>• blue-green algae<br>• vitamins A, B, $B_{12}$, C, D and E | • minerals: potassium |

# Glossary

**Abhyanga** – to smear, anoint; oil massage therapies, daily oilation

**Adharmic** – unrighteous

**Agni** – digestive fire, light, heat

**Agni homas** – fire ceremonies

**Agni swedhana** – a procedure designed to promote sweating and dilation of the srotas, nadis and dhatus

**Ahamkara** – ego, conception of one's individuality, identification with the sense of "I"

**Ahara** – food, that which goes in

**Ahara rasa** – the juice or essence of food, the final product of digested food that nourishes all dhatus (bodily tissues)

**Ahimsa** – non-violence, non-harming

**Ajna** – commanding or infinite power, the sixth chakra (also called the third eye chakra)

**Akash** – space, ether, sky, atmosphere

**Alochaka** – a subdosha of pitta that governs vision

**Ama** – a toxic material produced from undigested food, uncooked, raw, undigested

**Amavata** – a disorder caused when ama and vata enter the joints and cause arthritic-type diseases

**Ambuvaha srotas** – carries water

**Amla** – sour taste

**Anadi** – without beginning

**Anahata** – the unstruck sound, the fourth/heart chakra

**Ananda** – bliss

**Anandamaya kosha** – the bliss sheath

**Ananta** – infinite

**Annamaya kosha** – the food sheath

**Annavaha srotas** – the channels that transport food, the digestive system, alimentary canal

**Anupana** – the vehicle or medium for transporting herbal medicines into the body

**Anuvasana basti** – enema given with an oily substance

**Ap** – the element water, water

**Apana vata** – one of the subdoshas of vata, the downward and outward moving energy that is responsible for the elimination of waste (feces, gas, urine, menstrual blood, etc.)

**Aparigraha** – non-possessiveness, non-coveting, non-greediness

**Archana** – daily worship

**Arishtam** – naturally fermented herbal extracts

**Artavavaha srotas** – the channels for the female reproductive system

**Artha** – economy, money, object

**Asana** – posture, seat, position

**Asava** – medicated wines and juices of plants

**Ashtanga** – eight

**Ashtanga hrdaya** – an ancient ayurvedic text written by the rishi Vagabhatta

**Ashtanga Yoga** – eight-limbed yoga, Raja Yoga

**Asthayi** – unstable

**Asteya** – non-stealing

**Asthi** – bone

**Asthivaha srotas** – channels that carry nutrient material for bones

**Atma** – soul, spirit, true Self

**Atma nivedana** – surrender or dedication to God

**Atma vichara** – self-inquiry

**Aum (Om)** – primordial sound of universe; creation, preservation and dissolution

**Aushadhi** – ayurvedic management of disease

**Avalambaka** – Seated in the heart and lungs, this is one of the sub-doshas of kapha. It gives support and builds ojas and immunity.

**Avidya** – ignorance

**Ayu** – life

**Ayurveda** – the science of life

**Basti** – medicated enema

**Bhajans** – devotional songs in praise of God

**Bhakti** – devotion

**Bhasmas** – purified ash preparations

**Bhastrika** – a form of pranayama that engages rapid breathing

**Bhrajaka** – a subdosha of pitta that gives color or shining to the skin, is located in the skin

**Bhutagni** – the fire (enzyme) that digests the five elements/tastes

**Bodhaka** – one of the subdoshas of kapha that helps to determine various tastes, assists in the digestive process, is located in the mouth, tongue and throat

**Brahma** – the Creator, one of the Hindu trinity

**Brahmacharya** – celibacy, one that follows a strict spiritual life

**Brahma-muhurta** – the two-hour time period preceding sunrise

**Brahman** – the supreme reality

**Brahmananda** – the macrocosm

**Bruhana nasya** – medicated oil administered through the nostrils designed to nourish the brain and senses

**Buddhi** – intelligence, intellect

**Charaka** – considered to be the father and the foremost scholar of Ayurveda, original commentator on Ayurveda

**Charaka Samhita** – the first and primary ayurvedic text, Charaka's treatise on Ayurveda

**Chi** – the Chinese word for prana, life force

**Chikitsa** – treatment, a therapy to retain balance, practice or science of medicine

**Chitta** – the ability to know

**Churna** – herbal powders

**Dasa** – to become or adopt the attitude of a servant of God

**Dharana** – concentration of mind, to hold together

**Dharma** – righteousness, life purpose, right action

**Dhatu** – bodily tissue

**Dhatu-agni** – the digestive fire of the bodily tissue, the agni of the dhatus

**Dhauti** – the cleansing of the gastrointestinal tract

**Dhyana** – meditation

**Dinacharya** – daily routine

**Dosha** – bodily constitution (vata, pitta and kapha), fault, deficiency, that which contaminates

**Dosha sammurcchana** – the process where the dosha becomes increased or disturbed and enters into the dhatus, affecting its natural function

**Drava** – liquid

**Dusya** – that which is contaminated or adulterated, seat of disease manifestation in the body

**Dusa** – to vitiate

**Gandha** – odor or smell, the tanmatra that correlates to the earth element

**Gandusha** – retention of fluids in the mouth (Sesame oil is most frequently used.)

**Ghee** – clarified butter

**Ghrita** – medicated ghee

**Grahani** – small intestine

**Grishma** – summer

**Guna** – subtle quality of nature; sattva, rajas and tamas

**Guru** – teacher, heavy, weight, great, large

**Haridra** – tumeric, also called haldi in Hindi

**Hemanta** – winter

**Hima** – cold infusions

**Ida Nadi** – nadi beginning on left side, lunar nadi

**Indriya** – faculty of sense, organ of sense

**Ishta devata** – beloved form of God

**Ishvara Pranidhana** – surrender to the Divine will, devotion to God

**Jala** – water, fluid, liquid

**Jalaneti** – the yogic process of pouring water through the nostrils via a neti pot/cup, usually made of clay, copper or other metals

**Japa** – repetition of mantras

**Jathara** – stomach, abdomen

**Jatharagni** – digestive fire located in stomach, gastric juices, digestive enzymes

**Jiva** – the individual soul, consciousness

**Jnana** – knowledge

**Jnanendriya** – the organs of knowledge or perception

**Jyotish** – Vedic astrology

**Jyotishi** – Vedic astrologer

**Kala** – time period, season

**Kali Yuga** – the present age, the dark age of materialism

**Kalka** – herbal pastes

**Kama** – desire

**Kapalabhati** – skull shining; ayurvedic pranayama practice that cleanses the nasal sinus area, the lungs, blood, tissues and abdomen

**Kapha** – water and earth elements, phlegm, mucus, one of the three main biological energies (bodily humors) Karma – action

**Karmendriya** – organs of action

**Karnapurna** – medicated application to the ears, usually medicated oil or smoke

**Kasaya** – astringent

**Kathina** – hard, firm, stiff, harsh, inflexible, cruel

**Katti Basti** – external application of oil to the lower back region, pelvic girdle and sacral area

**Katu** – pungent taste or flavor

**Katu avastha paka** – the pungent stage of digestion that occurs in the fourth hour of digestion

**Kaya** – body, habitation

**Kayachikitsa** – treatment of body diseases through the use of internal medicine

**Khara** – hard, harsh, rough quality of food

**Kichari** – an ayurvedic dish made by cooking basmati rice and mung beans together, with spices

**Kirtan** – divine songs in praise of God

**Kledaka** – one of the subdoshas of kapha; wet, moist, phlegm in stomach; assists in the digestion of food by breaking them into small digestible particles

**Kosha** – sheath, a subtle energetic sheath that surrounds the human body

**Kriya** – action, practice, applying a remedy

**Krumi** – worms, parasites or infection

**Kumari** – aloe vera, also young female virgin

**Kundalini Shakti** – the purest form of divine spiritual energy in the form of the feminine

**Kvatha** – herbal decoctions

**Laghu** – light, small

**Lassi** – buttermilk, drink made by mixing water into yogurt and churning it

**Lavana** – salty taste

**Leham/avaleham** – medicated jellies

**Lepana** – application of herbal plaster on the skin

**Lila** – divine play

**Madhura** – sweet taste, pleasant, charming, delightful

**Madhuravastha** – the sweet stage of digestion, the final stage

**Mahabhuta** – the great elements, gross elements, space, air, fire, water and earth

**Mahat** – great, intellect, great principle

**Mahatma** – great soul

**Majja** – bone marrow

**Majjavaha srotas** – channels transporting bone marrow

**Mala** – metabolic waste material eliminated from the body, taint, impurity, dirt, filth

**Mala sanchaya** – the accumulation of the malas (waste materials in the body)

**Mamsa** – muscles, flesh, meat, fleshy part (pulp) of a fruit

**Mamsa dhatu– muscle**

**Mamsavaha srotas** – channels transporting muscles

**Manas** – mind

**Manda** – slow, or rice water (the first meal taken after completion of panchakarma)

**Mandagni** – slow, weakened state of digestive fire

**Manipura** – city of gems, the third/solar plexus chakra

**Manomaya kosha** – the mental sheath, that which is made from the mind

**Manovaha srotas** – channels that carries thought

**Mantra** – Vedic hymn, sacred or mystical verse, a prayer

**Marga** – the passage or pathway of travel

**Markava** – that which prevents premature graying

**Maya** – illusion

**Meda** – fatty/adipose tissue

**Medha** – mental power, intelligence, wisdom, prudence

**Medovaha srotas** – channels transporting fatty tissue

**Moksha** – Self-realization, to let flow, liberation

**Mridu** – soft, delicate, tender

**Mritu** – death

**Mudra** – a sign or hand position practiced in yoga and religious worship

**Mula** – root

**Muladhara** – first chakra, root chakra

**Mukha** – an opening, the mouth

**Mutra** – urine

**Mutravaha srotas** – channels transporting urine

**Nadi** – pulse, any tubular organ such as vein or artery

**Nadi swedhana** – application of herbalized steam through a hose to specific points (marmas) on the body

**Nadis** – rivers, the energy channels or pathways of the human body

**Namavali** – the repetition of the names of God through songs, sonnets or poetry

**Nasya** – nasal therapy, usually with oil

**Nauli** – intestinal washing or abdominal rolling

**Neti pot** – the pot that is used in perfoming jalaneti, nasal cleansing

**Netra basti** – localized application of herbalized ghee on the eyes

**Nidana** – cause of disease, investigation of cause of disease

**Nidra** – sleep

**Nirama** – the state of being without ama (toxins)

**Niruha basti** – an enema using an herbal decoction designed to remove ama

**Nirvichara** – without reflection

**Nirvikalpa** – without deliberation

**Nirvikalpa samadhi** – super-conscious state

**Niyama** – restrain, regulate, to fix upon, control, check

**Ojas** – vigor, strength, vitality, the essence of all tissues (dhatus)

**Pachaka** – one of the pitta subdoshas, is located in the small intestine and helps in digestion

**Pancha jnanendriyas** – the five sensory organs: mouth (taste), ears (hearing), eyes (sight), nose (smell), tongue (taste)

**Pancha karmendriyas** – the five organs of action: speech, grasping, walking, procreation and elimination

**Pancha mahabhutas** – the five great elements: space/ether, air, fire, water, earth

**Panchakarma** – five types of elimination therapies

**Paneer** – a type of fresh cheese made by curdling milk

**Paramatman** – Supreme Being

**Pariksha** – examination, inspection, investigation

**Paschatkarma** – "post action" therapies performed after panchakarma

**Peya** – rice gruel or any drink mixed with a small quantity of boiled rice

**Phanta** – hot herbal infusions

**Pinda swedhana** – a fomentation performed with a bolus of rice and hot milk designed to alleviate vata dosha by tonifying the muscles and improving circulation

**Pindanada** – the microcosm

**Pingala nadi** – right nadi, solar nadi

**Pisthis** – powders

**Pitta** – fire element, bile, one of the three main doshas

**Pizhichil** – the pouring of medicated oil all over the body

**Prabhava** – unique property or action of an herb

**Prajna** – wisdom, intelligence, knowledge

**Prajnaparadha** – not using intellect, wrong use of wisdom

**Prakriti** – nature, constitution, natural form, original nature

**Prana** – the breath of life, vital air, energy, power, consciousness

**Pranamaya kosha** – the sheath made from prana, the vital life force

**Pranavaha srotas** – channels carrying air, the respiratory system

**Prana vata** – one of the subdoshas of vata, is seated in the brain and governs respiration and sensory and mental functions

**Pranayama** – to control the breath, specialized breathing techniques

**Praspandanam** – to pulsate or throb

**Pratyahara** – withdrawal of senses from external objects

**Prithvi** – earth

**Puja** – ritualistic worship

**Purana** – to fill space

**Purisha** – feces, waste matter

**Purishavaha srotas** – channels transporting fecal matter, excretory system

**Purusha** – consciousness, the eternal witness

**Purvakarma** – preliminary actions administered before pancha-karma, preparation for the main action

**Purvarupa** – the pre-symptoms of disease, hidden signs of disease

**Rajahvaha srotas** – the channels that carry menstruation

**Rajas** – creative, passionate, active, mobile

**Rajasic** – passionate, active, sharp

**Rakta** – blood

**Rakta-moksha** – blood letting, usually by leaches

**Raktavaha srotas** – channels carrying blood, circulatory system

**Ranjaka** – one of the subdoshas of pitta, is located in the liver, spleen and stomach, and gives color

**Rasa** – taste, lymph, juice, flavor, essence, liquid, fluid

**Rasa dhatu** – plasma

**Rasavaha srotas** – channels carrying plasma or lymph

**Rasayana** – substances that prevent aging and promote longevity by nourishing and tonifying the whole body system

**Rishi** – seer, enlightened being, sage

**Ritucharya** – seasonal regimes, routine to be followed in various seasons

**Rtus** – seasons

**Ruksha** – dry, arid, not greasy, emaciated, thin

**Rupa** – form, sign, symptoms or mark of diseases

**Sadhak** – a spiritual aspirant, one who performs spiritual austerities or practices

**Sadhaka** – one of the subdoshas of pitta, located in the heart and governs circulation

**Sadhana** – spiritual practices

**Sadhya** – that which is desired to be attained, the goals of life

**Sahasrara** – seventh/crown chakra, "thousand-petaled"

**Sakhya** – friendship with God

**Samadhi** – state of absolute absorption in the Self, Divine Consciousness

**Samagni** – balanced state of digestive fire

**Samana** – one of the subdoshas of vata, is located in the small intestine and stomach, increases agni and digestive enzymes, and is the main site of digestion and equalization of air

**Samatva bhava** – the attitude of equal vision, mindful discrimination

**Samjna sthapana** – that which restores consciousness

**Samprapti** – pathogenesis, the complete route of manifestation of disease

**Samsara** – the repetitive cycle of death and rebirth

**Samskaras** – collected mental patterns, impressions

**Samyama** – control of the mind and its fluctuations

**Sananda** – with joy

**Sanatana Dharma** – the Eternal Truth

**Sandra** – dense

**Sankhya philosophy** – to know the truth, the order of creation in the universe, 24 cosmic principles

**Sanskrit** – the language of the Vedas
**Santosha** – contentment
**Sara** – essence, health, vitality of bodily tissue
**Sasmita** – with the sense of personality, individuality
**Satcidananda** – the nature of the true Self; truth-bliss-consciousness
**Sattva** – spiritual essence, qualities of purity, goodness, love, compassion
**Sattvic** – pure, genuine, spiritual, honest
**Satya** – truthfulness or non-lying
**Sauca** – cleanliness or purity
**Savichara** – with reflection
**Savikalpa** – with deliberation
**Seva** – selfless service
**Shabda** – sound, tone, voice
**Shakti** – divine feminine principle, supreme energy of the universe, power of consciousness
**Shamana** – palliation therapy
**Sharada** – autumn
**Sharira** – body, physical body
**Shastras** – Vedic scriptures
**Shiro basti** – basti of the head, the holding of medicated oil on the head inside of a cap
**Shiroabhyanga** – oil massage of the head
**Shirodhara** – pouring oil or any other liquid on forehead from a special pot
**Shishira** – late winter
**Shita** – cold
**Shiva** – pure consciousness, part of the Hindu trinity, the destroyer, the transformer
**Shivadruma** – the tree of Shiva
**Shodhana** – elimination therapy, purification
**Shravana** – listening to satsang or scriptures
**Shukra** – reproductive tissue, semen in men and ova in women
**Shukra artava** – male/female reproductive fluid

**Shukravaha srotas** – supplies the male reproductive system, including the testes, prostrate and semen

**Siddhis** – spiritual powers

**Sita** – cold, chilly, frigid

**Sleshaka** – one of the subdoshas of kapha, is located in the joints and assists in lubrication and protection, attaching, connecting

**Smarana** – constant remembrance of God

**Snehana** – medicated oil therapy, lubricating, anointing, rubbing with oil, unction

**Snigdha** – sticky, viscid, unctuous, smooth, adhesive

**Shodhana** – cleansing, purifying, refining

**Sparsha** – touch, sense or experience of touch

**Srotas** – channels, tubes, hollow vessels carrying substances

**Srota-dusti** – impurity of channels, impurity of srotas

**Stanyavaha srotas** – the lactation system, channel that carries breast milk

**Sthira** – stable, firm, hard, solid, compact, strong, immovable, fixed

**Sthula** – large, thick, gross, stout

**Sukravaha srotas** – channels transporting the reproductive tissue or fluid

**Sukshma** – subtle

**Surya namaskar** – sun salutations, a sequence of yoga asanas

**Sushruta** – one of the main founders of Ayurveda, the founder of ayurvedic surgical technique

**Sushruta samhita** – an ayurvedic text that primarily addresses surgical treatments

**Sushumna nadi** – the central nadi, or energy channel

**Sutraneti** – neti performed using a medicated thread

**Sutras** – thread, woven together

**Svadhyaya** – self-study

**Svadishtana** – the second chakra, the abode of the ego

**Svarasa** – juices

**Sveda** – sweat, sweating, warmth

**Svedavaha srotas** – the channels carrying sweat

**Swedana** – one of the main purvakarmas, sudation therapy, the use of heat to loosen toxins, herbal steam bath that induces sweating and brings toxins back to the gastrointestinal tract to be eliminated by panchakarma

**Tamas** – ignorance, darkness, illusion, dullness, inertia

**Tamasic** – ignorant, lazy, dark, stale

**Tanmatra** – primordial sensory perceptions, unmanifested form of the five elements

**Tantra** – a set of spiritual observances using mantra, yantra, puja, homas, alchemy and other esoteric techniques for Self-realization

**Tapas** – to purify by fire, austerities

**Tapasvi** – one who practices austerities

**Tarpaka** – one of the subdoshas of kapha, is found in the head and nourishes the senses; satisfying, fulfilling

**Tattvas** – 24 divine principles

**Tejas** – mental fire, the subtle essence of the fire element, light

**Thaila** – medicated oils

**Tikshna** – sharp, hot, fiery, pungent

**Tiksna agni** – strong digestive fire, increased activity of digestive fire, high pitta

**Tikta** – bitter taste

**Trataka** – concentration or gazing

**Tridosha** – the three doshas: vata, pitta and kapha

**Tridoshic** – balance of the three doshas

**Triguna** – the three qualities of nature: sattva, rajas and tamas

**Triphala** – a general laxative and colon cleanser, an ayurvedic formula made of three particular herbs/fruits (amalaki, bhibitaki, and haritaki)

**Udakavaha srotas** –channels transporting water or watery liquids in the body

**Udana** – one of the subdoshas of vata, the upward moving air responsible for exhalation, vomiting and speech

**Udvahana** – to move upward

**Udwartanam** – therapeutic massage using dry herbal powders to reduce kapha dosha

**Upadhatu** – a secondary tissue that supports the main tissue and is made from the primary dhatu

**Upanishads** – the written teachings of the Vedas and Vedanta

**Uro basti** – medicated oil placed on the chest and heart area

**Ushna** – hot, warm, passionate, expansive

**Vairagya** – dispassion or non-attachment

**Vajikarana** – the science of aphrodisiacs, producing virility, substances that strengthen the reproductive system

**Vamana** – vomiting, emesis using herbal formulations

**Vamana dhauti** – cleansing of the stomach by drinking salt water and vomiting

**Vandana** – praise of God, or prayer

**Varsha** – monsoon, rainy season

**Vasanas** – habits

**Vasanta** – spring

**Vata** – wind or air element, one of the three main biological humors of the body

**Vati** – herbal tablets and pills

**Vayu** – air, wind, one of the five elements

**Vedanta** – non-dual or unified consciousness, knowledge of the Self

**Vedas** – the ancient books of knowledge, sacred knowledge

**Vidya** – supreme knowledge

**Vijnanamaya kosha** – the sheath of knowledge

**Vikruti** – current imbalance of the doshas, sickness, alteration, change, imbalance, agitation

**Vipaka** – ripe, mature, state of food after digestion, the post-digestive taste

**Virechan** – purgation, a main therapy in panchakarma

**Virya** – potency of herbs or food, power, vigor, semen

**Vishada** – quality of clarity

**Vishama-agni** – irregular digestive fire, unstable digestive fire

**Vishnu** – one diety of the Hindu trinity, the preserver, the sustainer

**Vishuddha** – pure, the fifth chakra, throat chakra

**Viveka** – mindful discrimination, to separate, isolate or split

**Vrittis** – fluctuations or modifications of the mind

**Vyakta** – visible, manifested

**Vyana** – one of the subdoshas of vata, circulates throughout the body, governs blood circulation, musculo-skeletal and nervous system, responsible for all movements of reflex and joints

**Yagnas** – sacrifices (can include pujas, homas, agni hotras)

**Yamas** – disciplines, restraints, self-control, rules, instructions, guidelines

**Yang** – masculine form of energy, heat, positive, active

**Yantra** – sacred geometrical design correlated with a deity, mantra or planetary vibration

**Yin** – feminine form of energy, cool, negative, passive

**Yoga** – union, to link, to add, to join together, a progressive method to attain Self-realization

# Bibliography

Airola, Paavo. *How to Get Well: Handbook of Natural Healing.* Scottsdale, AZ:Health Plus Publishers, 1984.

American Dietetic Association and Dietitians of Canada, comp. "Vegetarian Diets." *Journal of the American Dietetic Association.* June 2003: Volume 103, Issue 6, Pages 748-765.

Atreya. *Ayurvedic Healing for Women.* New Delhi, India: Motilal Banarsidas, Pvt. Ltd., 2000.

Babu, Dr. Madham Shetty Suresh. *Yoga Ratnakara, Vol. I.* Varanasi, India: Chowkhamba Sanskrit Series, 2005.

Bachman, Nicolai. *The Language of Yoga: A Complete A to Y Guide to Asana Names, Sanskrit Terms and Chants.* Boulder, CO: Sounds True, Inc., 2004.

Barnard, Neal, M.D. "Doctor in the House." *PETA's Animal Times* Fall 2004:7.

---. *The Power of Your Plate.* Summertown, TN: Book Publishing Co., 1990.

Beckman, Howard. *Vibrational Healing with Gems.* New Delhi, India: Gyan Publishing House, 2000.

*Bhajanamritam 2010 Supplement.* Amritapuri, India: Mata Amritanandamayi Mission Trust, 2010.

Charak, Dr. K. S. *Subtleties of Medical Astrology,* New Delhi,India: Uma Publications, 2002.

---. *Essentials of Medical Astrology,* 4th Edition, New Delhi, India: Uma Publications, 2005.

Cole, Sebastian. *Ayurvedic Medicine: The Principles of Traditional Practice.* Philadelphia, PA: Elsevier, Ltd., 2006.

Dash, Vaidya Bhagwan and Sharma, R.K. *Caraka Samhita, Vol.I-VII.* Varanasi, India: Chowkhamba Sanskrit Series, 2005.

Devi, Sri Mata Amritanandamayi. *The Awakening of Universal Motherhood: An Address Given by Sri Mata Amritanandamayi Devi at the Global Peace Initiative of Women Religious and Spiritual Leaders at Palais des Nations,Geneva, October 7th, 2002.* Amritapuri, India: Mata Amritanandamayi Mission Trust, 2003.

---. *For My Children: The Teachings of Her Holiness Sri Mata Amritanandamayi Devi.* Amritapuri, India: Mata Amritanandamayi Mission Trust, 1995.

---. *Immortal Light: Advice to Householders.* Amritapuri, India: Mata Amritanandamayi Mission Trust, 2006.

---. *Living in Harmony: An Address Given by Sri Mata Amritanandamayi Devi at the Millennium World Peace Summit of Religious and Spiritual Leaders at the United Nations General Assembly, August 29th, 2000.* Amritapuri, India: Mata Amritanandamayi Mission Trust, 2005.

---. *May Peace and Happiness Prevail: Keynote Address by Sri Mata Amritanandamayi Devi during the Closing Plenary Session of the Parliament of World's Religions in Barcelona, Spain, on July 13th, 2004.* Amritapuri, India: Mata Amritanandamayi Mission Trust, 2004.

---. *May Your Hearts Blossom: An Address by Sri Mata Amritanandamayi Devi at the Parliament of the World's Religions, Chicago, September 1993.* Amritapuri, India: Mata Amritanandamayi Mission Trust, 2005.

---. *Unity is Peace: An Address by Sri Mata Amritanandamayi Devi at the Interfaith Celebration in Honor of the 50th Anniversary of the United Nations on October 21st, 1995, at the Cathedral of St. John the Divine, New York.* Amritapuri, India: Mata Amritanandamayi Mission Trust, 1996.

Essential Oils Desk Reference: Compiled by Life Science Publishing. Salt Lake City, UT: Life Science Publishing, 2006.

Fischer-Rizze, Susan. *Complete Aromatherapy Handbook.* New Delhi, India: Health Harmony, 2001.

Frawley, Dr. David. *Astrology of the Seers: A Guide to Vedic/Hindu Astrology.* Twin Lakes, WI: Lotus Press, 2000.

---. *Ayurveda and the Mind.* Twin Lakes, WI: Lotus Press, 1997.

---. *Ayurvedic Astrology: Self-Healing Through the Stars.* Twin Lakes, WI: Lotus Press, 2005.

---. *Ayurvedic Healing: A Comprehensive Guide.* Salt Lake City, UT: Passage Press, 1989.

---. *Vedantic Meditation: Lighting the Flame of Awareness.* Berkeley, CA: North Atlantic Books, 2000.

---. *Yoga and Ayurveda: Self-Healing and Self-Realization.* Twin Lakes, WI: Lotus Press, 1999.

---. *Yoga: The Greater Tradition.* Mandala Publishing, 2008.

Frawley, Dr. David and Kozak, Susan. *Yoga for Your Type*. Twin Lakes, WI: Lotus Press, 2001.

Frawley, Dr. David and Lad, Dr. Vasant. *The Yoga of Herbs*. Santa Fe, NM: Lotus Press, 1986.

Frawley, Dr. David and Ranade, Dr. Subhash and Lele, Dr. Avinash. *Ayurveda and Marma Therapy: Energy Points in Yogic Healing*. Twin Lakes, WI: Lotus Press, 2003.

Gerras, Charles. *The Complete Book of Vitamins.* Emmaus, PA: Rodhale Press, 1977.

Govindan, S.V. *Marma Treatment: Massage Therapy for Diseases of Vital Areas*. New Delhi, India: Abhinav Publishing, 2005.

Gupta, K.R.L. *Science of Sphygmica or Sage Kanda on Pulse*. New Delhi, India: Sri Satguru Publications, 2000.

Johari, Harish. *The Healing Power of Gemstones: In Tantra, Ayurveda and Astrology*. Rochester, Vermont: Destiny Books, 1996.

---. *Tools for Tantra*. Rochester, Vermont: Destiny Books, 1986.

Joshi, Binod Kumar, Joshi, Geeta, and Sah, Ram Lal. *Vedic Health Care System: Clinical Practice of Sushrutokta Marma Chikitsa and Siravedhan*. New Delhi, India: New Age Books, 2002.

Joshi, Sunil. *Ayurvedic Panchakarma: The Science of Healing and Rejuvenation*. Twin Lakes, WI: Lotus Press, 1997.

Kacera, Walter. *Ayurvedic Tongue Diagnosis*. Twin Lakes, WI: Lotus Press, 2006.

Lad, Dr. Vasant. *Ayurveda: The Science of Self-Healing*. Twin Lakes, WI: Lotus Press, 1984.

---. *Textbook of Ayurveda, Vol. I: Fundamental Principles*. Albuquerque, NM: The Ayurvedic Press, 2002.

---. *Textbook of Ayurveda, Vol. II: A Complete Guide to Clinical Assessment*. Albuquerque, NM: The Ayurvedic Press, 2006.

Lalwani, Dr. Neeraj. *Gem Therapy in Vedic Astrology*. New Delhi, India: Gyan Publishing House, 2002.

Lanou, Amy. "Healthy Eating for Life for Children." *Physicians'Committee for Responsible Medicine*. New York: John Wiley and Sons, 2002: 49.

Lappe, Frances Moore. *Diet for a Small Planet*. New York, NY: Ballantine Books, 1975.

Mahadevan, Dr. L. *Ayurveda for Beginners*. Kanyakumari, India: Sri Sarada Ayurveda Hospital, 2005.

Manoj, Dr. T. *Ayurveda*. Trivandrum, India: AIMS Health Publications, 2000.

Menon, C.V. Narayana, comp. *The Thousand Names of the Divine Mother: Sri Lalita Sahasranama.* Amritapuri, India: Mata Amritanandamayi Mission Trust, 2004.

Miller, Dr. Light. *Ayurvedic Remedies.* Twin Lakes, WI: Lotus Press, 1999.

Miller, Dr. Light and Dr. Brian. *Ayurveda and Aromatherapy: The Earth Essential Guide to Ancient Wisdom and Modern Healing.* Twin Lakes, WI: Lotus Press, 2005.

Murthy, Prof. K.R. Srikantha. *Vagbhata's Astanga Hrdayam.* Varanasi, India: Chowkhamba Krishnadas Academy, 2004.

"The Natural Resources Defense Council 25 Year Report." New York, NY: *Natural Resources Defense Council.*

Nibodhi. *Annapurna's Prasad: Ayurvedic Cooking for Health and Longevity.* Amritapuri, India: Mata Amritanandamayi Mission Trust, 2009.

Paranjpe, Dr. Prakash. *Ayurvedic Medicine: The Living Tradition.* New Delhi, India: Chaukhamba Sanskrit Pratishthan, 2003.

---. *Indian Medicinal Plants: Forgotten Healers: A Guide to Ayurvedic Herbal Medicine.* New Delhi, India: Chaukhamba Sanskrit Pratishthan, 2001.

Pitchford, Paul. *Healing with Whole Foods.* Berkeley, CA: North Atlantic Books, 2002.

Puri, Swami Amritaswarupananda. *From Amma's Heart: Conversations with Sri Mata Amritanandamayi Devi.* Amritapuri, India: Mata Amritanandamayi Mission Trust, 2005.

Puri, Swami Amritaswarupananda, trans. *Man and Nature.* Amritapuri, India: Mata Amritanandamayi Mission Trust, 2005.

Ranade, Dr. Subhash. *Natural Healing Through Ayurveda.* New Delhi, India: Motilal Banarsidas Pvt. Ltd., 1999.

Ranade, Dr. Subash and Lele, Dr. Avinash. *Ayurvedic Panchakarma.* New Delhi, India: Chaukhamba Sanskrit Pratishthan, 2003.

Reddy, Dr. K. Rama Chandra. *Ocean of Ayurvedic Pharmaceutics.* Varanasi, India: Chaukhambha Sanskrit Bhawan, 2007.

Reinfeld, Mark and Rinaldi, Bo. *Vegan Fusion.* Kapa'a, HI: Thousand Petals Publishing, 2005.

Robbins, John. *The Food Revolution.* Boston, MA: Conari Press, 2001.

Ros, Dr. Frank. *The Lost Secrets of Ayurvedic Acupuncture.* Twin Lakes, WI: Lotus Press, 1994.

Sadler, Julie. *Aromatherapy.* Delhi: Vision Books Pvt. Ltd., 1993.

Sah, Ram Lal, Joshi, Dr. Sunil and Joshi, Dr. Geeta. *Vedic Health Care System: Clinical Practice of Sushrutokta Marma Chikitsa and Siravedhan.* Delhi: New Age Books, 2002.

Saraswati, Swami Satyananda. *Kali Puja.* New Delhi, India: Devi Mandir Publications, 1996.

---. *Surya Namaskar: A Technique of Solar Vitalization.* Bihar, India: Yoga Publications Trust, 2007.

---. *Yoga Nidra.* Bihar, India: Yoga Publications Trust, 2006.

Shastri, V.V.Subramanaya. *Tridosha Theory: A Study on the Fundamental Principles of Ayurveda.* Malappuram Dist. Kerala, India: Kottakkal Arya Vaidya Sala Publications Dept., 2000.

Singer, Peter. *Animal Liberation: A New Ethic for Our Treatment of Animals* (2nd edition). New York: New York Review of Books, 1990.

Stiles, Mukunda.*Ayurvedic Yoga Therapy.* Twin Lakes, WI: Lotus Press, 2008.

---. *Structural Yoga Therapy.* New Delhi, India: Goodwill Publishing House, 2002.

Subramuniyaswami, Satguru Sivaya. *How to Win an Argument with a Meat Eater.* Kauai, HI: Himayalan Academy Publications, 2000.

Svoboda, Robert E. *Ayurveda: Life, Health and Longevity.* India: Penguin Books, 1992.

---. *Prakriti: Your Ayurvedic Constitution.* Twin Lakes, MI: Lotus Press, 1999.

Tirtha, Swami Sada Shiva. *The Ayurvedic Encyclopedia.* New Delhi, India: Health Harmony, 2006.

Tiwari, Maya. *Ayurveda Secrets of Healing.* Twin Lakes, WI: Lotus Press, 1995.

Winter, Ruth. *A Consumer's Dictionary of Food Additives.* New York, NY: Crown Publishers, Inc., 1989.

Yogananda, Paramahansa. *God Talks with Arjuna: The Bhagavad Gita: The Royal Science of God Realization, Vol. I and II.* Dakshineshwar, Kolkata, India: Yogada Satsanga Society of India, 2005.

## Website References

"E. Coli in up to Half of U.S. Cattle." *Associated Press* February 29, 2000. July 2000
<http://www.msnbc.com/news/376128.asp?cp1=1>

"Jesus was a Vegetarian." *People for the Ethical Treatment of Animals* Aug. 2000.
<http://www.jesusveg.com>

"Quotable Quotes." *American Vegetarian* January 28, 1998. Aug. 2000
<http://www.acorn.net/av/avquotes.html>

"Spiritual Basis." *American Vegetarian* 1998. Aug. 2000
<http://www2.acorn.net/doc/avspirit.doc>

"The Transformation of Animals into Food" *Vegan Outreach.*Aug. 2000.
<http://www.veganoutreach.org/wv/wv2.html>

"World Scientists' Warning to Humanity." *Union of Concerned Scientists*1992.
<http://www.earthednet.org>

# Resources

www.embracingtheworld.org (not-for-profit international collective of charities founded by renowned spiritual and humanitarian leader, Sri Mata Amritanandamayi Devi, also known as Amma)

www.amritapuri.org (homepage of Amma and Amritapuri Ashram)

www.amma.org (American website of Amma)

www.theammashop.org (products to support spiritual seekers)

www.amma-europe.org (European website of Amma)

www.iam-meditation.org (Integrated Amrita Meditation Technique®)

www.aimshospital.org (Amrita Institute of Medical Sciences)

www.ayudh.org (a movement of young people who want to lead a life as guided by Amma)

www.amrita.edu (Amrita University)

www.ayurveda.amrita.edu (Amrita School of Ayurveda and Amrita Ayurveda Hospital)

www.ayurveda.com (The Ayurvedic Institute)

www.veganoutreach.org (working to end cruelty to animals)

www.peta.org (People for the Ethical Treatment of Animals)

www.vegansociety.com (an educational charity)

www.vegetarian-nutrition.info (current information about the components of a healthful lifestyle)

www.happycow.net (the healthful eating guide)

www.veganfusion.com (workshops, vegan recipes)

www.world.org (World Environmental Organization™)

www.climateark.org (Climate Change and Global Warming Portal)

http://my.ecoearth.info (Environment Portal and Search Engine)

www.unep.org (United Nations Environment Programme)

www.edf.org (Environmental Defense Fund)

www.scorecard.goodguide.com (The Pollution Information Site)

www.ucsusa.org (Union of Concerned Scientists – Citizens and Scientists for Environmental Solutions)

www.ran.org (Rainforest Action Network)

www.emagazine.com (The Environmental Magazine)

www.purezing.com (List of the more widely known dangerous ingredients in body and food products)

www.thedailygreen.com (a consumer's guide to green)
www.foodnews.org (EWG's 2011 Shopper's Guide to Pesticides in Produce™)
www.Green-e.org (consumer protection program for the sale of renewable energy and greenhouse gas reductions)